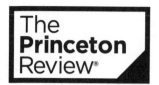

MCAT®

Critical Analysis and Reasoning Skills Review

3rd Edition

The Staff of The Princeton Review

Penguin
Random
House

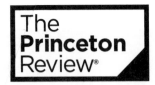

The Princeton Review
110 East 42nd St, 7th Floor

New York, NY 10017

Published in the United States by Penguin Random House LLC, New York, and in Canada by Random House of Canada, a division of Penguin Random House Ltd., Toronto.

Terms of Service: The Princeton Review Online Companion Tools ["Student Tools"] for retail books are available for only the two most recent editions of that book. Student Tools may be activated only once per eligible book purchased for a total of 24 months of access. Activation of Student Tools more than once per book is in direct violation of these Terms of Service and may result in discontinuation of access to Student Tools Services.

The material in this book is up-to-date at the time of publication. However, changes may have been instituted by the testing body in the test after this book was published.

If there are any important late-breaking developments, changes, or corrections to the materials in this book, we will post that information online in the Student Tools. Register your book and check your Student Tools to see if there are any updates posted there.

Every attempt has been made to obtain permission to reproduce material protected by copyright. Where omissions may have occurred the editors will be happy to acknowledge this in future printings.

ISBN: 978-0-593-51624-9
ISSN: 2332-404X

MCAT is a registered trademark of the Association of American Medical Colleges.

The Princeton Review is not affiliated with Princeton University.

Editor: Meave Shelton
Production Editor: Emma Parker, Sarah Litt
Production Artists: Deborah Weber, Shavon I. Serrano

Manufactured in China.

10 9 8 7 6 5 4 3 2 1

3rd Edition

The Princeton Review Publishing Team
Rob Franek, Editor-in-Chief
David Soto, Senior Director, Data Operations
Stephen Koch, Senior Manager, Data Operations
Deborah Weber, Director of Production
Jason Ullmeyer, Production Design Manager
Jennifer Chapman, Senior Production Artist
Selena Coppock, Director of Editorial
Aaron Riccio, Senior Editor
Meave Shelton, Senior Editor
Chris Chimera, Editor
Orion McBean, Editor
Patricia Murphy, Editor
Laura Rose, Editor
Alexa Schmitt Bugler, Editorial Assistant

Penguin Random House Publishing Team
Tom Russell, VP, Publisher
Alison Stoltzfus, Senior Director, Publishing
Brett Wright, Senior Editor
Emily Hoffman, Assistant Managing Editor
Ellen Reed, Production Manager
Suzanne Lee, Designer
Eugenia Lo, Publishing Assistant

For customer service, please contact
editorialsupport@review.com,
and be sure to include:

- full title of the book

- ISBN

- page number

CONTRIBUTORS

Jennifer S. Wooddell
Senior Author and Editor

Edited for Production by
Judene Wright, M.S., M.A.Ed.
National Content Director, MCAT Program, The Princeton Review

Jennifer and Judene would like to thank the following people for their contributions to this book:

Elizabeth Aamot (Fatith), John Bahling, M.D., Gary Bedford, Jessica Burstrem, M.A., Alix Claps, M.A., Cynthia Cowan, B.A., Sara Daniel, B.S., Cory Eicher, B.A., (James) Ben Gill, Jacqueline R. Giordano, Gina Granter, M.A., Corinne Harol, Christopher Hinkle, Th.D., Alison Howard, Paul Kugelmass, Jay Lee, Addie Lozjanin, Rohit Madani, B.S., Mike Matera, B.A., Ashleigh Menhadji, Katherine Montgomery, Don Osborne, Rupal Patel, B.S., Vivek Patel, Tyler Peikes, Nadia Reynolds, M.A., Maryam Shambayati, M.S., Angela Song, Kate Speiker, David Stoll, Jonathan Swirsky, Neil Thornton, Laura Tubelle de González, and David Weiskopf, M.A.

CONTENTS

Get More (Free) Content
at **PrincetonReview.com/prep**

As easy as **1·2·3**

1 Go to PrincetonReview.com/prep or scan the **QR code** and enter the following ISBN for your book:
9780593516249

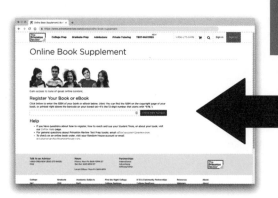

2 Answer a few simple questions to set up an exclusive Princeton Review account. *(If you already have one, you can just log in.)*

3 Enjoy access to your **FREE** content!

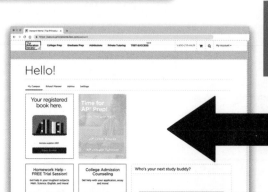

Once you've registered, you can...

- Take **3** full-length practice MCAT exams

- Find useful information about taking the MCAT and applying to medical school

- Check to see if there have been any corrections or updates to this edition

- Get our take on any recent or pending updates to the MCAT

Need to report a potential **content** issue?

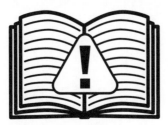

Contact **EditorialSupport@review.com** and include:

- full title of the book
- ISBN
- page number

Need to report a **technical** issue?

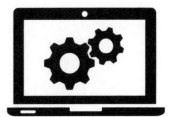

Contact **TPRStudentTech@review.com** and provide:

- your full name
- email address used to register the book
- full book title and ISBN
- Operating system (Mac/PC) and browser (Chrome, Firefox, Safari, etc.)

Chapter 1
MCAT Basics

SO YOU WANT TO BE A DOCTOR

So...you want to be a doctor. If you're like most premeds, you've wanted to be a doctor since you were pretty young. When people asked you what you wanted to be when you grew up, you always answered "a doctor." You had toy medical kits, bandaged up your dog or cat, and played hospital. You probably read your parents' home medical guides for fun.

When you got to high school you took the honors and AP classes. You studied hard, got straight As (or at least really good grades!), and participated in extracurricular activities so you could get into a good college. And you succeeded!

At college you knew exactly what to do. You took your classes seriously, studied hard, and got a great GPA. You talked to your professors and hung out at office hours to get good letters of recommendation. You were a member of the premed society on campus, volunteered at hospitals, and shadowed doctors. All that's left to do now is get a good MCAT score.

Just the MCAT.

Just the most confidence-shattering, most demoralizing, longest, most brutal entrance exam for any graduate program. At about 7.5 hours (including breaks), the MCAT tops the list...even the closest runners up, the LSAT and GMAT, are only about 4 hours long. The MCAT tests significant science content knowledge along with the ability to think quickly, reason logically, and read comprehensively, all under the pressure of a timed exam.

The path to a good MCAT score is not as easy to see as the path to a good GPA or the path to a good letter of recommendation. The MCAT is less about what you know, and more about how to apply what you know—and how to apply it quickly to new situations. Because the path might not be so clear, you might be worried. That's why you picked up this book.

We promise to demystify the MCAT for you, with clear descriptions of the different sections, how the test is scored, and what the test experience is like. We will help you understand general test-taking techniques as well as provide you with specific techniques for each section. In this book, we'll give you strategies for the Critical Analysis and Reasoning Skills (CARS) section, while our other MCAT subject books will review the science content. We'll show you the path to a good MCAT score and help you walk that path.

After all...you want to be a doctor. And we want you to succeed.

WHAT IS THE MCAT...REALLY?

Most test-takers approach the MCAT as though it were a typical college science test, one in which facts and knowledge simply need to be regurgitated in order to do well. They study for the MCAT the same way they did for their college tests, by memorizing facts and details, formulas, and equations. And when they get to the MCAT they are surprised…and disappointed.

It's a myth that the MCAT is purely a content-knowledge test. If medical school admission committees want to see what you know, all they have to do is look at your transcripts. What they really want to see is how you think, especially under pressure. That's what your MCAT score will tell them.

The MCAT is really a test of your ability to apply basic knowledge to different, possibly new, situations. It's a test of your ability to reason out and evaluate arguments. Do you still need to know your science content? Absolutely. But not at the level that most test-takers think they need to know it. Furthermore, your science knowledge won't help you on the Critical Analysis and Reasoning Skills (CARS) section. So how do you study for a test like this?

You study for the science sections by reviewing the basics and then applying them to MCAT practice questions. You study for the CARS section by learning how to adapt your existing reading and analytical skills to the nature of the test. (More information about the science sections can be found in their respective *MCAT Review* books.)

The book you are holding will teach you the strategies you need to do well on the MCAT CARS section. It includes many passages and questions designed to make you think about the material in a deeper way, along with full explanations to clarify the logical thought process needed to get to the answer. It also comes with access to three full-length online practice exams to further hone your skills. For more information on accessing those online exams, please refer to the "Get More (Free) Content" spread on page viii.

MCAT NUTS AND BOLTS

Overview

The MCAT is a computer-based test (CBT) that is *not* adaptive. Adaptive tests base your next question on whether or not you've answered the current question correctly. The MCAT is *linear*, or *fixed-form*, meaning that the questions are in a predetermined order and do not change based on your answers. However, there are many versions of the test, so that on a given test day, different people will see different versions. The following table highlights the features of the MCAT exam.

Registration	Online via www.aamc.org. Begins as early as six months prior to test date; available up until week of test (subject to seat availability).
Testing Centers	Administered at small, secure, climate-controlled computer testing rooms.
Security	Photo ID with signature, electronic fingerprint, electronic signature verification, assigned seat.
Proctoring	None. Test administrator checks examinee in and assigns seat at computer. All testing instructions are given on the computer.
Frequency of Test	Many times per year distributed over January, April, May, June, July, August, and September.
Format	Exclusively computer-based. NOT an adaptive test.
Length of Test Day	7.5 hours
Breaks	Optional 10-minute breaks between sections, with a 30-minute break for lunch.
Section Names	1. Chemical and Physical Foundations of Biological Systems (Chem/Phys) 2. Critical Analysis and Reasoning Skills (CARS) 3. Biological and Biochemical Foundations of Living Systems (Bio/Biochem) 4. Psychological, Social, and Biological Foundations of Behavior (Psych/Soc)
Number of Questions and Timing	59 Chem/Phys questions, 95 minutes 53 CARS questions, 90 minutes 59 Bio/Biochem questions, 95 minutes 59 Psych/Soc questions, 95 minutes
Scoring	Test is scaled. Several forms per administration.
Allowed/ Not allowed	No timers/watches. Noise reduction headphones available. Noteboard booklet and wet-erase marker given at start of test and taken at end of test. Locker or secure area provided for personal items.
Results: Timing and Delivery	Approximately 30 days. Electronic scores only, available online through AAMC login. Examinees can print official score reports.
Maximum Number of Retakes	The test can be taken a maximum of three times in one year, four times over two years, and seven times over the lifetime of the examinee. An examinee can be registered for only one date at a time.

Registration

Registration for the exam is completed online at www.aamc.org/students/applying/mcat/reserving. The Association of American Medical Colleges (AAMC) opens registration for a given test date at least two months in advance of the date, often earlier. It's a good idea to register well in advance of your desired test date to make sure that you get a seat.

Sections

There are four sections on the MCAT, all of which consist of multiple-choice questions:

Section	Concepts Tested	Number of Questions and Timing
Chemical and Physical Foundations of Biological Systems (Chem/Phys)	Basic concepts in chemistry and physics, including biochemistry, scientific inquiry, reasoning, research and statistics skills.	59 questions in 95 minutes
Critical Analysis and Reasoning Skills (CARS)	Critical analysis of information drawn from a wide range of social science and humanities disciplines.	53 questions in 90 minutes
Biological and Biochemical Foundations of Living Systems (Bio/Biochem)	Basic concepts in biology and biochemistry, scientific inquiry, reasoning, research and statistics skills.	59 questions in 95 minutes
Psychological, Social, and Biological Foundations of Behavior (Psych/Soc)	Basic concepts in psychology, sociology, and biology, research methods and statistics.	59 questions in 95 minutes

Most questions on the MCAT (44 in the science sections, all 53 in the CARS section) are passage-based; the science sections have 10 passages each and the CARS section has 9. A passage consists of a few paragraphs of information on which several following questions are based. In the science sections, passages often include equations or reactions, tables, graphs, figures, and experiments to analyze. CARS passages come from literature in the social sciences, humanities, ethics, philosophy, cultural studies, and population health, and do not test content knowledge in any way.

Some questions in the science sections are freestanding questions (FSQs). These questions are independent of any passage information and appear in four groups of about three to four questions, interspersed throughout the passages. 15 of the questions in the science sections are freestanding, and the remainder are passage-based.

Each section on the MCAT is separated by either a 10-minute break or a 30-minute lunch break. We recommend that you take these breaks.

Section	Time
Test Center Check-In	Variable, can take up to 40 minutes if center is busy.
Tutorial	10 minutes
Chemical and Physical Foundations of Biological Systems	95 minutes
Break (optional)	10 minutes
Critical Analysis and Reasoning Skills	90 minutes
Lunch Break (optional)	30 minutes
Biological and Biochemical Foundations of Living Systems	95 minutes
Break (optional)	10 minutes
Psychological, Social, and Biological Foundations of Behavior	95 minutes
Void Option	5 minutes
Survey (optional)	5 minutes

The survey includes questions about your satisfaction with the overall MCAT experience, including registration, check-in, etc., as well as questions about how you prepared for the test.

Scoring

The MCAT is a scaled exam, meaning that your raw score will be converted into a scaled score that takes into account the difficulty of the questions. There is no guessing penalty. All sections are scored from 118–132, with a total scaled score range of 472–528. Because different versions of the test have varying levels of difficulty, the scale will be different from one exam to the next. Thus, there is no "magic number" of questions to get right in order to get a particular score. Plus, some of the questions on the test are considered "experimental" and do not count toward your score; they are just there to be evaluated for possible future inclusion in a test.

At the end of the test (after you complete the Psychological, Social, and Biological Foundations of Behavior section), you will be asked to choose one of the following two options, "I wish to have my MCAT exam scored" or "I wish to VOID my MCAT exam." You have 5 minutes to make a decision, and if you do not select one of the options in that time, the test will automatically be scored. If you choose the VOID option, your test will not be scored (you will not now, or ever, get a numerical score for this test), medical schools will not know you took the test, and no refunds will be granted. You cannot "unvoid" your scores at a later time.

So, what's a good score? The AAMC is centering the scale at 500 (i.e., 500 will be the 50th percentile), and recommends that application committees consider applicants near the center of the range. To be on the safe side, aim for a total score of around 510. And remember that if your GPA is on the low side, you'll need higher MCAT scores to compensate, and if you have a strong GPA, you can get away with lower MCAT scores. But the reality is that your chances of acceptance depend on a lot more than just your MCAT scores. It's a combination of your GPA, your MCAT scores, your undergraduate course work, letters of recommendation, experience related to the medical field (such as volunteer work or research), extracurricular activities, your personal statement, etc. Medical schools are looking for a complete package, not just good scores and a good GPA.

GENERAL LAYOUT AND TEST-TAKING STRATEGIES

Layout of the Test

In each section of the test, the computer screen is divided vertically, with the passage on the left and the range of questions for that passage indicated above (e.g., "Passage 1 Questions 1–5"). The scroll bar for the passage text appears in the middle of the screen. Each question appears on the right, and you need to click "Next" to move to each subsequent question.

In the science sections, the freestanding questions are found in groups of 3–4, interspersed with the passages. The screen is still divided vertically; on the left is the statement "Questions [X–XX] do not refer to a passage and are independent of each other," and each question appears on the right as described above.

CBT Tools

There are a number of tools available on the test, including highlighting, strike-outs, the Flag for Review button, the Navigation and Review Screen buttons, the Periodic Table button, and of course, the noteboard booklet. All tools are available with both mouse control (buttons to click) or keyboard commands (Alt+ a letter). As everyone has different preferences, you should practice with both types of tools (mouse and keyboard) to see which is more comfortable for you personally. The following is a brief description of each tool.

1) **Highlighting:** This is done in the passage text (including table entries and some equations, but excluding figures and molecular structures), in the question stems, and in the answer choices (including Roman numerals). Select the words you wish to highlight (left-click and drag the cursor across the words), and in the upper left corner click the "Highlight" button to highlight the selected text yellow. Alternatively, press "Alt+H" to highlight the words. Highlighting can be removed by selecting the words again and in the upper left corner clicking the down arrow next to "Highlight." This will expand to show the "Remove Highlight" option; clicking this will remove the highlighting. Removing highlighting via the keyboard is cumbersome and is not recommended.

2) **Strike-outs:** This can be done on the answer choices, including Roman numeral statements, by selecting the text you want to strike out (left-click and drag the cursor across the text), then clicking the "Strikethrough" button in the upper left corner. Alternatively, press "Alt+S" to strike out the words. The strike-out can be removed by repeating these actions. Figures or molecular structures cannot be struck out, however, the letter answer choice of those structures can.

3) **Flag for Review button:** This is available for each question and is found in the upper right corner. This allows you to flag the question as one you would like to review later if time permits. When clicked, the flag icon turns yellow. Click again to remove the flag. Alternatively, press "Alt+F."

4) **Navigation button:** This is found near the bottom of the screen and is only available on your first pass through the section. Clicking this button brings up a navigation table listing all questions and their statuses (unseen, incomplete, complete, flagged for review). You can also press "Alt+N" to bring up the screen. The questions can be sorted by their statuses, and clicking a question number takes you immediately to that question. Once you have reached the end of the section and viewed the Review screen (described below), the Navigation screen is no longer available.

5) **Review Screen button:** This button is found near the bottom of the screen after your first pass through the section and, when clicked, brings up a new screen showing all questions and their statuses (either incomplete, unseen, or flagged for review). Questions that are complete are assigned no additional status. You can then choose one of three options by clicking with the mouse or with keyboard shortcuts: Review All (Alt+A), Review Incomplete (Alt+I), or Review Flagged (Alt+R); alternatively, you can click a question number to go directly back to that question. You can also end the section from this screen.

6) **Periodic Table button:** Clicking this button will open the periodic table (or press "Alt+T"). Note that the periodic table is large, covering most of the screen. However, this window can be resized to see the questions and a portion of the periodic table at the same time. The table text will not decrease, but scroll bars will appear on the window so you can center the section of the table of interest in the window.

7) **Noteboard Booklet (Scratch Paper):** At the start of the test, you will be given a spiral-bound set of four laminated 8.5″ × 14″ sheets of paper and a wet-erase black marker to use as scratch paper. You can request a clean noteboard booklet at any time during the test; your original booklet will be collected. The noteboard is only useful if it is kept organized; do not give in to the tendency to write on the first available open space! Good organization will be very helpful when/if you wish to review a question. Indicate the passage number, the range of questions for that passage, and a topic in a box near the top of your scratch work, and indicate the question you are working on in a circle to the left of the notes for that question. Draw a line under your scratch work when you change passages to keep the work separate. Do not erase or scribble over any previous work. If you do not think it is correct, draw one line through the work and start again. You may have already done some useful work without realizing it.

General Strategy for the Science Sections

Passages vs. FSQs in the Science Sections: What to Start With

Since the questions are displayed on separate screens, it is awkward and time consuming to click through all of the questions up front to find the FSQs. Therefore, go through the section on a first pass and decide whether to do the passage now or to save it for later, basing your decision on the passage text and the first question. Tackle the FSQs as you come upon them. More details are below.

Here is an outline of the procedure:

1) For each passage, write a heading on your noteboard with the passage number, the general topic, and its range of questions (e.g., "Passage 1, thermodynamics, Q 1–5" or "Passage 2, enzymes, Q 6–9"). The passage numbers do not currently appear in the Navigation or Review screens, thus having the question numbers on your noteboard will allow you to move through the section more efficiently.

2) Skim the text and rank the passage. If a passage is a "Now," complete it before moving on to the next passage (also see "Attacking the Questions" below). If it is a "Later" passage, first write "SKIPPED" in block letters under the passage heading on your noteboard and leave room for your work when you come back to complete that passage. (Note that the specific passages you skip will be unique to you; in the Bio/Biochem section, you might choose to do all Biology passages first, then come back for Biochemistry. Or in Chem/Phys you might choose to skip experiment-based or analytical passages. Know ahead of time what type of passage you are going to skip and follow your plan.)

3) Next, click on the "Navigation" button at the bottom to get to the navigation screen. Click on the first question of the next passage; you'll be able to identify it because you know the range of questions from the passage you just skipped. This will take you to the next passage, where you will repeat steps 1–3.

4) Once you have completed the "Now" passages, go to the review screen and double-click the first question for the first passage you skipped. Answer the questions, and continue going back to the review screen and repeating this procedure for other passages you have skipped.

Attacking the Questions

As you work through the questions, if you encounter a particularly lengthy question, or a question that requires a lot of analysis, you may choose to skip it. This is a wise strategy because it ensures you will tackle all the easier questions first, the ones you are more likely to get right. If you choose to skip the question (or if you attempt it but get stuck), write down the question number on your noteboard, click the Flag for Review button to flag the question in the Review screen, and move on to the next question. At the end of the passage, click back through the set of questions to complete any that you skipped over the first time through, and make sure that you have filled in an answer for every question.

General Strategy for the CARS Section

Ranking and Ordering the Passages: What to Start With

Ranking: Since the questions are displayed on separate screens, it is awkward and time consuming to click through all of the questions before ranking each passage as "Now" (an easier passage), "Later" (a harder passage), or "Killer" (a passage that you will randomly guess on). Therefore, rank the passage and decide whether or not to do it on the first pass through the section based on the passage text, by skimming the first 2–3 sentences.

Ordering: Because of the additional clicking through screens (or, use of the Review screen) that is required to navigate through the section, the "Two-Pass" system (completing the "Now" passages as you find them) is likely to be your most efficient approach. However, if you find that you are continuously making a lot of bad ranking decisions, it is still valid to experiment with the "Three-Pass" approach (ranking all nine passages up front before attempting your first "Now" passage).

Here is an outline of the basic Ranking and Ordering procedure to follow.

1) For each passage, write a heading on your scratch paper with the passage number and its range of questions (e.g., "Passage 1 Q 1–7"). The passage numbers do not currently appear in the Review screen, thus having the question numbers on your scratch paper will allow you to move through the section more efficiently.

2) Skim the first 2–3 sentences and rank the passage. If the passage is a "Now," complete it before moving on to the next. If it is a "Later" or "Killer," first write either "Later" or "Killer" and "SKIPPED" in block letters under the passage heading on your scratch paper and leave room for your work if you decide to come back and complete that passage. Then click through each question, flagging each one and filling in random guesses, until you get to the next passage.

3) Once you have completed the "Now" passages, come back for your second pass and complete the "Later" passages, leaving your random guesses in place for any "Killer" passages that you choose not to complete. Go to the Review screen and use your scratch paper notes on the question numbers. Double-click on the number of the first question for that passage to go back to that question, and proceed from there. Alternatively, if you have consistently flagged all the questions for passages you skipped in your first pass, you can use "Review Flagged" from the Review screen to find and complete your "Later" passages.

4) Regardless of how you choose to find your second pass passages, unflag each question after you complete it, so that you can continue to rely on the Review screen (and the "Review Flagged" function) to identify questions that you have not yet attempted.

Previewing the Questions

The formatting and functioning of the tools facilitates effective previewing. Having each question on a separate screen will encourage you to really focus on that question. Even more importantly, you can highlight in the question stem (but not in the answer choices).

Here is the basic procedure for Previewing the Questions:

1) Start with the first question, and if it has lead words referencing passage content, highlight them. You may also choose to jot them down on your scratch paper. Once you reach and preview the last question for the set on that passage, THEN stay on that screen and work the passage (your highlighting appears and stays on every passage screen, and persists through the whole 90 minutes).

2) Once you have worked the passage and defined the Bottom Line—the main idea and tone of the entire passage—work **backward** from the last question to the first. If you skip over any questions as you go (see "Attacking the Questions" below), write down the question number on your scratch paper. Then click **forward** through the set of questions, completing any that you skipped over the first time through. Once you reach and complete the last question for that passage, clicking "Next" will send you to the first question of the next passage. Working the questions from last to first the first time through the set will eliminate the need to click back through multiple screens to get to the first question immediately after previewing, and will also make it easier and more efficient to do the hardest questions last (see "Attacking the Questions" below).

3) Remember that previewing questions is a CARS-only technique. It is not efficient to preview questions in the science sections.

Attacking the Questions

The question types and the procedure for actually attacking each type will be discussed later. However, it is still important **not** to attempt the hardest questions first (you'll risk potentially getting stuck, wasting time, and discouraging yourself).

So, as you work the questions from last to first (see "Previewing the Questions" above), if you encounter a particularly difficult and/or lengthy question (or if you attempt a question but get stuck) write down the question number on your scratch paper (you may also choose to flag it) and move on backward to the next question you will attempt. Then click **forward** through the set and complete any that you skipped over the first time through the set, unflagging any questions that you flagged that first time through and making sure that you have filled in an answer for every question.

Pacing Strategy for the MCAT

Since the MCAT is a timed test, you must keep an eye on the timer and adjust your pacing as necessary. It would be terrible to run out of time at the end only to discover that the last few questions could have been easily answered in just a few seconds each.

In the science sections you will have about one minute and thirty-five seconds (1:35) per question, and in the CARS section you will have about one minute and forty seconds (1:40) per question (not taking into account time spent reading the passage before answering the questions).

Section	# of Questions in passage	Approximate time (including reading the passage)
Chem/Phys, Bio/Biochem, and Psych/Soc	4	6.5 minutes
	5	8 minutes
	6	9.5 minutes
CARS	5	8.5 minutes
	6	10 minutes
	7	11.5 minutes

When starting a passage in the science sections, make note of how much time you will allot for it, and the starting time on the timer. Jot down on your noteboard what the timer should say at the end of the passage. Then just keep an eye on it as you work through the questions. If you are near the end of the time for that passage, guess on any remaining questions, make some notes on your noteboard, Flag the questions, and move on. Come back to those questions if you have time.

For the CARS section, keep in mind that many people will maximize their score by *not* trying to complete every question or every passage in the section. A good strategy for test-takers who cannot achieve a high level of accuracy on all nine passages is to randomly guess on at least one passage in the section, and spend your time getting a high percentage of the other questions right. To complete all nine CARS passages, you have about ten minutes per passage. To complete eight of the nine, you have about 11 minutes per passage.

To help maximize your number of correct answer choices in any section, do the questions and passages within that section in the order *you* want to do them in. See "General Strategy" above.

Process of Elimination

Process of Elimination (POE) is probably the most useful technique you have to tackle MCAT questions. Since there is no guessing penalty, POE allows you to increase your probability of choosing the correct answer by eliminating those you are sure are wrong.

1) Strike out any choices that you are sure are incorrect or that do not address the issue raised in the question.
2) Jot down some notes to help clarify your thoughts if you return to the question.
3) Use the "Flag for Review" button to flag the question for review. (Note, however, that in the CARS section, you generally should not be returning to rethink questions once you have moved on to a new passage.)
4) Do not leave it blank! For the sciences, if you are not sure and you have already spent more than 60 seconds on that question, just pick one of the remaining choices. If you have time to review it at the end, you can always debate the remaining choices based on your previous notes. For CARS, if you have been through the choices two or three times, have reread the question stem and gone back to the passage and you are still stuck, move on. Do the remaining questions for that passage, take one more look at the question you were stuck on, then pick an answer and move on for good.
5) Special Note: if three of the four answer choices have been eliminated, the remaining choice must be the correct answer. Don't waste time pondering *why* it is correct; just click it and move on. The MCAT doesn't care if you truly understand why it's the right answer, only that you have the right answer selected.
6) More subject-specific information on techniques will be presented in the next chapter.

Guessing

Remember, there is NO guessing penalty on the MCAT. NEVER leave a question blank!

QUESTION TYPES

In the science sections of the MCAT, the questions fall into one of three main categories.

1) Memory questions: These questions can be answered directly from prior knowledge and represent about 25 percent of the total number of questions.
2) Explicit questions: These questions are those for which the answer is explicitly stated in the passage. To answer them correctly, for example, may just require finding a definition, or reading a graph, or making a simple connection. Explicit questions represent about 35 percent of the total number of questions.
3) Implicit questions: These questions require you to apply knowledge to a new situation; the answer is typically implied by the information in the passage. These questions often start "if… then…" (for example, "if we modify the experiment in the passage like this, then what result would we expect?"). Implicit style questions make up about 40 percent of the total number of questions.

In the CARS section, the questions fall into four main categories.

1) Specific questions: These either ask you for facts from the passage (Retrieval questions) or require you to deduce what is most likely to be true based on the passage (Inference questions).
2) General questions: These ask you to summarize themes (Main Idea and Primary Purpose questions) or evaluate an author's opinion (Tone/Attitude questions).
3) Reasoning questions: These ask you to describe the purpose of, or the support provided for, a statement made in the passage (Structure questions) or to judge how well the author supports his or her argument (Evaluate questions).

4) Application questions: These ask you to apply new information from either the question stem itself (New Information questions) or from the answer choices (Strengthen, Weaken, and Analogy questions) to the passage.

More detail on question types and strategies can be found in Chapter 4.

TESTING TIPS

Before Test Day

- Take a trip to the test center at least a day or two before your actual test date so that you can easily find the building and room on test day. This will also allow you to gauge traffic and see if you need money for parking or anything like that. Knowing this type of information ahead of time will greatly reduce your stress on the day of your test.
- During the week before the test, adjust your sleeping schedule so that you are going to bed and getting up in the morning at the same times as on the day before and morning of the MCAT. Prioritize getting a reasonable amount of sleep during the last few nights before the test.
- Don't do any heavy studying the day before the test. This is not a test you can cram for! Your goal at this point is to rest and relax so that you can go into test day in a good physical and mental condition.
- Eat well. Try to avoid excessive caffeine and sugar. Ideally, in the weeks leading up to the actual test you should experiment a little bit with foods and practice tests to see which foods give you the most endurance. Aim for steady blood sugar levels during the test: sports drinks, peanut-butter crackers, trail mix, etc. make good snacks for your breaks and lunch.

General Test Day Info and Tips

- On the day of the test, arrive at the test center at least a half hour prior to the start time of your test.
- Examinees will be checked into the center in the order in which they arrive.
- You will be assigned a locker or secure area in which to put your personal items. Textbooks and study notes are not allowed, so there is no need to bring them with you to the test center.
- Your ID will be checked, your palm vein will be scanned, and you will be asked to sign in.
- You will be given your noteboard booklet and wet-erase marker, and the test center administrator will take you to the computer on which you will complete the test. You may not choose a computer; you must use the computer assigned to you.
- Nothing is allowed at the computer station except your photo ID, your locker key (if provided), and a factory sealed packet of ear plugs; not even your watch.
- If you choose to leave the testing room at the breaks, you will have your palm vein scanned again, and you will have to sign in and out.
- You are allowed to access the items in your locker, except for notes and cell phones. (Check your test center's policy on cell phones ahead of time; some centers do not even allow them to be kept in your locker.)
- Don't forget to bring the snack foods and lunch you experimented with in your practice tests.
- At the end of the test, the test administrator will collect your noteboard.
- Definitely take the breaks! Get up and walk around. It's a good way to clear your head between sections and get the blood (and oxygen!) flowing to your brain.
- Ask for a clean noteboard at the breaks if you want a fresh one.

Chapter 2
Introduction to MCAT Critical Analysis and Reasoning Skills

GOALS

1) To understand the structure and scoring of the Critical Analysis and Reasoning Skills Section
2) To learn the fundamentals of Critical Analysis and Reasoning Skills strategies

Congratulations on choosing The Princeton Review for your MCAT preparation. You are well on your way to significantly raising your MCAT score and getting into your top-choice medical school. We understand that the Critical Analysis and Reasoning Skills (CARS) section presents many challenges to the typical MCAT student. We want our students to have every available tool, so we have devoted ourselves to developing the most rigorous CARS materials possible, based on intensive study of the MCAT itself and of the best strategies that lead to success on this test.

2.1 THE CRITICAL ANALYSIS AND REASONING SKILLS (CARS) SECTION

Structure

- CARS is the second section of the test.
- It consists of nine passages, which typically average 500–700 words each.
- Each passage is followed by 5–7 questions (with four answer choices per question), for a total of 53 questions.
- You will have 90 minutes to complete the section. You can do the questions and passages in any order that you choose within the 90-minute limit.
- You will be able to scroll up and down within the passage text. The questions are displayed one at a time on the right, with the passage (and any highlighting you have done in the passage text) always displayed on the left. Click on the Next and Previous buttons on the bottom of the screen to go back and forth between the questions and passages within the section. Clicking Next from the last question for a passage takes you to the next passage and the first question for that passage. Once the 90 minutes are up, however, you cannot go back to any of the CARS passages or questions.

Pacing

You do not necessarily need to complete all nine passages to get a competitive score. Many people will maximize their score by randomly guessing on at least one passage and focusing on getting a high percentage of the rest of the questions correct. Also, keep in mind that there is no guessing penalty. Never leave a question blank; always select a random guess for questions that you choose not to complete. You have a 25 percent chance of getting those questions right.

Content

The passages may be on any subject in the humanities and social sciences. Passage topics may include philosophy, ethics, archeology, economics, history, political science, literature and literary theory, psychology, sociology, anthropology, cultural studies, geography, population health, and art history and theory. This range of topics may seem overwhelming. However, unlike the other multiple choice sections of the test, CARS tests no outside knowledge of the subject. In fact, using your own factual knowledge or opinions of the subject can lead you to pick incorrect answers; the questions require you to use only the information provided in the passage. Clearly, you can't prepare for or approach this section of the test in the same way as physics or chemistry!

2.2 DEVELOPING YOUR CRITICAL REASONING SKILLS

The Critical Analysis and Reasoning Skills section can be intimidating for many people taking the MCAT. You have been studying hard for many years, packing your brain with lots of science knowledge and refining your memorization skills. But now, as you confront the CARS section, all those facts and mnemonics are useless, and you have to employ an entirely different approach. Even if you have taken a lot of humanities and social science courses and have been speaking and reading English for many years, you might find the CARS section to be challenging at first. This is because you need to adapt to the specific nature and requirements of this section of the MCAT.

There are many false beliefs regarding the CARS section, one of which is that your score depends on luck. That is, if you happen to get "good" passages, all is well, but if you don't, you are in trouble. However (and thankfully!), this is entirely untrue. There are ways that you can improve your CARS score regardless of the passages you happen to get on your test. BUT... to achieve this improvement, many, if not most, of you will need to fundamentally change how you read the passages and go about answering the questions. You will need to develop new skills that have little to do with memorization and everything to do with reading efficiently and thinking critically. The good news is that these are skills that everyone can develop and improve through practice and careful self-evaluation. These core skills fall into three basic categories.

Working the Passage
- **Reading the passage efficiently:** identifying the most important points made by the author while moving quickly through the details
- **Following the logical structure of the author's argument:** identifying such things as key shifts in direction, comparisons and contrasts, conclusions, and author's tone
- **Synthesizing the Bottom Line of the entire passage:** identifying the author's Main Idea and Attitude

Attacking the Questions

- **Correctly identifying and translating the questions:** knowing what each question is asking you to do in order to choose the correct answer
- **Using the passage (and only the passage) as a resource:** quickly locating the relevant passage information for each question
- **Answering in your own words:** predicting what the correct answer will do before considering the answer choices
- **Using Process of Elimination (POE):** eliminating down to the "least wrong" choice rather than just picking an answer that "sounds good"

General Test Strategy

- **Time management:** getting what you need from the passage without getting bogged down in irrelevant facts or spending too much time on one question
- **Pacing and accuracy:** not going so fast that you miss a high percentage of the questions that you complete, or so slow that you overthink the questions or do not complete enough questions to reach your target score
- **Stress management:** thinking clearly and working efficiently under stressful conditions

2.3 FUNDAMENTALS: THE SIX STEPS

Based on these core skills, here are the six steps to follow when working the CARS section.

■ STEP 1: RANK AND ORDER THE PASSAGES

Ranking

The passages are not necessarily, or even usually, presented in order of difficulty. There is no reason to waste time on the hardest passage or passages, only to skip or rush through an easy passage at the end of the section. So your first step, as you reach each new passage, is to decide if it is a Now (or easier) passage, a Later (or harder) passage, or a Killer passage (one that you will simply randomly guess on, or do last). To assign a rank, skim a few sentences of the passage and see if you can easily paraphrase it. If you can, it's most likely an easier passage to understand. If not, it is likely to be a harder passage that you should either come back to later during your 90 minutes or just randomly guess on.

Ordering

If a passage is a Now passage, go ahead and work it through, completing all of the questions. If it is a Later or Killer passage, click through each question, Flag it for review and fill in a random guess, and move on to ranking the next passage. Also note the passage number on your notepad. Once you have completed the Now passages in the section, come back through the section and complete the Later passages, and make sure that you have filled in your random guesses on your Killer passage or passages. (See Chapter 6 of this book for more information on Ranking and Ordering.)

■ STEP 2: PREVIEW THE QUESTIONS

Knowing what topics show up in the questions will help you work the passage more quickly and effectively. Before working the passage, read through the question stems from first to last (not the answer choices), identifying and highlighting any words or phrases that indicate important passage content. Do not worry at this stage about understanding the question or identifying the question type. (See Chapter 3 of this book for more information on Previewing the Questions.)

■ STEP 3: WORK THE PASSAGE

Stay on the screen for the last question and work the passage from here (your highlighting will stay and appear in the passage text regardless of which question for that passage you are working on). As you read through the passage, use the highlighting function (sparingly) to annotate the most important references in the text. This would include things like: question topics, topic sentences, shifts in direction or continuations, the author's tone, different points of view, and conclusions. As you read, articulate the Main Point of each chunk of information (usually, each paragraph). Use your notepad, especially on difficult passages, to jot down these main points. As you move through the passage, think about how these chunks relate to each other; that is, track the logical structure of the author's argument in the passage. (See Chapter 3 of this book for more information on Active Reading and Annotation.)

■ STEP 4: BOTTOM LINE

After you have read the entire passage, sum up the Bottom Line: the main idea and tone of the entire passage. For particularly difficult passages, write this down on your notepad to make sure that you have a reasonably clear idea of the point and purpose of the passage as a whole. (See Chapter 3 for more information on finding the Bottom Line.)

■ STEP 5: ATTACK THE QUESTIONS

This is how the question will be formatted on the screen.

1. When an argument is inductive, that argument:

A) is necessarily less conclusive than an argument that attempts to use deductive logic.

B) is based on probability, such that the likelihood that its premises are all true is no greater than the likelihood of the truth of its conclusion.

C) seeks to find or identify causes or explanations.

D) when valid, may be based on evaluation of a representative sample of a population.

Work through the questions backwards, so that you don't need to click back to the first question for that passage. As you work through each question, follow these steps:

- Read the question word for word and identify the question type.
- Translate the question task into your own words, thinking about what the question is asking you to do with or to the passage.
- When the question stem provides a specific reference to the passage, go back to the passage before reading the answer choices and find the relevant information (reading at least five lines above and below the reference).

- Paraphrase the passage information. Then, with the question type firmly in mind, think about what the correct answer will need to do.
- As you go through the choices, use POE actively. Look for reasons to strike out incorrect choices, and select the "least wrong" of the four. (See Chapters 4 and 5 of this book for more information on identifying and answering different question types.)
- If you hit a particularly difficult question, skip over it for the moment and complete the other easier questions. Then click forward through the questions towards the next passage, completing any questions that you initially skipped.

■ STEP 6: INSPECT THE SECTION

At or before the 5-minute mark (ideally, before you begin your last passage), double-check to make sure that you haven't left any incomplete questions. You can use the Review screen at this stage. Do NOT rethink questions you have already completed. Your goal in this step is simply to make sure that you have selected an answer for each question.

2.4   GUIDELINES FOR USING YOUR REVIEW MATERIALS

Focus on Accuracy

Whenever you're acquiring a new skill, you need to learn to do it well before learning to do it quickly. Many students feel that speed is their number one concern. This often leads them to rush through the initial "learning to do it well" phase. Unfortunately, this is entirely counterproductive and will ultimately keep you from scoring as highly as you possibly can.

As you begin working practice passages, do the passages untimed; focus on following the techniques and improving your accuracy. Once you become comfortable with these techniques, set a timer to count *up* as you do each passage (or, note your start and end times with a watch). Record how long it takes you to do a passage, but don't attempt to complete the passage within a set time limit. We will let you know when to begin using set time limits for individual passages or for full CARS sections.

Even after you have been studying for some time and have taken many practice tests, it is still useful to do some untimed passages, focusing on avoiding the types of mistakes you tend to make. Then bring that same focus into the next set of timed passages you complete or the next practice test that you take.

Build Endurance

At first, work on only a few passages at a time, developing the skills you've learned. Allowing yourself this time to practice slowly but accurately gives you a strong foundation for accurate timed practice. Always do passages at least two at a time to practice ranking and ordering them. After a couple of weeks, try to do a number of practice passages at once, and don't take any breaks between the passages. Also, at this stage, don't check your answers after every one or two passages. You need to get used to working through each new passage without the reassurance or feedback from knowing how you did on the previous passage. Build up your endurance over time, so that you can eventually maintain your concentration at its peak over the course of an entire 90-minute section. Set aside a daily time for CARS work and stick to your schedule. Keep in mind the particular strategies you should be focusing on depending on where you are in this book and in your preparation process.

Control Your Environment

Give your full attention to the passages when you practice. That is, don't do homework while watching TV or conversing with friends. However, when you take the actual MCAT, you'll be in a room full of people who are muttering to themselves, sniffling and coughing, typing loudly, standing up and sitting down at different times, and generally behaving in a distracting or annoying manner (unintentionally, we hope!). Therefore, practice working in less-than-ideal conditions. Go to a reasonably quiet coffeehouse, a room in the library where there are people moving around, or some other location with low-level distractions. Learn how to tune out what is going on around you and how to keep your focus on the passages in front of you. (Note: basic foam earplugs in a factory sealed package are allowed on the MCAT. You will also be provided with noise-reduction headphones in the testing center.)

Manage Your Stress

Managing your psychological and physical condition is just as important as studying and practicing. It doesn't do you any good to work all day every day if you are so burned out that your brain doesn't function any more. Build times for relaxation, including some kind of physical activity, into your schedule. Later in the book, we will discuss specific ways of reducing anxiety and stress as you study and on test day.

Evaluate Your Work

Constant self-evaluation is the key to continued improvement. Don't just answer the questions and tally your score at the end. Use the materials to teach yourself how to improve. What kinds of questions do you consistently miss? What kinds of passages slow you down? What kinds of answer traps do you tend to fall for? What caused you to pick the wrong answer to each question that you missed?

However, don't just think about the questions you got wrong—also analyze how you arrived at the credited response when your answers are correct. Did you avoid a common trap? Are there question types on which you are particularly strong? Did you successfully apply one of our techniques?

Use the charts and the Self-Evaluation Survey provided at the end of this chapter to identify patterns in the mistakes you are making. Only by identifying your mistakes can you learn to correct them. The next section provides you with guidance on how to use those resources.

2.5 SELF-EVALUATION

Every student has different strengths and weaknesses on the MCAT CARS section. To improve on your weaknesses, you must first recognize them. From now on, keep a log of every passage that you do (sample logs are provided later on).

The time you spend reviewing your work is just as important as the time spent working on the passages. After you complete a passage, go through each question and answer choice. Pay particular attention to those questions that you got wrong. In order to increase your score, you'll need to assess and change the way that you think. Often we continue to take the same steps or read in the same way, even when we've seen that this way is not successful. You may not even realize that you're making the same mistake over and over again until you see it logged into your chart several times. Look for patterns in your mistakes and successes; based on those patterns, define ways in which you need to change how you read and think in order to raise your score.

There are three resources provided at the end of this chapter to help you with the self-evaluation process.

I. Individual Passage Log

Fill out this log for every passage that you do, and for every question within each passage that you miss. Also fill out the log for every question that you got right but were unsure of the correct answer when you picked it (for example, you were down to two choices and then guessed).

At the end of each chapter there are two Individual Passage Logs to use on the practice passages for that chapter. To use the Individual Passage Logs on other practice materials (such as online practice passages), make clean copies of the logs or follow the same structure on notebook paper or in an Excel spreadsheet.

II. Test Assessment Log

Fill out this log for each full CARS test section that you do. Complete it as soon as you can after the test; once a few hours have passed, it will be difficult to remember why you made the choices that you did. As with the Individual Passage Log, either make multiple clean copies of the log for future use, or follow the same structure on notebook paper or in a spreadsheet.

Following the blank version of that log you will find a filled-out sample log. It doesn't correspond to any particular test; it is provided to give you an idea of how you should be filling out your own logs.

III. Self-Evaluation Survey

Complete the Self-Evaluation survey for every full CARS test section that you do. It consists of a series of questions to help you to analyze your overall performance on the section and on each question within it. It is generally best to fill out the Test Assessment Log first, while the questions are still fresh in your mind, and then use the Survey to sum up your analysis and set goals for future tests.

I. Individual Passage Log

Key for Passage Log

Passage # and Time spent on passage

Indicate the location of the passage and how long it took you to complete it (once we have instructed you to begin timing the passages).

Q # and Q type

For each question you miss in a passage, indicate the number and the type of question. Refer to the list of question types in Chapter 4.

Attractors

For the first 15 individual logs that you fill out, list what was wrong with every wrong answer, including the ones that you did not pick. After that, you can list only the wrong answers that you chose or seriously considered choosing.

Refer to the Attractors described and listed in Chapters 4 and 5.

What did you do wrong?

Describe the error that led you down the path to the wrong answer, and how you will avoid making that same mistake in the future. Below is a (non-exhaustive) list of common mistakes. Choose one or more items from this list (there may be more than one misstep involved in picking a wrong answer), or, if none fits, describe the error in your own words. If, time after time, you cannot figure out why you chose the wrong answer, it is very likely that you are working too quickly and/or too carelessly. Did you

- misread the question?
- fail to go back to the passage?
- fail to read all four of the answer choices?
- fail to read the entire answer choice?
- over-interpret the passage or the answer choice?
- forget the "EXCEPT/LEAST/NOT" in the question?
- pick an answer choice that was
    - …out of scope or not the issue?
    - …too extreme or absolute?
    - …from the wrong part of the passage?
    - …half right, half wrong?
    - …strengthening when it should have been weakening (or vice versa)?
    - …too narrow on a general question?

Using the Individual Passage Log, take the time to assess how your current thought processes led you to a tempting but wrong answer choice, and how a different way of thinking on the question would have been more successful. The log will help you to see how the test is constructed, and most importantly, how you are responding to it. **You can't change the test, but you can change your responses to it.** This process will allow you to work through the MCAT CARS section more quickly and with greater accuracy.

Individual Passage Log

Passage # _2 P1_   Time spent on passage _____

Q#	Q type	Attractors	What did you do wrong?
#1	inference		I selected something I thought & didnt go back
#3	inference		did not notice time diff
#6	structure		did not read except

Revised Strategy _read more carefully._

Passage # _M2. P1_   Time spent on passage _____

Q#	Q type	Attractors	What did you do wrong?
#5	structure		Confusing q. again- tried to use reasoning instead of looking at passage & clear evidence

Revised Strategy _look 4 clear evidence._

2.5

II.   Test Assessment Log

Use this worksheet to record and monitor your performance on full nine-passage sections, as well as to continue the self-evaluation process. In particular, use it to see if you are spending the time you need on the easier passages in order to get most of those questions right. Keep track of how much time you spent (roughly) on the Now passages and on the Later passages. If you find that you are spending the bulk of your 90 minutes on the harder passages with a low level of accuracy, you need to reapportion your time. You should also evaluate your ranking; are you choosing the right passages?

2.5

Now Passages

Now Passage #	Q # and Type (for questions you got wrong)	Attractors (for wrong answers you picked or seriously considered)	What did you do wrong?

Approximate time spent on Now passages _____

Total Now passages attempted _____

Total # of Qs on Now passages attempted _____

Total # of Now Qs correct _____

% correct of Now Qs attempted _____

Later Passages

Later Passage #	Q # and Type (for questions you got wrong)	Attractors (for wrong answers you picked or seriously considered)	What did you do wrong?

Approximate time spent on Later passages _____

Total Later passages attempted _____

Total # of Qs on Later passages attempted _____

Total # of Later Qs correct _____

% correct of Later Qs attempted _____

Final Analysis

Total # of passages attempted (including partially completed) _____

Total # of questions attempted _____

Total # of correct answers _____

Total % correct of attempted questions _____

Revised Strategy

Pacing	
Passage choice/ranking	
Working the Passage	
Attacking the Questions	

2.5

Sample Completed Test Assessment Log—Now Passages

Now Passage #	Q # and Type (for questions you got wrong)	Attractors (for wrong answers you picked or seriously considered)	What did you do wrong?
1	None	N/A	Spent a bit too much time—was *overly* cautious
3	Q12: Main Point	Q12 D: too narrow	Q12: got it down to two and guessed—didn't compare choices or reread the question stem
4	Q23: Inference	Q23 A: out of scope	Q23: Got it right but took too much time—should have gone back to the passage before POE (almost talked myself into an answer that was clearly wrong once I went back to passage)
7	Q39: Weaken Q41: New Information Q42: Inference	Q39 B: opposite Q41 C: opposite Q42 C: reversal	All three: shouldn't have done this passage at all—it was a killer. Didn't understand the passage at all (very abstract and confusing), and got the author's argument all turned around.
9	None!	N/A	Nothing!

Approximate time spent on Now passages **a little less than an hour**

Total Now passages attempted **5**

Total # of Qs on Now passages attempted **28**

Total # of Now Qs correct **23**

% correct of Now Qs attempted **82%**

Sample Completed Test Assessment Log—Later Passages

Later Passage #	Q # and Type (for questions you got wrong)	Attractors (for wrong answers you picked or seriously considered)	What did you do wrong?
2	Q7: Analogy Q10: New Information/Weaken	Q7 A: half right, half wrong Q10 D: opposite	Q7: didn't read the whole choice (or the rest of the answer choices) carefully—made up my mind too fast Q10: lost track of question type—picked what would be strengthened, not weakened
5	Q26: Retrieval	Q26 B: words out of context	Q26: didn't read carefully enough when went back to passage. Easy question.
6	Q33: Evaluate Q35: Analogy Q37: Inference	Q33 A: half right, half wrong Q35 D: out of scope Q37 C: too extreme	Q33: didn't make sure that the description matched Q35: panicked and didn't think about the logic/theme of the relevant part of the passage Q37: saw the strong language but picked it anyway because was rushed
8	Q43: Inference Q44: Weaken Q46: Structure Q47: Retrieval	Q43 B: too extreme Q44 C: opposite Q46 D: right answer wrong question Q47 A: words out of context	Q43: didn't pay enough attention to strength of language Q44: forgot the question type and picked something supported by the passage (as if was answering Inference question) Q46: forgot the question type and picked answer that was supported by passage but not the purpose of the reference Q47: picked answer because sounded like what I remembered from the passage—in reality, was never mentioned Overall: was rushing, running out of time

Approximate time spent on Later passages **35 minutes**

Total Later passages attempted _____**4**_____

Total # of Qs on Later passages attempted _____**25**_____

Total # of Later Qs correct _____**15**_____

% correct of Later Qs attempted _____**60%**_____

Final Analysis

Total # of passages attempted (including partially completed) _____9_____

Total # of questions attempted _____53_____

Total # of correct answers _____38/53_____

Total % correct of attempted questions _____72%_____

Revised Strategy

Pacing	Slow down—only do 8 passages.
Passage choice/ranking	Skip over more Later/Killer passages in first pass. Take difficulty of abstract passage texts seriously—skip or do Later.
Working the Passage	Pay more attention to author's opinion, and to contrasting points of view (so that I don't mix them up later). Write down the main points and Bottom Line on harder passages.
Attacking the Questions	Read the question carefully and reread it when down to two answer choices. Go back to the passage more, and read more carefully when I do. Read THE WHOLE answer choice word for word and para-phrase it. Compare choices to each other when down to two. Pay more attention to strength of language and tone.

III. CARS Self-Evaluation Survey

This section consists of a series of questions intended to help you evaluate your performance on each practice test.

Before answering the questions in this section, you should review your score report, go back over the questions that you missed, and fill out your Self-Evaluation Passage Logs or Test Assessment Logs. You may wish to look through the questions in this survey first and then review your exam using the score report. Finally, come back and select your answers for the survey and read the feedback corresponding to your responses.

Do this one exam at a time—i.e., answer these survey questions after each exam you take. Don't answer them for multiple exams in a group. The survey is extensive; you may even wish to break up your evalu-ation of a single exam into two or more chunks of time. Note that it is important to answer the survey questions, especially those regarding the reasons why you missed particular questions, as soon as possible after taking the exam, when your reasoning is fresh in your mind. Therefore, answer the questions in Part III within a day of taking the practice test. However, you can fill in your responses for Parts I and II a day or two later.

There is space under each question to list the answer choice or choices (for some of the survey questions, you may be selecting more than one choice). Compare your responses for each practice test to look for trends.

After completing the survey for each test that you take, write down at least three things that you will focus on during your next practice test, or during your next set of practice passages. Space is provided at the end of the survey for you to write down these goals.

PART I: OVERALL ACCURACY AND PACING

1. Approximately what percentage of the 53 questions did you get correct?

Test 1 _____

Test 2 _____

Test 3 _____

Test 4 _____

Test 5 _____

A. 85–100%

Your accuracy is excellent. Define the strategies that led to your correct answers and apply them to the practice MCATs that you take in the future. If you missed any questions, carefully diagnose the reasons why, so that you can achieve an even higher level of accuracy in the future.

B. 70–84%

Your accuracy is reasonably good. Make a list of at least three reasons why you missed the questions that were incorrect, and focus on not making those same kinds of mistakes on the practice passages and MCATs that you take in the future. Define some of the strategies that led to correct answers, and apply those to future practice tests as well.

C. 55–69%

You need to work on improving your accuracy, especially if you are on the low end of this range. Make a list of at least three reasons why you missed the questions that were incorrect and focus on not making those same kinds of mistakes on the practice MCATs you take in the future. Compare the questions you got wrong to the questions that you got right in order to diagnose the strategies that were and were not working for you.

D. 40–54%

Your accuracy is relatively low. In the prep you do in the near future, focus on getting a higher percentage of the questions that you complete correct, even if that means slowing down for now and not answering all of the questions. Make a list of at least three reasons why you missed the questions that you got incorrect and focus on not making those same kinds of mistakes on the practice MCATs you take in the future.

Compare the questions you got wrong to the questions that you got right in order to diagnose the strategies that were and were not working for you.

E. Less than 40%

Your accuracy is low. You will need to significantly increase your percentage correct in order to get a competitive score. That will likely involve slowing down and randomly guessing on at least one passage in the section. Make a list of at least three reasons why you missed the questions that were incorrect and focus on not making those same kinds of mistakes on the practice MCATs you take in the future.

2. Is your accuracy:

Test 1 _____

Test 2 _____

Test 3 _____

Test 4 _____

Test 5 _____

A. highest in the beginning of the section and falling off toward the end?

Work on building up your endurance by studying for longer and longer periods of time. Taking as many mock MCATs as you can will also help you keep your concentration at a high level throughout a test. You may also have been lingering too long on the questions in the beginning, and then rushing the questions at the end.

Many test-takers will maximize their score by randomly guessing on a certain percentage of the questions in a CARS section. If you had to rush through many of the questions and if you got many of those questions wrong, this is an indication that, at this point in your preparation process, you should not be trying to work through all of the passages or questions.

B. highest in the middle of the section?

It is likely that it took you some time to warm up in the beginning, and then you tired out (or got impatient or rushed) at the end. Try warming up a bit by working through a passage before you take your next test. Take little 5-10 second breaks every 10-15 minutes during a test so that you can maintain your energy and focus at the end of the section.

C. highest at the end of the section?

It is likely that you gradually warmed up as you went through the test. The good news is that endurance was not a problem for you. To achieve a high level of accuracy from beginning to end, try warming up by working through a passage before you take your next practice test.

D. about the same all the way through the section?

Good work, if your accuracy was relatively good. On the MCAT, your goal is to hit the ground running and to keep your focus and energy high through the entire test.

2.5

3. **For the questions that you missed, on average, what was your level of confidence as you answered those questions?**

Test 1 _____

Test 2 _____

Test 3 _____

Test 4 _____

Test 5 _____

2.5

A. Fairly high

If you commonly felt very confident while picking answers that were in fact incorrect, and if you answered those questions relatively quickly, you may have been answering based on memory rather than by using the passage actively. If this is the case, in the future go back to the passage, find the relevant information, and base your answer closely on the passage text. Alternatively, you may have misread the question stem and/or answer choices, or selected a response before reading through all four choices. Look back at the questions you missed to determine if this was the case. Make a conscious effort to slow down when you read the question stem and answer choices, and read all four choices before selecting your response.

However, if you spent a great deal of time on the questions before picking the wrong answer, and if you read through the answer choices multiple times or spent a lot of time debating between two choices, you may have been overthinking the question and talking yourself into a wrong answer. In the future, limit yourself to two careful passes through the answer choices, select an answer (based on the passage information and question task), and then move on.

B. Moderate

It is normal to have a moderate level of confidence on most of the questions that you miss. If you missed quite a few questions (more than 16), however, your confidence and accuracy will increase if you read the question, the answer choices, and the relevant passage text more carefully, and if you base your answers more closely on the information in the passage. Use the feedback for your responses to the survey, especially questions 8–10, to diagnose specific reasons for your mistakes.

C. Fairly low

If you only missed a few questions, it is normal to have a low level of confidence on those questions; they were likely among the hardest questions in the test. However, if you missed many questions (more than 16), it is likely that you were not using the passage information actively enough. If you read the question stem and answer choices more carefully and go back to the passage text more consistently to find the relevant information, your level of confidence and your accuracy (and potentially your speed as well) will increase.

4. **For the questions that you got correct, what was your average level of confidence while answering the question?**

Test 1 _____

Test 2 _____

Test 3 _____

Test 4 _____

Test 5 _____

2.5

A. Fairly high

If you completed the section in the time allowed, and if you had excellent accuracy (that is, missed 8 or fewer), a high level of confidence is a sign that your approach to the questions was solid. However, if you had trouble completing the section (that is, did not get to one or more passages and/or had to rush at the end and missed many of those final questions), you may have been overly cautious. If your experience fits this scenario, don't double or triple check your answers. Once you have eliminated three of the choices and have a reasonable answer left, select that choice and move on.

B. Moderate

If your accuracy was fairly good (that is, you missed 12 or fewer), a moderate level of confidence on the questions that you got correct is normal. However, if your accuracy was significantly lower than this, it can improve through a combination of reading the passage text more carefully (at least the part that is relevant to the question), thinking through the question task more carefully, and paying attention to every word in each answer choice. Use the feedback for your responses to this survey, especially questions 8–10, to diagnose specific reasons for your mistakes.

C. Fairly low

If your accuracy was fairly good (you missed 12 or fewer questions and you completed the section), having a low level of confidence is not necessarily a bad thing. You do not need to understand every idea or detail in the passage in order to get most questions correct. If your accuracy was significantly lower, however, it most likely means that in general you may not be reading the questions carefully enough, using the passage actively enough, or reading and analyzing the answer choices closely enough. Focus on reading the question stem and answer choices word for word, as well as on finding specific information in the passage to support your response.

PART II: GENERAL TESTING STRATEGIES

5. **Did you read the question stems (not the choices) before you read the passage text?**

   Test 1 _____

   Test 2 _____

   Test 3 _____

   Test 4 _____

   Test 5 _____

A. Yes

This is an effective approach for most test-takers. When you preview the questions, don't worry about the question type. Rather, look for words in the question that relate to passage content to help you focus in on the key parts of the passage as you read it the first time through.

B. No

On the MCAT, Previewing the Questions (just the stem, not the choices) can be a very useful technique. If you haven't tried it, or if you have only tried it a few times and then abandoned the technique, it is worth practicing to see if it will pay off for you. On your next set of practice passages or practice test, try quickly reading through the question stems before reading the passage. Don't worry about the question type at that stage. Instead, pick out and highlight the words and phrases that relate to the content of the passage. This will allow you to focus on the most important parts of the passage, and to highlight words in those sections to help you go back efficiently to find the necessary information as you answer the questions.

However, if you have in fact practiced it for a month or more, and if you have implemented it on several tests without seeing a payoff in accuracy and/or speed, then not Previewing the Questions is a reasonable choice for you.

6. **Did you use notepad as you took the test?**

   Test 1 _____

   Test 2 _____

   Test 3 _____

   Test 4 _____

   Test 5 _____

A. No

Using notepad (provided by the test center on the real MCAT) is a very useful strategy. Writing down a few words to express the main point of each paragraph or big chunk of information, as well as the main point or Bottom Line of the whole passage, can help you to understand and keep track of the key parts of the author's argument, especially on the harder passages. It can also be quite helpful to keep track of your Process of Elimination on Roman numeral and EXCEPT/LEAST/NOT questions. If you are not used to using notepad, try it on several practice passages and then on at least two practice tests. Once you practice it, you will most likely find that it improves both your accuracy and your speed.

B. Yes

If you are using notepad already, the next step is to think about how you can use it even more effectively than you are now. In particular, make sure that it is well organized and that you are writing clearly. If you are writing quite a bit, work on paring it down (for example, limiting yourself to 4-5 words to express the main point of a paragraph or of the passage as a whole). You may not need to write down the main point of every paragraph for every passage. If the passage is easy to follow and understand, you might define some or all of the main points as a mental step without writing them all down. If you are making notes on the passage but never on the questions, try using it (sparingly) to write down brief notes to help you clarify and organize your thought process on difficult questions.

PART III: ATTACKING THE QUESTIONS AND POE

7. **When you went back over the questions that you missed, which of the following reactions did you often have? Select all that apply and read the feedback for those responses.**

   Test 1 _____

   Test 2 _____

   Test 3 _____

   Test 4 _____

   Test 5 _____

A. "The correct answer looks obvious in retrospect, and I don't know why I didn't pick it."

If the correct answer looks obvious in retrospect and/or if you don't remember why you made the choices that you did during the test, this is often due to going too fast and choosing based on intuition rather than on test-appropriate reasoning. Don't just pick the first answer that "sounds good." Instead, base your answer closely on the question task and the passage text.

B. "I see why the right answer could be right, but I still think the answer I picked is right too."

In MCAT CARS, many wrong answers are written to sound very good, but they have something, sometimes something fairly subtle, in them that makes them worse than the credited response. The correct answer is the "least wrong" answer. That is, it may not be perfect, but the other three are even worse. Furthermore, the correct answer must be based on the passage, not on outside knowledge or your own opinion. Go back to the questions that you missed, compare the right answers to your wrong answers, and identify the differences between them that make the credited response the best of the four choices.

C. "I see why the right answer is right and the wrong answer is wrong, but I think that I would still pick the wrong answer in the future."

A big part of maximizing your CARS score is learning the logic of the test itself. Each time you break down the logic of a question that you missed, you prepare yourself to get similar questions right in the future. Always review questions that you missed, not only to see why the right answer was right, but to diagnose what caused you to disregard it. Your ultimate goal is to get points; if you understand the logic of the test, you can begin to answer more strategically and avoid picking wrong answers in the future.

2.5

D. "I still don't get it."

Make sure to read the explanations for these questions especially carefully. Then go back through the question step by step: paraphrase what the question is really asking, identify and paraphrase the relevant information in the passage text, and go through the choices one more time, comparing them to each other and identifying differences between them. Even if this process takes some time, on most questions you will come to see the logic of the test, and questions will make more and more sense to you in the future.

8. **For which of the following question types did you miss two or more questions? Select all that apply and read the corresponding feedback below each response.**

   Test 1 _____

   Test 2 _____

   Test 3 _____

   Test 4 _____

   Test 5 _____

A. Inference and Retrieval questions

The key to getting these questions right is sticking as closely as possible to the information in the passage. Compare your wrong answers to the credited responses and identify how the right answers are better supported by the text. In the future, whenever possible, answer in your own words (based only on the passage text) before you evaluate the answer choices.

B. Main Point, Primary Purpose, and Tone/Attitude questions

The answers to these general question types must include, explicitly or implicitly, the whole passage, not just a part of it. Commonly, wrong answers for these types will be too narrow, too strong, or have a word or phrase within them that is inconsistent with the passage. Identify the Bottom Line of the passage (including the author's tone) before you go through the answer choices. Make sure to track the author's tone or attitude throughout the passage and highlight the relevant words. When you are down to two answers, look for differences in tone and scope.

2.5

C. Structure and Evaluate questions

To get these questions right, you need to identify the logical structure of the relevant part of the passage. You must see how different statements in the passage relate to each other, which includes separating the author's claims or conclusions from the support for those claims. Often, wrong answers are true based on the passage, but do not answer the question being asked. When attacking these questions, generate an answer in your own words, based not just on content but also on the logical structure of the passage, before you go through the answer choices.

D. New Information questions

These questions require you to summarize the theme of the new information in the question stem, and then apply it to the relevant information in the passage text. When you get these questions wrong, identify whether or not you correctly understood the point of the new information. If you did, see if you might have lost track of the relevant issue in the passage, and/or picked an answer that took the wrong direction (e.g., it was inconsistent with the passage, but the question asked how the author would respond). In the future, first identify the theme of the new information, then describe its relationship to the passage, including whether the question requires an answer consistent or inconsistent with the passage. Keep track of this direction as you evaluate each answer choice.

9. **For which of the following question types or formats did you miss two or more questions? Select all that apply and read the corresponding feedback below each response.**

    Test 1 _____

    Test 2 _____

    Test 3 _____

    Test 4 _____

    Test 5 _____

A. Strengthen and Weaken questions

These questions require you to accept the new information in the answer choices as true, and to find the correct answer that goes in the right direction. The answer must be strong enough to have a significant impact on the relevant part of the author's argument. Look at your wrong answers and identify if they were too weak to "most strengthen" or "most undermine" the passage, if they went in the opposite direction (for example, strengthened instead of weakened), or if they were not directly relevant to the passage. In the future, define what the correct answer needs to do before evaluating the answer choices. You may benefit from jotting this on your notepad, especially on Weaken questions.

B. Analogy questions

These questions ask you to find an answer with the same logic as the relevant part of the passage. In most cases, the correct answer will not be about the same subject matter as the passage. Look at your wrong answers to see if they match the content/topic but not the passage logic, or if they are part right/part wrong (one piece matches, another does not). In the future, describe the logic of the relevant part of the passage in generic terms before looking at the answer choices (e.g., if the passage states "increased food production led to a population explosion," you could write "an increase in A led to a large increase in B").

C. Roman Numeral questions

These questions provide you with three statements, and ask you to select the answer choice that includes all the statements that correctly answer the question and none that do not. Look at your wrong answers. Did you include too many (you were not strict enough) or too few (you eliminated statements that were not quite as good as those most obviously correct, but that were still good enough)? In the future, use your notepad to keep track of your evaluation of each statement as you go. Also, if you are sure that a statement is correct, eliminate answer choices that do not include it, and compare the remaining choices. If you are sure a statement is incorrect, eliminate choices that do include it and compare what remains.

D. EXCEPT/LEAST/NOT questions

These questions ask you to select the "worst" answer. For example, when a question asks "All of the following can be inferred EXCEPT," the three wrong answers will be supported by the passage, and the correct answer will not. Look at the questions you missed to see if you lost track of the EXCEPT, LEAST, or NOT. In the future, use your notepad to keep track of why you are eliminating each choice as you go.

10. **For which of the following reasons did you miss one or more questions? Select all that apply and read the suggestions below each selection.**

     Test 1 _____

     Test 2 _____

     Test 3 _____

     Test 4 _____

     Test 5 _____

A. "I misunderstood the question."

Read the question stem word for word and put it into your own words before you read the answer choices.

B. "I misunderstood the passage."

If you read the passage text very quickly, slow down a bit and (at least!) pay more attention to the most important statements. When you go back to the passage while answering the question, read the relevant part carefully and paraphrase it. If you spent quite a bit of time reading the passage, however, you may have overthought it. Stick to what is explicitly stated, and don't waste time speculating about what the author might have meant.

C. "I answered from memory, and my memory was inaccurate."

Go back to the passage and read the relevant part carefully when answering the questions.

D. "I based my answer on the wrong part of the passage."

Make sure to keep track of the precise issue raised in the question stem, and to identify all the parts of the passage that may be relevant to it. Previewing the Questions before you work the passage will help you to do this most effectively and efficiently.

2.5

E. "I misunderstood or misread one or more of the answer choices."

Read each answer choice word for word the first time through. Paraphrase complicated choices to make sure that you understand what they are saying.

F. "I talked myself into the wrong answer."

The correct answer should not take a lot of effort to justify. Stick to the question task, the passage, and the exact wording of the answer choice. Use process of elimination aggressively; look for reasons to strike out choices.

G. "I got it down to two and then picked the wrong one."

This happens because there is often at least one wrong answer that is written to be very attractive. When you are down to two choices, reread the question, compare the two choices to each other, and if needed, go back to the passage again. Remember to pick the "least wrong" answer, not just the answer that "sounds best."

11. **On average, how often did you read all or part of the passage before answering a question?**

Test 1 _____

Test 2 _____

Test 3 _____

Test 4 _____

Test 5 _____

A. Once

This is fine if you had a high level of accuracy. If you had a low level of accuracy, use the passage more actively (as if you are taking an open book test).

B. Twice

This is usually appropriate. Most of the time, you will read the passage as a whole once, and then go back at least once to the relevant section or sections as you answer each question.

C. Three times

This can be appropriate for harder questions. However, make sure that you are both reading the relevant section thoroughly enough and pausing to paraphrase it. Often, reading the appropriate part of the passage more completely and thoughtfully earlier on (during the process of answering the question) will eliminate the need to go back to it again and again. Focus more on answering the question in your own words in order to increase your efficiency and speed.

D. Four or more times

You may be reading and rereading bits and pieces of the passage out of context, which then requires you to go back and forth between the answer choices and the passage too often. Focus on reading and paraphrasing the entire relevant chunk, as well as on answering in your own words so that you can increase your efficiency and speed.

Ask yourself if you are overworking the questions, rethinking them or rereading parts of the passage over and over, even when you have a solid basis for picking an answer and moving on. If so, give yourself a limit on the number of times you can go back to the passage (for example, twice). Once you have hit that limit, select an answer and go on to the next question.

> **12. On average, how many times did you read through the set of answer choices before making a final selection?**
>
> Test 1 _____
>
> Test 2 _____
>
> Test 3 _____
>
> Test 4 _____
>
> Test 5 _____

A. Once

This was appropriate if you had a high level of accuracy (you missed 8 or fewer questions). If your accuracy was significantly lower, take two passes through the choices, at least on the more difficult questions. Eliminate the one or two most clearly wrong answers the first time through, and then compare the remaining choices before making a final selection.

B. Twice

This is usually appropriate. In most cases, you will eliminate one or two choices the first time through, and then compare the remaining answers in order to make a final decision.

C. Three times

This can be necessary on the more difficult questions. However, if you are going through the choices three times on most questions, you can increase your efficiency (and accuracy) by answering in your own words first whenever possible, and by reading the choices word for word (and paraphrasing complicated statements) the first time through.

D. Four or more times

If you are often reading through the choices four or more times, you need to work on attacking the questions more efficiently. Make it a goal to eliminate at least one or two choices on your first read through, based on the question task and the relevant passage information. Whenever possible, answer the question in your own words first so that you have more information in hand up front. When you are down to two choices, compare them to each other, reread the question, and go back to the passage rather than just rereading the choices over and over. Keep your focus on what is wrong with each choice, and on selecting the "least wrong" answer.

2.5

Goals for Test 2:

1)

2)

3)

Goals for Test 3:

1)

2)

3)

Goals for Test 4:

1)

2)

3)

Goals for Test 5:

1)

2)

3)

Goals for Real MCAT:

1)

2)

3)

2.6   STRESS MANAGEMENT

Most students feel some level of stress before an important exam. A certain level of anxiety, while uncomfortable, is beneficial: it sharpens your attention, keeps you alert, and intensifies your focus. However, if you find that your stress and anxiety gets out of control to the point where your performance suffers, there are ways to manage it and reduce it to a reasonable level. Some of these methods (see I, II, and IV below) involve scheduling your time and acclimating yourself to the experience of taking the test: these are important for everyone to implement from the beginning of your preparation. Other methods (see III below) involve reducing anxiety through relaxation and other exercises. You will find that some of these techniques work better for you than others. Try them all out, settle on some that work for you, and then use them consistently up to, and on, the day of the test.

I. Preparing for the Test

Develop and Implement a Clear Strategy

Anxiety comes in part from feeling as if you are unable to control a situation. Identify the aspects of the test, the testing conditions, and the importance of the test that instill fear in you, and do things that will help you confront and minimize those fears.

- **Build up your stamina.**
  It is difficult to maintain concentration over many hours under normal circumstances, let alone under stressful conditions. Prepare for test day by working passages over longer and longer periods with shorter and shorter breaks, until you can comfortably concentrate for a few hours at a time.

- **Take as many full practice tests as possible.**
  Experience builds confidence. Once you have practiced doing several passages at a stretch, take on doing more and more practice tests. Complete full tests in one sitting, taking breaks between sections. Don't have any food or water during the test except during the breaks. If you get cold or hot, don't put on or take off clothing unless you're on a break. That is, take your practice tests under the same conditions as the real MCAT. On test day, you can walk in to the testing center knowing that you know how to do this—this is just one more test in a long line of tests you've already completed.

- **Practice dealing with distraction.**
  Do passages or practice tests under less-than-ideal conditions. Go to a reasonably quiet coffee house, or an area of the library where people are moving around (but not talking loudly). Practice tuning out your surroundings while you work.

II. Taking the Test (including Practice Tests)

- **Take a breath.**

  The more tense we get, the more shallow our breathing becomes. Lack of oxygen can then contribute to your anxiety in a feedback loop. Stop this process as soon as you realize that your muscles are tightening or your focus is fading. Sit back in your chair and take three deep breaths. Take your eyes off the screen for 10-15 seconds, and move your arms and shoulders around to release the muscles. Don't force yourself onward to the next question if you realize that you're not working at your peak. Rather than wasting a big chunk of time getting questions wrong because you can't think straight, take a few seconds to relax and regroup, and make the most of the rest of your time.

- **Don't obsess about time.**

  Of course you are going to check the timer while you work, but checking the time constantly will distract you and make things more stressful. Doing lots of practice tests will help you develop a sense of timing while you work, so you know how long it takes you to read passages and get through questions. Only check the clock between passages; otherwise, immerse yourself in the task of working passages and attacking questions efficiently and effectively.

- **Take the breaks you are given.**

  The MCAT is designed to give you a feeling of burnout. The test makers give you as little help as possible during your test day, so make good use of what they DO give you! Just as you should use the annotation tools provided, such as highlighting and strikeout, you must also take advantage of the breaks you are offered. Use them for the basics (eating, using the restroom, etc.) but also to clear your mind, breathe deeply, get your eyes away from the screen, and shift gears for the next session.

III. Reducing Anxiety

Use Positive Reinforcement

- When we place high demands on ourselves, it's easy to fall into negative thinking at moments of frustration. You may find yourself thinking self-critical thoughts while studying or doing a practice test. Do "How could I miss that question!", "I'm so stupid!", or "I'm never going to get this!" sound familiar?

- Recognize these responses for what they are: a reaction to stress, not a representation of reality. Find words and phrases to replace the negative thoughts, such as "I know I'm smart, I'm working hard, and it will all pay off in the end." It may sound goofy, but it works.

MCAT CRITICAL ANALYSIS AND REASONING SKILLS REVIEW

Reward Yourself

- Don't let yourself burn out over the next month or two (or three). Yes, study and practice are crucial, but so is maintaining peace of mind. If you are so overworked and tired that you cannot concentrate on what you're doing, give yourself a break. If you can't commit to scheduling your time as extensively as recommended below, just make sure to nip feelings of being overworked in the bud as soon as you feel them coming on: set a goal (i.e., a certain number of hours of study time, or a particular number of practice passages). Once you achieve that goal, go to a movie, hang out with friends, go to the gym: do whatever you enjoy most for a few hours.

Practice Creative Visualization

- Creative visualization, if practiced over time, can offer significant long-term anxiety reduction. Lie on the floor (at home, not during the test!) on your back, with your arms and legs stretched out. Adjust your position until you feel comfortable and relaxed. Then close your eyes and picture the most wonderful, relaxing place you have ever visited or would like to visit, or a situation that makes you feel safe and at peace. It may be a tropical island, a quiet forest, a deserted beach, or a gathering at home with friends and family. See your surroundings clearly, smell the air, hear the birds, or picture the faces of the people who make you happy. When you are ready to stop, picture the most relaxing part of the scene one last time. Count to three slowly, then open your eyes. If you practice this regularly for a few weeks, especially at times when you feel tense, you should begin to feel less anxious. Then, if you do find yourself becoming anxious during the test, breathe deeply and imagine yourself back in that peaceful place. You will find yourself relaxing quickly, because you've trained yourself to respond that way.

- While creative visualization of relaxing escapes are great for managing stress, if you're going to think about the aftermath of the test, it is helpful to focus on positive outcomes, imagining success. Who will be the first person you tell about your MCAT score? How will that person react to the good news? Imagine the look on your parent's face, the hugs you will get, and the feeling of accomplishment you will have as you share news of your score. Thinking of these things as part of your goal, rather than simply focusing on the numerical score you want to achieve, can help you feel more motivated.

IV. Managing Your Time

- Just as a clear pacing strategy will help you to work more methodically and stay calm during the test, pacing yourself in your preparation will help you feel more in control and will help ensure that you still make time to relax and spend time with friends and family (and therefore maintain your sanity).

- Consider how many hours of MCAT preparation you should do in a week and create a daily schedule of the hours of the day you will dedicate to it. Be practical in your estimation of hours: you may feel like you should be studying all the time but you likely have other responsibilities and commitments, plus you need time to eat, rest, exercise, and unwind.

- Below are two sample schedules. Both are for days when you don't have to go to class or work: the first is for a day dedicated to reading and passage drills, and the second is for days on which you are taking full practice tests. Both entail 8–9 hour prep days. Notice how much time is left to do other things.

- You may only be able to manage two hours of MCAT prep if you have a heavy day with classes, work, or other commitments—set your schedule accordingly. And, if you can manage it, having one day a week that is completely, or at least significantly, free of MCAT study can be restorative (and help you to get even more out of the other six days of the week). A great benefit of creating a schedule to manage your time is that when you are not scheduled to study, you don't have to feel guilty about not studying!

- Your schedule should be personalized based on when you tend to wake, eat, sleep, and on your own individual activities. Do make sure to adjust your sleep and study schedule to correspond to the time of day you are taking the MCAT, at least in the last few weeks before your test.

Construct your own agenda for the weeks or months remaining before the MCAT, using these sample schedules as guidelines.

Sample Schedule: No Full Practice Test

6:30 A.M.–8:00 A.M.: Wake up, breakfast, quick morning walk/run or workout, shower.

8:00 A.M.–11:30 A.M.: MCAT prep (this could be half a practice test, practice questions and passages, test review, or some chapter reading for various subjects)

11:30 A.M.–1:00 P.M.: Lunch and leisure time (read a magazine, check social media news, meet with a friend, dance to your favorite song)

1:00 P.M.–4:00 P.M.: MCAT prep

4:00 P.M.–5:00 P.M.: Snack, stretch, unwind

5:00 P.M.–7:00 P.M.: MCAT prep

7:00 P.M.–10:30 P.M.: Dinner and leisure time

10:30 P.M.–11:00 P.M.: Go to bed

Sample Schedule: Full Practice Test

6:30 A.M.–7:30 A.M.: Wake up, breakfast, quick morning walk/run or workout, shower.

7:30 A.M.–9:00 A.M.: Warm up for the test (do a few practice questions and passages to get your mind going)

9:00 A.M.–4:30 P.M.: Full practice MCAT (including break times)

4:30 P.M.–6:00 P.M.: Dinner/snack, relax

6:00 P.M.–8:00 P.M.: Test review (always review your performance as soon as possible; review CARS on the same day as the test so that you can remember your thought process during the test)

8:00 P.M.–10:30 P.M.: Relax, do whatever else needs to be done

10:30 P.M.–11:00 P.M.: Go to bed

2.6

Chapter 2 Summary

Your preparation for the MCAT CARS section should include familiarization with passage structure, question types, and answer traps, as well as training in the efficient and effective use of passage information.

In addition to reading practice passages and answering the questions, smart preparation includes a careful, continuing analysis of your performance.

CHAPTER 2 PRACTICE PASSAGES

Individual Practice Drills

Do the following two passages untimed. Focus on implementing the six steps you learned in this chapter. After you have checked your answers, fill out an Individual Passage Log for each passage.

CHAPTER 2 PRACTICE PASSAGE 1

"To live as our fathers and grandfathers lived will not do. The village resident more and more feels that his life is connected by thousands of invisible threads not only with his fellow villagers, with the nearest rural township, but this connection goes much farther. He dimly perceives that he is a subject of a vast state, and that events taking place far from his place of birth can have a much greater influence on his life than some event in his village." –Petr Koropachinskii, Ufa Provincial Zemstvo Chairman, 1906

When Koropachinskii wrote these words, he viewed the "invisible threads" connecting the villager with the state as a new political consciousness gained primarily through the political mobilization of the 1905 revolution. Salient features of this mobilization, such as political parties, their programs, and a freer press, drew the attention of political actors at the time and, subsequently, of historians of late imperial Russia. We might consider these connections from another perspective, however: that of the state and the "invisible threads" it used to connect with its subjects. Furthermore, many of these connections were not so much invisible threads as paper trails—written documents found in the files of bureaucracies staffed by officials who sought to extend the regime's knowledge about its population.

[One such method,] registration through the state church, presented complications in an empire composed of many religious groups. Not all of the tsar's subjects were Orthodox. What to do about the rest? As Gérard Noiriel has pointed out, the Old Regime in France had faced a similar problem. Registration by Catholic priests left many Jews and Protestants without civil status. In 1792, the revolutionary Republic addressed this situation by secularizing registration and requiring municipal authorities to register all French citizens. This option held little attraction for the Russian state, where an autocrat ruled an empire organized by legal estates. Tsar Nicholas had no interest in creating citizens. As protector of the Orthodox Church, Nicholas I did not desire to eliminate religious registration, either.

Nonetheless, Nicholas I and his officials did seek to identify the tsar's subjects and to include them in the civic order. The tsarist regime attempted to achieve the civic inclusion of the non-Orthodox by insisting that they register with their own religious institutions. Between 1826 and 1837, the tsar decreed that Catholic priests, Muslim imams, Lutheran pastors, and Jewish rabbis must keep metrical registers. These laws did not extend civil status to all religious groups. Religious dissenters known as Old Believers, numbering as much as 10 percent of the empire's population, and animist peoples were notable exceptions. The Orthodox Church

claimed Old Believers as part of its flock, but the dissenters had rejected seventeenth-century reforms in the liturgy and generally wanted nothing to do with the Orthodox clergy. Furthermore, the expansion of metrical registration came at the expense of uniformity. Muslim imams did not report estate status. Religious leaders who did not know Russian could maintain the books in their native languages—the imams could use Tatar, for instance. Nonetheless the expansion of metrical books in the 1820s and 1830s represented a major step toward the inclusion of the empire's non-Orthodox residents into legally recognized subjecthood.

[Decades later, under a different regime,] the Great Reform era brought a new governing ethos to the empire, one that changed the role of metrical registration. Reform-minded bureaucrats sought to increase the population's participation in the administration of the empire and to reduce the importance of estate distinctions. The state emancipated the peasantry, introduced a new court system, and allowed elected units of self-administration (zemstvos) a limited role in local affairs. The military service reform of 1874 marked a shift toward the equalization of male subjects in law. Before 1874, military service was an obligation for those of lower status. The military reform of 1874 made males of all estates liable for military service. A universal military obligation, with reduced burdens based on educational achievement, replaced an estate-based system. After the Great Reforms, the autocracy took the first, halting steps toward a more inclusive, less particularistic civic order.

Material used in this particular passage has been adapted from the following source:
C. Steinwedel, "Making Social Groups, One Person at a Time: The Identification of Individuals by Estate, Religious Confession, and Ethnicity in Late Imperial Russia," *Documenting Individual Identity: The Development of State Practices in the Modern World.* © 2001 by Princeton University Press.

1. Nicholas I's regime ordered inhabitants of Russia to register with their particular religious institutions because: p4

A) the Orthodox Church would have required registrants to convert. (no suggestion)

B) the tsar did not want to extend civil rights to all people by having the state register them.

C) some political parties, such as the Old Believers, rejected the authority of the Catholic Church.

D) the military service reform of 1874 had not yet been enacted to equalize the status of the male population.

2. Suppose a Russian peasant in the early 20th century returning home from a day's work first told his wife of rumors from St. Petersburg that the tsar had been deposed and only later mentioned to her, as an afterthought, that the local Orthodox Church had new priest. Based on the information in the passage:

A) the peasant's conversation with his wife supports the claim that Old Believers did not value the Orthodox Clergy.

B) the tsar's hope of including subjects in the civic order through registration had been fulfilled.

C) the peasant is likely part of a minority religious group not recognized by the Orthodox Church.

D) the peasant's behavior may strengthen Koropachinskii's assertions in paragraph 1.

3. Which of the following is LEAST supported by the passage?

A) Nicholas I's new court system sought to increase the population's participation in the administration of his empire. P 6

B) Some residents of Russia were not citizens prior to the reign of Nicholas I.

C) Nicholas I had an interest in maintaining the power of the Orthodox Church. p 3

D) Not all Russian residents understood the official language.

P5

4. Which of the following events, if it occurred, would most support the author's description of the changes happening in Russian society and politics in the 1870s?

A) Old Believers and animists united to oppose registration and were granted independent civil status in 1835.

B) A peasant attended university in 1880 and was then elected chairman of the zemstvo. P6

C) A man in early 20th century Russia had a life different from his father's.

D) The progress of the so-called Great Reform era was reversed upon Nicholas II's ascent to the throne.

5. The author's discussion of Koropachinskii's assertions most supports which of the following statements?

A) The changes Koropachinskii identified were possible only after the advent of political parties and a freer press.

B) Religion was less important in people's lives than were the affairs of government.

C) Koropachinskii did not believe the threads were actually invisible.

D) Part of the chairman's statement may not be entirely accurate.

6. 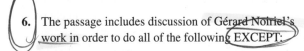 The passage includes discussion of Gérard Noiriel's work in order to do all of the following EXCEPT:

A) help place events in Russia in a broader context.

B) provide a precedent for the author's analysis of Nicholas I's policies.

C) offer one solution Nicholas I declined to pursue.

D) illustrate another situation where the Orthodox Church served a majority but not all of the population.

CHAPTER 2 PRACTICE PASSAGE 2

People's facility with numbers ranges from the aristocratic to the Ramanujanian, but it's an unfortunate fact that most are on the aristocrats' side of our old Mainer. I'm always amazed and depressed when I encounter students who have no idea what the population of the United States is, or the approximate distance from coast to coast, or roughly what percentage of the world is Chinese. I sometimes ask them as an exercise to estimate how fast human hair grows in miles per hour, or approximately how many people die on earth each day, or how many cigarettes are smoked annually in this country. Despite some initial reluctance (one student maintained that hair just doesn't grow in miles per hour), they have often improved their feel for numbers dramatically.

Without some appreciation of common large numbers, it's impossible to react with the proper skepticism to terrifying reports that more than a million American kids are kidnapped each year, or with the proper sobriety to a warhead carrying a megaton of explosive power—the equivalent of a million tons (or two billion pounds) of TNT.

And if you don't have some feeling for probabilities, automobile accidents might seem like a relatively minor problem of local travel, whereas being killed overseas by terrorists might seem to be a major risk when going overseas. As often observed, however, the 45,000 people killed annually on American roads are approximately equal to all American dead in the Vietnam War. On the other hand, the seventeen Americans killed by terrorists in 1985 were among the 28 million of us who traveled abroad that year—that's one chance in 1.6 million of becoming a victim. Compare that with these annual rates in the United States: one chance in 68,000 of choking to death; one chance in 75,000 of dying in a bicycle crash; one chance in 20,000 of drowning; and one chance in 5,300 of dying in a car crash.

Confronted with these large numbers and with the correspondingly small probabilities associated with them, the innumerate will invariably respond with the non sequitur, "Yes, but what if you're that one," and then nod knowingly, as if they've demolished your argument with their penetrating insight. This tendency to personalize is, as we'll see, a characteristic of many people who suffer from innumeracy. Equally typical is a tendency to equate the risk from obscure and exotic malady with the chances of suffering from heart and circulatory disease, from which about 12,000 Americans die each week.

There's a joke I like that is marginally relevant. An old married couple in their nineties contact a divorce lawyer, who pleads with them to stay together. "Why get divorced now after seventy years of marriage? Why not last it out? Why now?" The little old lady finally pipes up in a creaky voice: "We wanted to wait until the children were dead."

A feeling for what quantities or time spans are appropriate in various contexts is essential to getting the joke. Slipping between millions and billions or between billions and trillions should in the sense be equally funny, but it isn't, because we too often lack an intuitive feeling for these numbers. Many educated people have little grasp for these numbers and are even unaware that a million is 1,000,000; a billion is 1,000,000,000; and a trillion, 1,000,000,000,000.

A recent study by Drs. Kronlund and Phillips of the University of Washington showed that most doctors' assessments of the risks of various operations, procedures, and medications (even in their own specialties) were way off the mark, often by several orders of magnitude. I once had a conversation with a doctor who, within approximately twenty minutes, stated that a certain procedure he was contemplating (a) had a one-chance-in-a-million risk associated with it; (b) was 99 percent safe; and (c) usually went quite well. Given the fact that so many doctors seem to believe that there must be at least eleven people in the waiting room if they're to avoid being idle, I'm not surprised at this new evidence for their innumeracy.

Material used in this particular passage has been adapted from the following source:

J.A. Paulos, *Innumeracy: Mathematical Illiteracy and Its Consequences.* © 1988, 2001 by John Allen Paulos.

1. Which of the following best describes the author's primary purpose?

A) To explain the causes of innumeracy and provide options on how to prevent it
B) To demonstrate that Americans are, on the whole, undereducated
C) To provide data concerning probabilities of various causes of death
D) To describe innumeracy and some of its consequences

2. It can be inferred that, as used in paragraph 1, the term *aristocratic*:

A) describes individuals with better-than-average mathematical skill.
B) refers to the traditional ruling class.
C) represents people with only a limited facility with numbers.
D) refers to an inability to understand the difference between a million and a billion.

3. The author would most likely agree with which one of the following statements?

A) A megaton describes an unimpressive amount of explosive power.
B) It is unlikely that more than a million American children are kidnapped each year.
C) Driving an automobile is less dangerous than swimming.
D) Numbers such as a billion or a trillion are often amusing.

4. Which of the following, according to the passage, may characterize the innumerate?

I. Inability to improve their understanding of numbers
II. Personalizing improbable but tragic outcomes
III. Inaccurate assessments of the probabilities of possible outcomes of medical procedures

A) I only
B) II only
C) I and III
D) II and III

5. The author most likely included the joke about the old married couple in order to:

A) provide further evidence of innumeracy in the elderly.
B) argue that couples in their nineties should not seek divorce.
C) illustrate the significance of an understanding of apt quantities based on context.
D) further support a point made in paragraph 3.

6. Which of the following is NOT included as evidence of innumeracy among doctors?

A) Personal experience in the form of an anecdote
B) Statistics regarding the frequency of death due to heart disease
C) Recent academic research
D) A humorous exaggeration of a common experience

SOLUTIONS TO CHAPTER 2 PRACTICE PASSAGE 1

1. **B** This is an Inference question.

    A: No. The passage does not suggest that the Orthodox Church would *require* conversion.

    B: **Yes. See the end of paragraph 3 and the beginning of paragraph 4. Nicholas rejects the French solution, municipal registration, because "Nicholas had no interest in creating citizens…Nicholas I and his officials did seek to identify the tsar's subjects and to include them in the civic order. The tsarist regime attempted to achieve the civic inclusion of the non-Orthodox by insisting that they register with their own religious institutions."**

    C: No. The Catholic Church is not the church from which the Old Believers (who also aren't described as a political party) dissented—they rejected the Orthodox Church (paragraph 4).

    D: No. Even though this choice includes an accurate description of the military service reform of 1874, lack of equality is not, according to the passage, the reasoning behind Nicholas's religious registration.

2. **D** This is a New Information question.

    A: No. The peasant and his wife were not identified as Old Believers. Furthermore, there is no suggestion in the new information that the actions of the peasant indicate anything about ideas of Old Believers regarding the value of the Orthodox Church.

    B: No. This situation doesn't specifically relate to the issue of religious registration.

    C: No. The peasant and his wife were not identified with any fringe or minority religious group.

    D: **Yes. Koropachinskii notes that a Russian villager, "dimly perceives that he is a subject of a vast state and that events taking place far from his place of birth can have a much greater influence on his life than some event in his village." The fact that the peasant reports rumors regarding the distant tsar before he reports more concrete news about his own village could support Koropachinskii's assertion.**

3. **A** This is an Inference/EXCEPT question (for more on EXCEPT questions, see Chapter 4, page 142).

    A: **Yes. The correct answer will be the statement that is NOT supported by the passage. The author does not state that Nicholas I instituted a new court system. This came "decades later, under a different regime" (paragraph 5).**

    B: No. In paragraph 3 and paragraph 4, the author states that "Nicholas had no interest in creating citizens" through registration. Note that although the passage doesn't say that Nicholas made everyone citizens, this choice is still correct in saying that not everyone was a citizen before his reign (even if during and after his reign that may still have been the case).

    C: No. The end of paragraph 3 says, "As protector of the Orthodox Church, Nicholas I did not desire to eliminate religious registration, either." If Nicholas sought to protect a function of the Church, this suggests that he had an interest in maintaining the Church's power.

    D: No. The end of paragraph 4 states that some religious groups in Russia whose leaders "did not know Russian could maintain the books in their native languages."

4. **B**   This is a Strengthen question (for more on Strengthen questions, see Chapter 4, page 132).

   A: No. This would likely undermine the author's description of events; the passage indicates in paragraph 4 that Nicholas I was opposed to extending civil recognition to these groups.

   B: **Yes. If a peasant had access to higher education and was then able to rise to a position of power in local government, it supports the claim in paragraph 5 that eventually measures were taken to promote a "more inclusive, less particularistic civil order."**

   C: No. This is consistent with Koropachinskii's description of Russian life in paragraph 1, but the question asks you to support the author's description, not Koropachinskii's.

   D: No. Ultimately, this choice is irrelevant to the author's description. The passage never argues or suggests that the changes were temporary. Furthermore, the passage never discusses the reign of Nicholas II, only that of Nicholas I.

5. **D**   This is an Inference question.

   A: No. The author does say that the changes Koropachinskii noted occurred as a result of shifts in 1905 that included the advent of a freer press and political parties, but the author never says that those were the *only* things that could have led to these changes. This choice is too extreme.

   B: No. The author's discussion does not suggest that religion became less important than government, just that the state's actions served to make people aware that they were part of something larger than simply their individual townships.

   C: No. While the author notes in paragraph 2 that "these connections were not so much invisible threads as paper trails—written documents," this is the author's belief, not Koropachinskii's.

   D: **Yes. The author states in paragraph 2 that "these connections were not so much invisible threads as paper trails—written documents."**

6. **D**   This is a Structure/EXCEPT question.

   A: No. When the author says "the Old Regime in France had faced a similar problem," he's announcing a parallel between Old France and the events in Russia, creating a broader context.

   B: No. The events in France occurred prior to the events in Russia. Therefore, the case of France can be seen as a precedent.

   C: No. This choice is in line with the author's analysis of Noiriel's parallel: that the French option "held little attraction" for Nicholas (paragraph 3).

   D: **Yes. The correct answer will be the statement that doesn't explain why the author cited Noiriel. The Orthodox Church was never mentioned as being in France—the only cited French religious authority is the Catholic Church (paragraph 3).**

SOLUTIONS TO CHAPTER 2 PRACTICE PASSAGE 2

1. **D**   This is a Main Idea/Primary Purpose question.

    A: No. The author addresses neither the causes of innumeracy, nor any options for preventing it.

    B: No. While the passage does suggest that most Americans have a relatively poor understanding of numbers, it does not address the overall level of American education. Lack of education is not described as a cause of innumeracy, nor is innumeracy used as an example for a more general critique of the educational system.

    C: No. This choice is too narrow. The author provides data and probabilities in paragraph 3 as examples supporting the broader point of the passage. That is, the purpose of the passage as a whole is not limited to providing death statistics.

    D: Yes. The passage describes innumeracy in the first paragraph and discusses its consequences through the rest of the passage.

2. **C**   This is an Inference question.

    A: No. The passage uses the term "unfortunate" to refer to the aristocrats' side of the spectrum measuring people's facility with numbers (paragraph 1), indicating that their facility with numbers is NOT better-than-average.

    B: No. There is no reference to an actual social or ruling class in the passage. Always stick to the context of the passage and beware of applying outside knowledge to MCAT questions, especially where vocabulary is concerned, since this is a common trap.

    C: Yes. The author states in paragraph 1 that "it's an unfortunate fact that most [people's facility with numbers is]…on the aristocrats' side," and then goes on to discuss students' lack of understanding of numbers.

    D: No. This answer choice is too specific. This is only one example of innumeracy; while the "aristocrats" might not understand the difference between a million and a billion, the word itself does not refer specifically to the lack of understanding of that difference.

3. **B**   This is an Inference question.

    A: No. The author uses the phrase "proper sobriety" to describe the appropriate reaction to a warhead carrying a megaton of explosive power, indicating his belief that this is a serious amount of power.

    B: Yes. The author's use of the phrase "proper skepticism" provides strong support for this answer choice by indicating his opinion that such figures are likely exaggerated.

    C: No. While, in paragraph 3, the author cites statistics on the likelihood of drowning and dying in a car crash, he does not explicitly relate these to swimming or being the driver of a car.

    D: No. The passage states in paragraph 6 that slipping between millions and billions or between billions and trillions should be funny but isn't, not that the numbers themselves are funny.

4. **D** This is an Inference/Roman numeral question.

   I: False. This statement is too extreme. The last sentence of paragraph 1 states that students "have often improved their feel for numbers dramatically."

   II: True. This is discussed in paragraph 4.

   III: True. This paraphrases the findings of the recent study referenced in the last paragraph.

5. **C** This is a Structure question.

   A: No. The passage never discusses innumeracy specifically in the elderly.

   B: No. The author makes no personal judgment on whether or not people should divorce.

   C: Yes. This answer choice paraphrases the first sentence of paragraph 6, which explicitly refers to the joke.

   D: No. Paragraph 3 discusses errors in judging risks. The joke in paragraph 5 relates to understanding appropriate quantities and times, as the author indicates in the paragraph immediately following the joke itself.

6. **B** This is a Retrieval/EXCEPT question.

   A: No. The author describes a conversation he had with a doctor, which qualifies as a personal anecdote.

   B: Yes. The correct answer will contain a statement that is NOT given as an example of innumeracy among doctors. Death due to heart and circulatory disease is mentioned in paragraph 4 as an example of the tendency to "equate the risk from obscure and exotic malady" with the chances of acquiring a common disease. There is no connection made here to risk assessments made by doctors.

   C: No. The "recent study" referenced in paragraph 7 is given as an example of doctors' inaccurate risk assessments.

   D: No. The author speculates that in order to avoid being idle, doctors seek to have at least eleven people in the waiting room. The author intends this as a humorous exaggeration of the common experience of waiting in a doctor's office—the last sentence of the passage links the example to the issue of innumeracy.

Chapter 3
Active Reading

GOALS

1) To develop new—and more effective—active reading habits
2) To read for logical structure and get to the Bottom Line
3) To use annotation in order to be able to retrieve information quickly and accurately

3.1   BASIC APPROACH: THE SIX STEPS

First, here is a review of the six basic steps to approaching the CARS section that we discussed in Chapter 2. In the rest of this chapter, we will focus on steps two, three, and four.

STEP 1: RANK AND ORDER THE PASSAGES

Decide whether to do the passage Now, Later, or Never, based on the difficulty level of the passage text.

STEP 2: PREVIEW THE QUESTIONS

Read through the question stems from first to last (not the answer choices) before you read the passage. Look for and highlight words and phrases that indicate important passage content. Do not worry at this stage about identifying the question type.

STEP 3: WORK THE PASSAGE

As you read through the passage (staying on the screen that includes the last question of the set for that passage), use the highlighting function (sparingly) to annotate the most important references in the passage, especially words that indicate the logical structure of the author's argument and references that appeared in your preview of the questions. Notice topic sentences that help you to identify conclusions made by the author. Articulate the Main Point of each chunk of information (usually, each paragraph). Use your noteboard, especially on difficult passages, to jot down these main points. As you read, think about how these chunks relate to each other, and identify the structure of the passage.

STEP 4: BOTTOM LINE

After you have read the passage, sum up the Bottom Line: the main point and tone of the entire passage.

STEP 5: ATTACK THE QUESTIONS

Start with the last question in the set for that passage. Read the question word for word, identifying the question type and translating the question task into your own words. Go back to the passage before reading the answer choices and find the relevant information (reading at least five lines above and below the reference). Think about what the correct answer will need to do, and generate an answer to the question in your own words. Use Process of Elimination (POE) actively. Select the "least wrong" answer.

Move backwards through the set of questions. If a question looks especially difficult, skip over it the first time through, and answer it after the easier questions as you click forward through the questions towards the next passage.

STEP 6: INSPECT THE SECTION

At or before the 5-minute mark (ideally, before you begin your last passage), double-check to make sure that you haven't left anything blank. You can use the Review function at this stage. Do NOT rethink questions you have already completed.

3.2 ACTIVE READING: READING FOR STRUCTURE AND THE BOTTOM LINE

What Is the Bottom Line?

When you read a CARS passage for the first time, you must read it in a very different way than you would read most other texts. For example, when you are studying for a bio exam for a class, you are trying to understand and memorize every fact and detail in the course material. If you read a CARS passage in that way, however, you will not only waste a great deal of precious time, but you will also overlook the things that are really important: the main points being made by the author, and how they fit together to communicate the core idea, or Bottom Line, of the entire passage. In this chapter, we will first discuss what you are reading FOR the first time through a passage: the logical structure and core ideas of the passage. Then we will lay out HOW you should be working the passage by using your highlighter and noteboard to map out those basic aspects of the passage.

As you've no doubt noticed, MCAT CARS passages are often dense, convoluted, and full of details that you ultimately don't need to know in order to answer the questions. Such passages are impossible to read as closely as you would read a text for school, especially given the time constraint. On the MCAT, your goal is not to develop a deep understanding of every aspect of the passage; your goal is to find the information you need to answer the questions, and to pay as little attention as possible to everything else.

Therefore, do not attempt to understand or memorize every detail. This is time-consuming and counterproductive. Instead, visualize the passage as comprised of several large chunks of information. Each chunk, which may span part or all of a paragraph, has a Main Point and serves a particular function within the passage as a whole.

As you read, separate the central point of each paragraph from the evidence used to support that point. Translate the Main Point of each paragraph into your own words. What is the author trying to prove? Pay close attention to words that indicate the author's opinion or attitude. Jot down a few words or a short sentence indicating the Main Point of the chunk and/or paragraph on your noteboard. Link this theme with the Main Points of the previous paragraphs. Imagine that you are reading a mystery novel, following a twisty plot line and adding up the major clues to the story as you go.

After you have read and identified the Main Point of the last paragraph, define the main idea and tone of the passage as a whole: this is the Bottom Line of the entire passage.

How to Get the Bottom Line

In order to read the passages effectively (that is, quickly and with a reasonable degree of comprehension), you must become an *active reader*. Don't read passively; imagine yourself attacking and taking control over each passage. Think of the passage as an argument that you are breaking down into its most basic parts.

Here are the basic principles for active reading.

1) Preview the questions for content (not for question type). Predict what issues will be especially important in the passage you are about to read.
2) Note the author's tone and purpose. What side is the author on? Why is he or she writing this passage?
3) Notice pivotal words and other transitions: use them to identify the "chunks" of an argument and how those chunks relate to each other.
4) Highlight the words that indicate the logical structure of the passage—that is, how the parts of the passage relate to each other. Also highlight topics that appeared in the questions.
5) Translate the Main Point of each paragraph or chunk of information into your own words. Link it to what you've already read and predict what will come next.
6) Articulate the Bottom Line of the whole passage to yourself before answering the questions.

Reading For Structure

The structure of a passage can be identified on three levels.

- **Level 1:** The structure of individual sentences. Look for how the parts of the sentence work together, and how the words used by the author indicate the meaning of that sentence. Don't get caught up in parsing out the structure of every line of every paragraph. But, when sentences contain **indicator words** like *however, although, therefore, on one hand, for example*, etc., it is important to use those words to figure out the meaning of that sentence.

  For example, pivotal words such as *however* or *but* signal a shift in meaning or subject. When you identify a pivotal word in the sentence, ask, "What is it shifting from, and what is it shifting to? How do the two parts of a sentence (or the pair of sentences, if the indicator words come at the beginning of a sentence) relate to each other, and what does this tell me about the author's argument?" Or, if you see the word *therefore*, your immediate question should be, "What is the conclusion or claim being made and where is the evidence supporting that claim?" (especially important for answering Reasoning questions). The words *for example* should raise the question, "what larger claim is being supported by this example, and how does it connect to the author's argument in the passage as a whole?"

  By paying attention to indicator words, you can identify the sentences that will play a particularly important role in constructing the author's argument and skim over the sentences that are less important at this stage.

- **Level 2:** The structure of a paragraph or chunk of information. If you ask these questions about individual sentences, it naturally leads you to the structure and intent of the entire paragraph. Did it introduce an opposing point of view? Did it provide specific evidence and support for a conclusion drawn earlier? Does it introduce another stage of development, or continue to develop a description of a particular phase?

  Separate the paragraph into **claims** and **evidence**. The claims being made are important in understanding the main point of the paragraph, whereas the details of the evidence supporting those claims are usually important only when answering the questions.

  Look for **topic sentences.** Often (but not always) the author uses the first or last sentence of the paragraph to sum up the theme or main point of the paragraph as a whole.

- **Level 3:** The structure of the passage as a whole. The relationship between the individual paragraphs creates or constructs the logical structure of the author's argument. This leads you naturally into an understanding of the Bottom Line (the author's overall argument). Having this map of the passage in mind also helps you to quickly locate the information you need as you are answering the questions.

Some common passage structures are

- compare and contrast
- cause and effect
- thesis with evidence
- rebuttal
- narration or description
- analysis of different aspects of an issue or idea
- old and new theory
- chronology

3.3 THE MAPS OF A PASSAGE

There are four basic components to any passage that, when clearly identified and articulated, give you a firm grounding in the text and build a foundation for the process of answering the questions.

These components are the **MAPS** or

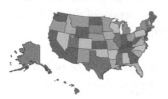

Main Point

Attitude

Purpose

Support

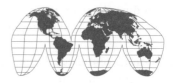

1) The **MAIN POINT** of each paragraph encapsulates the core of *what* the author is trying to communicate. It includes the main idea of each paragraph or chunk of information, and defines and delimits the scope of the passage. The **MAIN POINT** of the passage is the Bottom Line.

2) The **ATTITUDE** expresses *who* the author is through the tone of the passage. Is the author presenting himself or herself as a critic? An advocate? A neutral observer?

3) The **PURPOSE** is the intent of each chunk of the passage and of the passage as a whole. *Why* did the author write it? Was it to compare and contrast two theories? To propose a new theory? To trace the evolution of an idea? To describe a process?

4) The **SUPPORT** is the evidence the author uses to support his or her claims. *How* does the author construct the passage?

Think about a real map. It is constructed in a particular way with a particular purpose: to guide you to your destination. When you use a map, you don't need to pay attention to every street or highway or reference; you only need to find the streets and the connections between those streets which are relevant to your particular goal at that particular time. Memorizing the entire map is not only unnecessary, it's impossible. If you look at the entire picture without separating out the important from the unimportant sections, you will be lost—it's just too much information!

By breaking a passage down into MAPS, you define both Logic and Location. The Logic gives you the Bottom Line, which is crucial for all questions. Location "labels" the different parts of the passage, enabling you to use your map to find the specific information you need as you are answering each question.

So, let's look at our four MAPS components in more detail in connection to passage structure. To follow the process you actually go through as you work a passage, we will reverse the components to SPAM, starting at the lowest level and working up to the Main Point.

Support

How does the passage use evidence to support the author's larger claims?

All passages, even neutral explanatory passages, are made up of big claims and specific evidence support-ing those claims. As we discussed above, your main goal the first time through a passage should be to identify the author's main points and overall purpose; the evidence or support should be skimmed or read more quickly so that you don't get bogged down in the details. So, you need to be able to identify the support used by the author in order to 1) decide to skim through it in your first read-through, as it is less important to the logic of the passage, and 2) re-locate it, if and when it becomes relevant to the questions. Many CARS questions also require you to enumerate or to characterize evidence presented in a passage. While you should not dwell on the support during your first reading of the passage, you should ask your-self, "What larger point is being supported here?"

So, how do you recognize the support?

There are many ways to support a Main Point. The following are the most common:

1) **Examples:** The author illustrates the Main Point with an example from the real world or with a hypothetical example meant to reflect the real world. Examples are often introduced with standard words or phrases that help you to identify them: *in this case, in illustration, for example.*

2) **Generalizations:** To make a point about Christmas, for example, an author might generalize about something larger—like holidays in general. Or the author might make a point about Christmas by discussing Christmas trees. In other words, a generalization supports a main idea by giving an example of something larger—or something smaller—than the subject.

3) **Steps/stages:** Many passages describe the development of an idea, a historical time line, or an evolutionary process. Generally, each paragraph will describe one of those stages. Or, a passage may describe how one thing preceded another in order to support a larger claim about cause and effect.

4) **Comparisons/contrasts:** An effective way to explain something is to compare it to, or con-trast it with, something else. Through differences and similarities, the specific characteristics of an idea can be highlighted. A specific type of comparison is an *analogy*, where one situation is described in order to communicate something about another, supposedly similar situation.

5) **Statistics:** Statistics can be any type of numerical information—percentages, ratios, prob-abilities, populations, prices, etc. It is especially important to avoid getting bogged down in these details. You will be able to find them again later, if you need to.

6) **Studies:** The author cites studies, research, or polling data to support a conclusion.

7) **Definitions:** The author defines key terms in order to communicate something about the context or issues within which those terms are used.

8) **Quotes or citation of others:** The passage includes either direct quotes or citation of other works. It is important to ask yourself if the author is agreeing or disagreeing with these other writers or speakers.

9) **General opinion:** The author describes a past or present common belief. Authors often do this in order to introduce a different or alternative idea. Always define whether the common belief is consistent or inconsistent with the author's point of view.

10) **Anecdotes:** The author tells a story, often from his or her personal experience.

Purpose

Why was the passage written?

Purpose is closely related to structure, and it can be broken down to three levels in a similar way.

1) What is the purpose of the support provided by the author? What larger claim is being supported? Answering this question will lead you to the next level.
2) What is the purpose of the paragraph? What role does it play within the logical structure of the passage? How do the different paragraphs connect to each other? Answering this question leads you to the final level.
3) What is the purpose of the passage as a whole? Why did the author write it? What overall claim or point is being made?

The purpose of the passage as a whole includes the author's attitude. The intent of neutral passages is to describe or explain something. In a purely descriptive passage, it is likely that each paragraph will deal with a different characteristic of the thing being described.

An explanatory passage often includes both generalizations as well as specific examples as illustrations of those generalizations. Identify transition words to ascertain when the author is moving from one point to another (*additionally, also, furthermore,* etc.) or from a generalization to a specific case or illustration (*for example*).

On the other hand, evaluative, critical, or persuasive passages often present one idea or position, a contrasting idea or position, and the author's opinion, which may involve choosing one of those sides over the other or presenting a separate alternative altogether. A common purpose is to contrast old with new theories, or to present and evaluate a debate or controversy.

Keep in mind the strength of the tone and the language. For example, the author may be rejecting the validity of a claim, or may simply be raising questions about or problems with that claim. Keep track of pivotal words (*however, but, yet, conversely, although,* etc.) that indicate when the author is shifting in the discussion from one side to the other, or introducing a qualification. (Pivotal words, however, are not limited to opinionated passages, just as transitional words do not appear exclusively in neutral passages.) Difficult passages may have several such shifts.

Attitude

Who wrote the passage? What is the author's tone?

When asking yourself "who wrote the passage," don't take the question literally, and don't speculate about what kind of person the author might be in real life. Rather, connect this to the purpose of the passage and to how the author presents himself or herself through the passage text. An author may position himself or herself as a neutral observer, simply describing or explaining without expressing an opinion. The author may even describe a debate or conflicting points of view without directly entering into that debate.

In other passages, the author is more present—speculating, evaluating, criticizing, praising, or advocating. To define the attitude of the author, look for words that indicate the tone of the passage (e.g., *unfortunately, shamefully, at last, thankfully*, etc.), or statements that embody the voice or opinion of the author. If the author does have an opinion, evaluate how strongly negative or positive it is. Look out for qualifying language (e.g., *might, could, in some cases, while it is sometimes true that*, etc.) that authors often use to moderate their tone.

Occasionally, a question will directly ask for the attitude or tone of the author. However, attitude can play a role in any question type. It is particularly central to Main Point or Primary Purpose questions, to any question that asks how the author would respond to new information, and to Strengthen and Weaken questions.

Main Point

What is the passage trying to prove?

Articulating the main point or main idea (that is, the Bottom Line of the passage) is one of the most important steps you can take to maximize both your accuracy and your speed in working through the questions. A question may directly ask for the main point or central thesis. However, even if there is no such question, the main point can be used on a variety of question types to quickly eliminate answer choices that are out of scope or not the issue of the passage. The main point may be summarized in the first or last paragraph of the passage, but this is not always the case. In many passages, parts of the main point are scattered throughout, and it can be defined only by synthesizing or piecing together the main idea of each chunk of information.

Students often fall into one of two traps when attempting to identify the main point. On the one hand, they might state it too broadly, as a vague category or idea that includes—but goes beyond—the passage. On the other hand, they may define it too narrowly, focusing on only one among several of the points made by the author.

3.4 CARS EXERCISES: MAPS

Exercise 1: Separating Claims from Evidence

Read and highlight each of the following paragraphs. As you read, identify the evidence used and the claims made based on that evidence. Note the wording and/or paragraph structure used by the author to distinguish the evidence from the main point. Note any topic sentences (sentences that express the main point of the paragraph). Finally, answer the three questions following each paragraph. Answers follow at the end of the Exercise.

Paragraph 1

Drug activity was the life force of Coco's new building. There was no pretense of security: doors were propped open, and the interior hallway made for a nerve-wracking trip from the sidewalk to the hall. Pigeon droppings formed a putrid sand castle in the building's crumbling fountain. The mailboxes were bashed in, their little doors dented and askew. People snatched the light bulbs from the hallways.

1. What is the Main Point? Is it expressed in a topic sentence?

    Yes, how drug life formed coco's building the ⬆ describes the building conditions

2. What is the evidence supporting that Main Point, and what is the nature of that evidence?

    anecdotal evidence

    → evidence of how there wasn't security
    → " " the pigeon chopping
    → " " violence + stealing

3. What language or paragraph structure did the author use to distinguish the ⬭evidence⬭ from the ⬭claims⬭?

    claim: evidence

    assertion to description

Paragraph 2

To assert, as one is tempted to, whether friendly or hostile to Nietzsche, that his results were flashes of poetic insight, or brilliant intuition, misses, I think, the real thrust and importance of his position. The fundamental intention of Nietzsche's work must be to recover and make manifest these underlying presuppositions which were the foundations of the coherence of Greek culture. It is apparent, for instance, that he does not intend a historical portrait of Greece shortly after the Cliesthenian reforms. In another context, speaking of Myerbeer's opera, he will argue that "it is *now* a matter of *indifference*" that the founders of opera were revolting against the Church, and that "it is *enough* to have perceived" that they were in fact engaged in *sub rosa* glorification of natural man.

1. What is the Main Point? Is it expressed in a topic sentence?

    How one may miss Nietzches imp. for if they look @ his poetry or intuition just

2. What is the evidence supporting that Main Point, and what is the nature of that evidence?

    quotes from Nietzche but not sure if they are his... — so weak evidence

3. What language or paragraph structure did the author use to distinguish the evidence from the claims?

    It is apparent —
    in another context
    starts w assertion contradicting
    asserts his own
    uses Nietzche's quotes

Paragraph 3

English serfs were not slaves—human chattels—as in the Roman Empire and American South. They had legal rights to strips of arable land of their own to work (after putting in around two-thirds of their time working the lord's personal lands, called his demesnes). The serf villagers had a right to pasturage of a modest number of domesticated animals. They could hunt for boar and rabbits (not deer, which were reserved for the ruling class) in the neighboring forests or haul fish out of a nearby stream to eat on Catholic Fridays and during Lent. They could plant vegetable gardens next to their houses. The lord had to provide in each village a mill to grind the peasant's grain for their heavily cereal diet.

1. What is the Main Point? Is it expressed in a topic sentence?

   English serfs were not slaves

2. What is the evidence supporting that Main Point, and what is the nature of that evidence?

   assertion to description, could hunt
   → legal rights to land
   → right to pasturage   → plant vegetables

3. What language or paragraph structure did the author use to distinguish the evidence from the claims?

   claim to description of evidence
   claim in topic & rest was used to
   support the claim

Paragraph 4

The *Nude Descending a Staircase* is now one of the most celebrated milestones of modern art, but when the show's organizers saw it, far from being dazzled, they were horrified. Their view of what Cubism was, or ought to be, centered increasingly narrowly upon the mathematics of the Golden Section. Marcel's *Nude* owed nothing to this. In fact, it was clearly influenced as much by the Futurists as the Cubists. The Futurists were concerned with speed, noise, movement: their works had been exhibited the previous month at Bernheim Jeune's gallery, an exhibition which Duchamp visited several times. He was at this time concerned not with pure form, but with the problem of describing movement on a static canvas: he said later that the idea had come from Marey's serial photographs of people and animals in movement, and described its geometry a 'sport of distortion other than Cubism.'

3.4

1. What is the Main Point? Is it expressed in a topic sentence?

   yes, the nude descending staircase influenced by futurists as the cubist

2. What is the evidence supporting that Main Point, and what is the nature of that evidence?

   concerned w/ speed & noise, author's
   claim about his inspiration
   contrast of how it was viewed & how it is   viewed

3. What language or paragraph structure did the author use to distinguish the evidence from the claims?   *now*

   a an anecdote followed by
   the claim followed by
   description followed by
   the artists more inspiration for
   painting

   historical & general evidence

Paragraph 5

The discrepancy between people who had rats and people who did not was underscored in 1959. It was a time when Americans and New Yorkers were thinking pretty highly of themselves, when people on Park Avenue felt safe from rats. It was during the Cold War, and Soviet officials were in Manhattan visiting a technology show that highlighted Soviet inventions. A headline in the *Daily News* boasted U.S. EXPERTS WANDER AT RED SHOW AND WONDER AT NOTHING. The same week, however, a three-year old baby died in Coney Island. His mother had heard him crying in the night and thought he wanted a bottle but soon discovered he was being bitten by rats…. Between January of 1959 and June 1960, 1,025 rat bites were reported in New York…. Sixty thousand buildings were identified as rat harborages by the city's health department—buildings constructed before 1902 that had been designed to house a few families and were now housing dozens. In 1964, nine hundred thousand people were reported living in forty-three thousand old tenements.

1. What is the Main Point? Is it expressed in a topic sentence?

   Yes, by stating that more people had rats in their house than initially thought

2. What is the evidence supporting that main point, and what is the nature of that evidence?

   contrasts people in park ave vs. tenements

   claim → time → story anecdotal
   in history ↑ evidence

3. What language or paragraph structure did the author use to distinguish the evidence from the claims?

   contrast statement → pivotal phrase story = evidence

Answers to Exercise 1: Separating Claims from Evidence

Paragraph 1:

1. Topic sentence: "Drug activity was the life force of Coco's new building."
2. The paragraph uses anecdotal evidence to illustrate the Main Point.
3. The paragraph flows from the assertion into the description.

Paragraph 2:

1. Topic sentence: "The fundamental intention of Nietzsche's work must be to recover and make manifest these underlying presuppositions which were the foundations of the coherence of Greek culture."
2. The author quotes from Nietzsche's work to support his position.
3. The author starts by contradicting the "tempting" position, then asserting his own, and supporting that assertion with evidence from Nietzsche's writings.

Paragraph 3:

1. Topic sentence: "English serfs were not slaves…"
2. The author lists the legal rights that the English serfs did have, as evidence that they were not outright slaves.
3. The claim is presented in the topic sentence, and the rest of the paragraph works to support that claim.

Paragraph 4:

1. The Main Point of this passage is that Marcel Duchamp's painting, *Nude Descending a Staircase*, was influenced by Futurism as much as, or more than, by Cubism. There is no single topic sentence in this paragraph.
2. The author uses general evidence about the artistic philosophy of the Cubists and the Futurists to prove his point about this painting. The contrast between how the painting was seen at the time and how it is now viewed reinforces this point.
3. The author's claim needs to be pieced together from the historical and general evidence she provides. The initial contrast between the painting's reception in its time and now introduces the point, however.

Paragraph 5:

1. The Main Point of the passage is that rats were an identifiable city-wide problem for many people in New York in 1959. There is no single topic sentence in this paragraph.
2. The author uses both anecdotal evidence (the baby on Coney Island) and statistical evidence to demonstrate the rat problem. He also contrasts people on Park Avenue with people living in tenements to show that some people did not have to worry about the rat problem, while others were severely affected by it.
3. An initial contrast is suggested ("The discrepancy…"), and then developed by discussion of the complacency of many people as opposed to the rat-related suffering of others. The latter is introduced by a pivotal phrase: "The same week, however…".

Exercise 2: MAPS Exercise

Read the following passage in 3–4 minutes, and then write down the Main Point, Attitude, Purpose, and Support. Don't just think about the answers; *write them down* to ensure that you have clearly articulated each component. Explanations follow the exercise.

3.4

Race relations and racial attitudes in the United States have changed dramatically over the past quarter of a century. Although many of these changes are well documented, controversies persist about whether, in fact, race has declined in its significance as a determinant of social, economic, and political statuses and outlooks.

An intriguing argument which attempts to reconcile and make sense of the discrepant findings about the status of Blacks vis-à-vis whites is the "polarization thesis." William Julius Wilson, for example, argues that the Black community is becoming socially, politically, and economically polarized. He points out that a number of Blacks are completing college educations and moving into the kinds of prestigious jobs that provide economic security, higher standards of living, and homes in the suburbs. These Blacks, he argues, have been able to take advantage of the opportunities which emerged as a result of the civil rights movement. On the other hand, many other Blacks are trapped in inner-city ghettos where schools are poor and where opportunities for employment and advancement are limited. As the Black community becomes more socioeconomically differentiated, race becomes a less important determinant of the life chances and outlooks of individual Blacks than does socioeconomic status. Implicit in this argument is the idea that as race decreases in importance as a stratifying agent, Blacks will become more similar to non-Blacks with the same socioeconomic position than they will be to other Blacks with vastly different socioeconomic statuses.

When it was first published in 1978, Wilson's *Declining Significance of Race* touched off much controversy and debate. Critics of the book marshaled a great deal of evidence and numerous counter-arguments to undermine Wilson's declining significance of race thesis. Charles V. Willie, for example, basing his arguments on data concerning income, education, and housing, put forth the idea that not only was race not declining in its import, but it was actually increasing as a determinant of the quality of life for Blacks.

Similarly, Robert Hill argued that conditions for Blacks as a group were not improving, and on some fronts things were actually getting worse. For example, he pointed out that recessions continued to affect Blacks disproportionately. Unemployment rates for Blacks remain twice those of whites. The number of Blacks living in poverty continued to rise at the same time that the number of whites living in poverty decreased.

Recent empirical investigations have provided both support for Wilson's declining significance hypothesis and evidence against this position. For example, through the 1960s and 1970s, Blacks improved their relative standings in education, occupational status, and personal income, but failed to make substantial gains when compared with whites in such areas as family income, unemployment rates, housing patterns, and rates of poverty. To date, however, no study has indicated whether changes in stratification patterns have simultaneously led to a convergence between Blacks and non-Blacks in their social, political, and economic outlooks and a polarization among Blacks.

Material used in this particular passage has been adapted from the following source:

C. Herring, "Convergence, Polarization, or What? Racially Based Changes in Attitudes and Outlooks," *Sociological Quarterly.* © 2005, Midwest Sociological Society.

Main Point: findings on ye how
Blacks have gained done better in
society and the contrast on how they
have been worse

Attitude: neutral — the author
states both positions — interest in
wilsons theory but finds
evidence & counter arg + wilson

Purpose: to talk about wilsons thesis
how blacks here are higher
in society are less diff by race and
counter arguments
wilsons thesis, counter arguments,
end w/ no resolution

Support: recessions affect
poverty ↑
1960s & 70s improved edu, occ, ...
cites authors on both sides w/
evidence

Analysis of the Passage

Here is one possible MAPS outline for the preceding passage.

Main Point:	Although Black people have made gains in some areas and suffered losses in others, it is difficult to know whether polarization has occurred, and if it has, what its effect might be.
Attitude:	Interested in Wilson's thesis, but not convinced without empirical evidence
Purpose:	To describe a promising theory, present critics of the theory, and suggest there is no clear resolution to date
Support:	Illustrates a controversy by citing authors on both sides, and describes how they back up their claims. Cites own evidence showing that empirical support exists for both sides.

Exercise 3: Putting It All Together

To break down and explore each of these components in more detail in the context of tracking the structure of the passage, let's visit a sample MCAT CARS Passage, which is reproduced on the following pages.

3.4 Preview the questions and work the passage. For each example provided, ask yourself why the author uses that example. Identify wording that indicates the author's tone. For each paragraph, identify how that paragraph relates to the rest of the passage. Articulate the Bottom Line of the passage.

Then answer the questions, specifically looking for how your understanding of MAPS and passage structure applies. Finally, read through the explanation that follows.

From Romania to Germany, from Tallinn to Belgrade, a major historical process—the death of communism—is taking place. The German Democratic Republic does not exist anymore as a separate state. And the former GDR will serve as the first measure of the price a post-Communist society has to pay for entering the normal European orbit. In Yugoslavia we will see whether the federation can survive without communism, and whether the nations of Yugoslavia will want to exist as a federation. (On a larger scale, we will witness the same process in the Soviet Union.)

One thing seems common to all these countries: dictatorship has been defeated and freedom has won, yet the victory of freedom has not yet meant the triumph of democracy. Democracy is something more than freedom. Democracy is freedom institutionalized, freedom submitted to the limits of the law, freedom functioning as an object of compromise between the major political forces on the scene.

We have freedom, but we still have not achieved the democratic order. That is why this freedom is so fragile. In the years of democratic opposition to communism, we supposed that the easiest thing would be to introduce changes in the economy. In fact, we thought that the march from a planned economy to a market economy would take place within the framework of the *nomenklatura* system, and that the market within the Communist state would explode the totalitarian structures. Only then would the time come to build the institutions of a civil society; and only at the end, with the completion of the market economy and the civil society, would the time of great political transformations finally arrive.

The opposite happened. First came the big political change, the great shock, which either broke the monopoly and the principle itself of Communist Party rule or simply pushed the Communists out of power. Then came the creation of civil society, whose institutions were created in great pain, and which had trouble negotiating the empty space of freedom. And only then, as the third moment of change, the final task was

undertaken: that of transforming the totalitarian economy into a normal economy where different forms of ownership and different economic actors will live one next to the other.

Today we are in a typical moment of transition. No one can say where we are headed. The people of the democratic opposition have the feeling that we won. We taste the sweetness of our victory the same way the Communists, only yesterday our prison guards, taste the bitterness of their defeat. And yet, even as we are conscious of our victory, we feel that we are, in a strange way, losing. In Bulgaria the Communists have won the parliamentary elections and will govern the country, without losing their social legitimacy. In Romania the National Salvation Front, largely dominated by people from the old Communist *nomenklatura*, has won. In other countries democratic institutions seem shaky, and the political horizon is cloudy. The masquerade goes on: dozens of groups and parties are created, each announces similar slogans, each accuses its adversaries of all possible sins, and each declares itself representative of the national interest. Personal disputes are more important than disputes over values. Arguments over labels are fiercer than arguments over ideas.

1. Which of the following best expresses the main idea of the passage?

A) Communism will never completely vanish from the Earth.
B) Democracy is the highest good that any Eastern European country can ever hope to achieve.
C) Market economies do not always behave as we might predict.
D) Although many formerly Communist countries are now "free," this does not always mean that they have a democracy.

economy → civil insh → political

2. The author originally thought that the order of events in the transformation of society would be represented by which of the following?

A) The totalitarian structure would collapse, leaving in its wake a social structure whose task would be to change the state-controlled economy into a free market.

B) The transformation of the economy would destroy totalitarianism, after which a different social and political structure would be born.

C) The people would freely elect political representatives who would then transform the economy, which would then undermine the totalitarian structure.

D) The change to a democratic state would necessarily undermine totalitarianism, after which a new economy would be created.

3. Which of the following best represents the relationship between freedom and democracy, as it is described by the author?

A) A country can have freedom without having democracy.

B) If a country has freedom, it necessarily has democracy.

C) A country can have democracy without having freedom.

D) A country can never have democracy if it has limited freedom.

4. Which of the following best describes the author's attitude toward what has taken place in communist society?

A) He is relieved that at last the democratic order has surfaced.

B) He sees the value of returning to the old order.

C) He is disappointed with the nature of the democracy that has emerged but nevertheless pleased with the victory of freedom.

D) He is confident that a free economy will ultimately provide the basis for a true democracy.

5. When the author mentions "the same process" (paragraph 1), it can be inferred from the passage that he is most likely referring to:

A) the gradual shift away from authoritarian politics.

B) the potential disintegration of the Soviet Union.

C) the possible breakdown in the general distribution systems in the Soviet Republic.

D) the expected sale of state-owned farms to private enterprise.

6. Which of the following does the author imply has contributed to the difficulties involved in creating a new democratic order in Yugoslavia?

I. The people who existed under a totalitarian structure did not have the experience of "negotiating the empty space of freedom."

II. Mistaking the order in which political, economic, and social restructuring would occur.

III. Changes in the economy were more difficult than anticipated.

A) II only

B) I and III only

C) II and III only

D) I, II, and III

7. It can be inferred from the passage that the democratic opposition feels that it is "in a strange way, losing" (paragraph 5) because:

A) some of the old governments are still unwilling to give in to freedoms at the individual level.

B) the new governments are not strong enough to exist as a single federation.

C) newly elected officials have ties to old political parties.

D) no new parties have been created to fill the vacuum created by the victory of freedom.

3.4

Answers to Exercise 3: Putting It All Together
1. **D**
2. **B**
3. **A**
4. **C**
5. **B**
6. **B**
7. **C**

Support

This passage supports its main thesis by contrasting what *actually* happens with the expectation that formerly communist nations would evolve into democracies, and then cites specific cases in the first and last paragraphs to illustrate the point. Your paragraph-by-paragraph outline might look like this.

1) Examples of the death of communism
2) Generalization and contrast nature of freedom and democracy
3) Expected progression
4) Real progression
5) Examples of incomplete transition

Knowing where and how the author supports his claims is particularly important in answering questions 2, 5, 6, and 7.

Purpose

In this passage, the purpose is to analyze how and why sociopolitical transformation in the formerly communist nations did not follow the expected path, and to express regret that this has left their evolution into democracies incomplete.

Take a look at questions 2 and 5, and consider the role played by the Purpose of the author in each of the credited responses.

Attitude

The author is clearly present in this passage. Note the repeated use of the word "we"; the author presents as a participant (paragraph 3) as well as an informed expert (paragraph 1), not as a disinterested outsider. Note also the tone and language of the passage. Democracy is something to be "achieved," from which we can infer that it is a desirable thing. The author speaks of the "sweetness of our victory," telling us that freedom, in this sense, while limited, is greatly appreciated. Yet at the same time the author feels that "we are, in a strange way, losing." This indicates the author's discontent with the incomplete nature of the transformation.

Now take a look at question 4, which directly asks for the author's attitude. Choices A and D are too positive (and A is wrong for other reasons as well; it is inconsistent with the author's analysis). Choice B is too negative. The author appreciates the changes that have occurred, and wants the transformation to continue. Only choice C reflects the mixture of appreciation and regret that defines the author's attitude in this passage.

Main Point

In this passage, the author argues that many formerly communist nations have overthrown totalitarian regimes and achieved political freedom. However, because the transformation of the economy and civil society of these countries is as yet incomplete, true democracy does not exist. A student without a firm grasp on the driving theme and scope of the argument might incorrectly identify the main point as, "One can have freedom without democracy," which is too broad. A student who gets too caught up in one part of the passage might say the Main Point is that, "In Bulgaria and Romania, members of the old communist order still hold positions of power." A student who gets it just right, however, might say that the Main Point is something like this: "Many countries have overthrown communism and are now free, but they have not yet achieved democracy."

Now take a look in particular at questions 1, 3, and 4. Notice how useful it is to have a clear statement of the Main Point as a tool to eliminate traps and choose the correct answer.

3.4

Exercise 4: Practice MAPS

Use this log as a template to outline the MAPS for at least 8 passages from online or from other resources. **While you do not need to actually write down the MAPS of a passage during an MCAT,** by practicing this technique, you will improve your ability to characterize and evaluate the passage's central thesis, its logical structure, and the nature and strength of its claims.

MAPS Log

Passage #

MAIN POINT:

ATTITUDE:

PURPOSE:

SUPPORT:

3.5 PASSAGE ANNOTATION AND MAPPING

Now that we have broken down what you are reading for during your first time through a passage, let's get into the mechanics of working a passage. That is, what you should be doing with your pencil and the highlighter in order to keep your focus on the logic and structure of the passage, and to set up the process of answering the questions as accurately and efficiently as possible.

3.5

Why Annotate?

Annotation is a crucial part of active reading. Like any successful traveler, you need a *map* to help you navigate the passage. Intelligent annotation can help you to create this map. A smart annotation system is neither too sparse nor too elaborate.

In the course of your undergraduate studies, you may have become accustomed to highlighting large chunks of text. However, this approach is not going to help you on the MCAT. If you highlight everything that "looks important" in the passage, in the end, all you will have is some big blocks of yellow text. This won't help you to understand the logic of the argument as you read, and you will have to reread huge chunks of text to find the relevant information as you answer the questions.

You must have a specific strategy for annotating or mapping the text of the passage. While you do not need to write down all aspects of the four parts of MAPS that we discussed above, your physical mapping of the passage is based on the logical structure of the passage that you identified through reading for MAPS. Mapping is an active process that keeps you engaged with the text. It forces you to decide which points are most crucial to the author's argument, and how those points relate to each other to create the Bottom Line. It also marks the breaks between logically important chunks of the passage, which helps you locate information necessary for answering the questions.

Mapping

There are two tools you have to map the passage: *making notes on your noteboard* and *highlighting the passage*.

Making Notes

Use your noteboard to jot down the Main Point of each paragraph and the Bottom Line of the passage. Do this for every passage now; eventually, you may only need to write it down for the harder passages. Do NOT, however, use your noteboard to list every fact mentioned in each paragraph; your goal is to identify the core idea of that chunk, not to write down a detailed outline of it. Also, if there is a complicated timeline in the passage, write it down so that you can use your notes as you answer the questions. You can also use your noteboard to write down translations of difficult questions and answer choices.

What to Highlight

Question Topics   When you see words or phrases that you recognize from your preview, highlight them. However, don't jump out of the passage to answer the question at this point (you don't know yet what else the author might have to say about that subject!). By highlighting them, you make it easy to come back and find them when you do answer the question.

Transitions: Pivotal Words   Pivotal words are especially important, so let's discuss them in more detail.

MCAT CARS passages rarely contain a single point reiterated over and over again. Rather, a chain of reasoning is more likely to change direction one or more times. These turns in the overall direction of a passage are often marked by **pivotal words**. Here are some common pivotal words and phrases.

but	although	however
yet	despite	nevertheless
nonetheless	except	admittedly
in spite of the fact that	in contrast	even though

These words indicate *change* or *contrast*. Pivotal words signal that the author is about to shift the course of the argument by

- placing a condition on the argument;
- introducing an antithetical point;
- shifting from a simple to a more complex level of argument;
- making a concession to an opposing viewpoint.

Think of pivotal words as signposts that appear at crucial turns or refinements in the argument. Highlight them as you work through the passage. Highlighting pivotal words serves at least two functions.

- First, it increases the visibility of the parts of the passage that are likely to contain key ideas.
- Second, stopping to highlight a pivotal word lets you know that you need to determine *why* a transition is occurring at that point. In other words, the most valuable aspect of highlighting pivotal words—indeed, of annotating in general—is that it alerts you to the parts of the passage to which you need to pay the most attention, and it helps you track the logic of the author's argument.

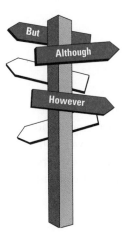

3.5

Transitions: Continuations   These words indicate that the author is further developing or ex-plaining the point he or she has just made. Noticing and highlighting them will help you to distinguish different parts of the author's argument from each other. Here are words commonly used to indicate continuations.

furthermore
additionally
also
moreover

Conclusions   Authors use these words to sum up their Main Points. Finding and highlighting these words will help you to do the same. Here are some common conclusion indicators.

therefore	thus
so	consequently
clearly	hence
for this reason	

Opinion Indicators   One of the most important aspects of the Bottom Line is the author's tone. To accurately identify the author's point of view, look for and highlight phrases that express opinion, and words like

finally
fortunately
thankfully
unfortunately
sadly

Emphasis Words   Authors use words like these to catch your attention, because what follows is especially important. Here are some examples of emphasis words.

most important
primarily
chiefly
key
crucial

Comparisons and Contrasts   Not only are these words important to the logical structure of the passage; they also alert you to potential traps in the questions. When the passage describes two things as different, a wrong answer will describe them as similar, and vice versa. When the author discusses a change over time, wrong answers will reverse the chronology. By locating and highlighting comparison/contrast indicators, you are already helping yourself get the questions right. Here are some examples.

similarly	like
analogy	unlike
in contrast	later
the difference between	before/after

All of the categories of words discussed above indicate that something important to the Bottom Line is being discussed by the author; that is, major claims that deserve some attention on your first reading of the passage. These last three categories, however, tend to indicate details or support for those major claims. Highlight these markers to indicate location of the support, but read through what follows them in the text more quickly. You can follow your highlighting back to the relevant part of the passage if you need to as you are answering the questions.

Examples   These words tell you that what follows is an example or illustration of a larger, more important point. Highlight them so that you can find these details if they become important to the questions. These markers are especially useful for answering questions that ask you if, or how well, the author's claims are supported. What you should be *thinking* about now as you read, however, is the conclusion being supported by the example. This is what will give you the Main Point of the chunk and eventually the Bottom Line of the passage. Here are some common example indicators.

> for example
> because
> since
> in this case
> in illustration

List Markers   When the author provides a string of claims or examples, it can be difficult to pull out the relevant item from that list when you are answering the questions. Highlight just the markers, not the entire list. But, just as with example indicators, define what this list is illustrating as you read: what is it a list of? List markers include

> first   There are three aspects
> second
> thirdly

Names   Highlight names now so that you don't have to reread large chunks of text to find them when they show up in the question stems and answer choices.

3.6 CARS EXERCISES: ACTIVE READING

Exercise 1: Working the Passage

Previewing the Questions

Read through the five questions below. Identify the words and phrases that indicate the issues in the passage that will be relevant to answering these questions. Don't try to identify the question type at this stage; focus only on clues to passage content. After we preview these questions, we will move on and read the passage attached to them.

1. According to the author, which of the following constitutes a fundamental human characteristic?

2. Which of the following, based on information in the passage, would most strengthen the author's claim in paragraph 6 that the work of economists is necessary to the advancement of civilization?

3. The author claims that human beings find it difficult to survive. What explanation is offered in support of this conclusion?

4. According to the passage, why do economists have such significant influence over society?

5. It can be inferred from the passage that economists are relatively unknown because:

Summing it up: What will this passage be about? _how economists have_
influence over civilization even though they are relatively
unknown. Prob also talks about human behavior

The questions you have just previewed are about the passage (presented paragraph by paragraph) on the following pages. As you work through those paragraphs, keep in mind what you learned from these questions.

Defining the Main Points and the Bottom Line

What we have here is an entire passage. These paragraphs have already been highlighted for you, as an illustration of what you should be (and shouldn't be) highlighting. As you read, think about *why* those words have been highlighted, and what those highlighted words tell you about the important parts of the author's argument.

For each paragraph, define the Main Point of that chunk. Write down the Main Point in the space provided before you move on to the next paragraph. Don't make a list of all the information included. Focus on the claims being made, not the evidence supporting those claims. At the end, we will articulate the Bottom Line of this passage.

3.6

> The very fact that man has had to depend on his fellow man has made the problem of survival extraordinarily difficult. Man is not an ant, conveniently equipped with an inborn pattern of social instincts. On the contrary, he is preeminently the creature of his will-o'-the-wisp whims, his unpredictable impulses, and his selfishness. Man is torn between a basic need for gregariousness—to coexist peaceably with his neighbors—and a pronounced tendency toward greediness. Often, his tendency to guard his own interest is at odds with his need to survive in a community. And it is to this clash and conflict that the first great economists addressed themselves.

Main Point: <u>Man has contradictory behaviors – generous & greedy</u>

> One would think that in a world torn by economic problems, a world in which we constantly worry about economic affairs and talk of economic issues, the great economists would have an important place in history and be as familiar to us as the great philosophers or statesmen. Yet they seem to be only shadowy figures of the past. In the 1760s an educated traveler in England would probably have heard of Adam Smith, a professor at the University of Glasgow, but today a great many educated people do not know that this gentleman was the father of economics.

Main Point: <u>Economists should be more famous bc our society focuses on them but blep! no one knows them.</u>

No economist has ever been either a national hero or a national villain. Yet what economists have done has been more decisive for history than many acts of statesmen who basked in brighter glory. Often their deeds have been more profoundly disturbing than the shuttling of armies back and forth across frontiers, more powerful for good and bad than the edicts of kings and legislatures. Since economists have shaped and swayed men's minds they have necessarily shaped and swayed the world.

Main Point: economists have a large influence!

Few economists ever lifted a finger in action. They worked, in the main, as scholars: quietly, inconspicuously, and without much regard for what the world had to say about them.

Main Point: economists are more behind the scenes

Economists are not well known because most people do not understand the significance of economics and believe it to be a rather uninteresting academic pursuit. But a man who thinks that economics is only a matter for professors forgets that this is the science that has sent men to their battle stations. A man who has looked into an economics textbook and concluded that economics is boring is like a man who has read a primer on logistics and decided that the study of warfare must be dull.

Main Point: they arent well known but this is due to fallible reasons

To be sure, not all the economists were titans. Adam Smith was a stunningly interesting character. But thousands of his followers wrote texts, some of them monuments of dullness, and explored minutiae with all the zeal of medieval scholars. Nonetheless, economists are the worldly philosophers, and their work is essential to the growth and continuation of advanced civilizations. Economists have sought to embrace in a scheme of philosophy the most worldly of man's activities: his drive for wealth. It is not, perhaps, the most elegant kind of philosophy, but there is no more intriguing or important[1].

3.6

Main Point: to say that not all economists made such a huge impact but their work is still sig.

Bottom Line of the passage as a whole: economists are important members of society that help w the generous/greed issue even if they are not rec. in society

---

[1] Material used in this particular passage has been adapted from the following source: R. L. Heilbroner, *The Worldly Philosophers.* © 1999 by Simon & Schuster Inc.

Answers for Exercise 1: Mapping the Passage

Previewing the Questions

Summing it up: What will this passage be about?

This passage will be about human nature and survival, economists and their relationship to society, and why economists are not well known.

Defining the Main Points and the Bottom Line:

3.6

NOTE: Your own notes may be briefer; these are written out in more complete terms than you may need for your own understanding.

1) Man's independence conflicts with his need to be part of a group for survival.
2) Economists surprisingly fade into the background of history.
3) Economists have great influence over history.
4) Economists are scholarly, removed from the world.
5) People don't "get" economics, and so don't know economists.
6) Economists are vital to civilization.

Bottom Line of the passage as a whole: Although they fade into history, economists are crucial to the advancement of society.

Exercise 2: Annotation and Active Reading—Putting It All Together

Read and annotate the following passage. As you read, stop and write down the Main Point of each paragraph on your noteboard. When you have read the whole passage, write down the Bottom Line. Then, turn the page and read through the sample annotations and explanation of the passage. The sample passage also indicates what sections of the passage you should skim or move through more quickly.

Passage for Annotation Exercise 2

There are two major systems of criminal procedure in the modern world—the adversarial and the inquisitorial. The former is associated with common law tradition and the latter with civil law tradition. Both systems were historically preceded by the system of private vengeance in which the victim of a crime fashioned his own remedy and administered it privately, either personally or through an agent. The vengeance system was a system of self-help, the essence of which was captured in the slogan "an eye for an eye, a tooth for a tooth." The modern adversarial system is only one historical step removed from the private vengeance system and still retains some of its characteristic features. Thus, for example, even though the right to institute criminal action has now been extended to all members of society, and even though the police department has taken over the pretrial investigative functions on behalf of the prosecution, the adversarial system still leaves the defendant to conduct his own pretrial investigation. The trial is still viewed as a duel between two adversaries, refereed by a judge who, at the beginning of the trial, has no knowledge of the investigative background of the case. In the final analysis the adversarial system of criminal procedure symbolizes and regularizes punitive combat.

By contrast, the inquisitorial system begins historically where the adversarial system stopped its development. It is two historical steps removed from the system of private vengeance. Therefore, from the standpoint of legal anthropology, it is historically superior to the adversarial system. Under the inquisitorial system the public investigator has the duty to investigate not just on behalf of the prosecutor but also on behalf of the defendant.

Additionally, the public prosecutor has the duty to present to the court not only evidence that may lead to the conviction of the defendant but also evidence that may lead to his exoneration. This system mandates that both parties permit full pretrial discovery of the evidence in their possession. Finally, in an effort to make the trial less like a duel between two adversaries, the inquisitorial system mandates that the judge take an active part in the conduct of the trial, with a role that is both directive and protective.

Fact-finding is at the heart of the inquisitorial system. This system operates on the philosophical premise that in a criminal case the crucial factor is not the legal rule but the facts of the case and that the goal of the entire procedure is to experimentally recreate for the court the commission of the alleged crime.

Material used in this particular passage has been adapted from the following source:

M. A. Glendon, *Comparative Legal Traditions in a Nutshell.* © 1982 by West Academic Publishing.

P1: adversarial vs. inquisitorial
(+ how)
private vengeance

P2: why inquisitorial is better

P3: more info

P4: A more ex

private = self help
adversarial: common law
came next
inqui-
P2: came after " "
superior bc less bias
greater role
P3: inqui- more facts based

Sample Annotation (Annotation Exercise 2)

There are two major systems of criminal procedure in the modern world—the adversarial and the inquisitorial. The former is associated with common law tradition and the latter with civil law tradition. Both systems were historically preceded by the system of private vengeance in which the victim of a crime fashioned his own remedy and administered it privately, either personally or through an agent. The vengeance system was a system of self-help, the essence of which was captured in the slogan "an eye for an eye, a tooth for a tooth." The modern adversarial system is only one historical step removed from the private vengeance system and still retains some of its characteristic features. Thus, for example, even though the right to institute criminal action has now been extended to all members of society, and even though the police department has taken over the pretrial investigative functions on behalf of the prosecution, the adversarial system still leaves the defendant to conduct his own pretrial investigation. The trial is still viewed as a duel between two adversaries, refereed by a judge who, at the beginning of the trial, has no knowledge of the investigative background of the case. In the final analysis the adversarial system of criminal procedure symbolizes and regularizes punitive combat.

skim this section

By contrast, the inquisitorial system begins historically where the adversarial system stopped its development. It is two historical steps removed from the system of private vengeance. Therefore, from the standpoint of legal anthropology, it is historically superior to the adversarial system. Under the inquisitorial system the public investigator has the duty to investigate not just on behalf of the prosecutor but also on behalf of the defendant. Additionally, the public prosecutor has the duty to present to the court not only evidence that may lead to the conviction of the defendant but also evidence that may lead to his exoneration. This system mandates that both parties permit full pretrial discovery of the evidence in their possession. Finally, in an effort to make the trial less like a duel between two adversaries, the inquisitorial system mandates that the judge take an active part in the conduct of the trial, with a role that is both directive and protective.

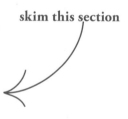

skim this section

Fact-finding is at the heart of the inquisitorial system. This system operates on the philosophical premise that in a criminal case the crucial factor is not the legal rule but the facts of the case and that the goal of the entire procedure is to experimentally recreate for the court the commission of the alleged crime.

Explanation of the Passage

This passage presents a clear argument, using detailed descriptions to support it. The trick to understanding this argument is to keep track of the three kinds of legal systems: the adversarial, the inquisitorial, and the system of private vengeance, and the differences among them.

Notice that there are three major chunks of information here. They roughly correspond to the three legal systems, but they do not correspond to the three paragraphs; paragraph 1 contains two chunks: a description of the system of private vengeance and of the adversarial system. Paragraphs 2 and 3 work together as one chunk to describe the features of the modern inquisitorial system. Your annotation and summation of the Main Points in the passage should focus on the contrast drawn by the author between the three different systems. Good annotation and "chunking" will help you to get to the Bottom Line of a passage and to find the details necessary to answer the questions.

Your understanding of the Bottom Line of the passage should be something like: "The adversarial system of criminal law is similar to the traditional system of private vengeance and is therefore less developed than the modern inquisitorial system."

On the next page is an example of what your noteboard might look like. You will notice that these notes are very brief. Remember that you may be expressing the main points and Bottom Line with just a few words; only you—no one else—needs to be able to understand your notes.

3.6

P1: *Private vengeance: self-help

*Adversarial came next: similar features

P2: Inquisitorial more developed: public actors greater role

P3: Inquisitorial: goal of discovering facts

BL: Inquisitorial more developed than adversarial

—less like private vengeance

3.7 HABITS OF EFFECTIVE READERS

Here are some suggestions for learning to read not only faster but more efficiently, the first time through the passage.

- **Focus on big ideas and skim the details.** Don't get bogged down in long descriptions. Practice using the clues provided in the author's wording to distinguish the major claims from the (potentially irrelevant) details.
- **Hit the right pace.** If you read too fast, you won't get anything out of the passage, and will end up rereading the entire passage as you answer the questions. If you go too slowly, however, you will lose focus and/or overthink what you are reading.
- **Don't try to memorize.** Remember: this is essentially an open book test. You will be going back to the passage for the facts you need for the questions.
- **Practice reading in chunks of words.** Rather than "sounding out" each word in your mind as if you were reading out loud, think about seeing the words in groups of two or three to get a sense of what is being said. When you are answering the questions, however, always read word-for-word.
- **Push your eyes forward towards the end of the sentence.** Keep your momentum; don't linger on or ponder every word.
- **Visualize as you read.** When you hit an important point in the passage, create an image in your mind that captures the author's meaning.
- **Sit back and relax!** If you have your nose up against the screen, it is harder to think about the "big picture." You will get tired and stiff, and it will be harder to keep focused.

3.7

Outside Reading

Many MCAT students feel uncomfortable with the kind of material they encounter in the CARS section. You may not have much experience reading texts from the social sciences and humanities. To further develop your active reading skills, use some of the sources and resources listed on the next page. Use these sources not to learn more about the subject, but to practice active reading and annotation. If you are using a hard copy source, photocopy a chapter or article or two from a few different books or periodicals. Treat each page as a passage. Highlight the key words and phrases that fall into the categories we have discussed in this chapter. Articulate the Main Point of each paragraph and write it down. Think about how the paragraphs fit together logically to come up with the Bottom Line (including the author's tone) for each page or two.

Suggested Supplemental Reading List

Books

1) Wellek, Rene and Warren, Austin (1955), *Theory of Literature*
2) Bate, Walter Jackson (1991), *The Burden of the Past and the English Poet*
3) Campbell, Joseph (1949), *The Hero with a Thousand Faces*
4) Durant, Will (1935), *The Story of Civilization*
5) Giroux, Henry A. (1988), *Schooling and the Struggle for Public Life: Critical Pedagogy in the Modern Age*
6) Lakoff, George and Johnson, Mark (1980), *Metaphors We Live By*
7) Panofsky, Erwin (1955), *Meaning in the Visual Arts*
8) Bronowski, Jacob (1962), *The Western Intellectual Tradition*
9) Sontag, Susan (1983), *A Susan Sontag Reader*
10) Stanovich, Keith (2009), *How to Think Straight About Psychology*

Periodicals

Make sure to choose articles that are written at a fairly high level (that is, not a simple news article or movie review).

The New Yorker
Atlantic Monthly
The Economist
The American Scholar
Legal Affairs
Harper's
Foreign Affairs

Online Sources

If you find that you have more difficulty doing passages online than on paper, make sure to do as much of your outside reading as possible online. Many of the periodicals listed above allow some degree of free online access. There are also two websites that provide non-copyright material for free.

Gutenberg.org
Authorama.com

Make sure to choose nonfiction texts that are at a fairly high level of difficulty (that is, at MCAT CARS level). Here are some appropriate texts that will give you practice with reading challenging passage material.

1) Plato, *The Republic*
2) Friedrich Wilhelm Nietzsche, *Beyond Good and Evil*
3) Henry David Thoreau, *Walden*
4) Edward Gibbon, *The History of the Decline and Fall of the Roman Empire*
5) Ludwig Wittgenstein, *Tractatus Logico-Philosophicus*
6) Friedrich Wilhelm Nietzsche, *Thus Spake Zarathustra*
7) Adam Smith, *An Inquiry into the Nature and Causes of the Wealth of Nations*

3.7

3.8 DOS AND DON'TS FOR ACTIVE READING

Do

- Highlight key words and phrases.
- Link and predict major themes.
- Take notes on your noteboard.
- Keep it simple.
- Translate the main idea of each paragraph into your own words.
- Summarize the main point and tone of the whole passage before attacking the questions.

Don't

- Focus on the details.
- Read parts of the passage text over and over (instead, move on!).
- Memorize.
- Copy words or phrases on to your noteboard without knowing what they mean.

Chapter 3 Summary

- Read actively! Take control of the passage. Don't let the passage control you.

- Read efficiently! If a detail is important for a question, you'll find it when you go back to the passage text to answer that question. If it isn't important, don't waste your time.

- Limit your highlighting to words and phrases that relate to the logical structure of the author's argument and to your preview of the questions.

- Find the annotation style that works best for you and stick to it. It may seem to slow you down at first, but it will save you time and increase your accuracy in the long run.

CHAPTER 3 PRACTICE PASSAGES

Individual Passage Drills

Do the following two passages untimed. Separate the claims (Main Points of each chunk) from the evidence used to support them (details). Use a yellow highlighter to annotate the words and phrases that appeared in your preview of the questions or that related to the logical structure of the author's argument.

As you answer the questions, uses your annotation (notes and highlighting) actively.

Once you have completed the passages, use the Individual Passage Log to evaluate your performance. Think in particular about how, and how well, you worked the passage, and how that affected your performance on the questions. Did you miss any questions because you didn't get the Bottom Line? Could more effective annotation have helped you find the information you needed? Did you highlight too much or too little, and then didn't know where to go back to in the passage?

NOW

CHAPTER 3 PRACTICE PASSAGE 1

Nothing short of this curious sympathy could have brought into close relations two young men so hostile as Roony Lee and Henry Adams, but the chief difference between them as collegians consisted only in their difference of scholarship: Lee was a total failure; Adams a partial one. Both failed, but Lee felt his failure more sensibly, so that he gladly seized the chance of escape by accepting a commission offered him by General Winfield Scott in the force then being organized against the Mormons. He asked Adams to write his letter of acceptance, which flattered Adams's vanity more than any Northern compliment could do, because, in days of violent political bitterness, it showed a certain amount of good temper. The diplomat felt his profession.

If the student got little from his mates, he got little more from his masters. The four years passed at college were, for his purposes, wasted. Harvard College was a good school, but at bottom what the boy disliked most was any school at all. He did not want to be one in a hundred—one per cent of an education. He regarded himself as the only person for whom his education had value, and he wanted the whole of it. He got barely half of an average. Long afterwards, when the devious path of life led him back to teach in his turn what no student naturally cared or needed to know, he diverted some dreary hours of faculty-meetings by looking up his record in the class-lists, and found himself graded precisely in the middle. In the one branch he most needed—mathematics—barring the few first scholars, failure was so nearly universal that no attempt at grading could have had value, and whether he stood fortieth or ninetieth must have been an accident or the personal favor of the professor. Here his education failed lamentably. At best he could never have been a mathematician; at worst he would never have cared to be one; but he needed to read mathematics, like any other universal language, and he never reached the alphabet.

Beyond two or three Greek plays, the student got nothing from the ancient languages. Beyond some incoherent theories of free-trade and protection, he got little from Political Economy. He could not afterwards remember to have heard the name of Karl Marx mentioned, or the title of "Capital." He was equally ignorant of Auguste Comte. These were the two writers of his time who most influenced its thought. The bit of practical teaching he afterwards reviewed with most curiosity was the course in Chemistry, which taught him a number of theories that befogged his mind for a lifetime. The only teaching that appealed to his imagination was a course of lectures by Louis Agassiz on the Glacial Period and Paleontology, which had more influence on his curiosity than the rest of the college instruction altogether. The entire work of the four years could have been easily put into the work of any four months in after life.

Harvard College was a negative force, and negative forces have value. Slowly it weakened the violent political bias of childhood, not by putting interests in its place, but by mental habits which had no bias at all. It would also have weakened the literary bias, if Adams had been capable of finding other amusement, but the climate kept him steady to desultory and useless reading, till he had run through libraries of volumes which he forgot even to their title-pages. Rather by instinct than by guidance, he turned to writing, and his professors or tutors occasionally gave his English composition a hesitating approval; but in that branch, as in all the rest, even when he made a long struggle for recognition, he never convinced his teachers that his abilities, at their best, warranted placing him on the rank-list, among the first third of his class. Instructors generally reach a fairly accurate gauge of their scholars' powers. Henry Adams himself held the opinion that his instructors were very nearly right, and when he became a professor in his turn, and made mortifying mistakes in ranking his scholars, he still obstinately insisted that on the whole, he was not far wrong. Student or professor, he accepted the negative standard because it was the standard of the school.

Material used in this particular passage has been adapted from the following source:

H. Adams, *The Education of Henry Adams.* © 1918 by Houghton Mifflin Co.

[handwritten top margin: Adams college main occupation vy adam]

1. Which of the following best characterizes the author's opinion of Adams' college experience?

A) Positive, because Harvard College was a good school
B) Negative, because the four years at college were a complete waste
C) Mixed, because while Adams learned little, there was some value to the experience
D) It cannot be determined from the passage because the opinions expressed are Adams', not the author's

2. The author's claim that in mathematics "failure was so nearly universal that no attempt at grading could have had value" is most *inconsistent* with which of the following statements also made in the passage?

A) "Instructors generally reach a fairly accurate gauge of their scholars' powers."
B) "The four years passed at college were, for his purposes, wasted."
C) "The entire work of the four years could have been easily put into the work of any four months in after life."
D) "He regarded himself as the only person for whom his education had value, and he wanted the whole of it."

3. Which of the following statements is/are supported by information in the passage?

    I. Adams was a man beholden to vanity regarding his appearance.
    II. Adams returned to teach and was motivated by instilling a new generation with useful information that was well received by his students.
    III. Adams had a predilection for politics and literature.

A) I only
B) III only
C) I and III only
D) I, II, and III

4. All of the following are suggested as occupations or interests held by Adams EXCEPT:

A) college professor.
B) paleontology.
C) chemistry.
D) military officer.

5. The author's primary purpose in the passage is to:

A) detail the academic life of a subpar college student's experience and lobby for changing the system of education.
B) argue for the necessity of a liberal arts education in order to create a well-educated citizenry.
C) critically recount Adams' college experiences.
D) recount the positive and negative experiences of students at Harvard.

[handwritten notes:]

#1: adams + lee relationship
        lee asked adams 4 are

P2: lee was a bad student +
      he couldnt pass math for
      anything

P3: he sucked at school but
      was curious abt chem +
      fothers

P4: Adams was not favored in
      school + saw his failures as
      correct + a didnt learn.

B1: adams + lee were both failures

CHAPTER 3 PRACTICE PASSAGE 2

A college class on the American novel is reading Alice Walker's *The Color Purple* (1982). A student raises her hand and recalls that the Steven Spielberg film version (1985) drew angry responses from many African American viewers. The discussion takes off: Did Alice Walker "betray" African Americans with her harsh depiction of Black men? Did Spielberg enhance this feature of the book or play it down? Another hand goes up: "But she *was* promoting lesbianism." "Spielberg *really* played that down!" the professor replies. A contentious voice in the back of the room: "Well I just want to know what a serious film was doing with Oprah Winfrey in it." This is answered by another student, "Dude, she does have a *book* club on her show!" Class members respond to these points, examining interrelationships among race, gender, popular culture, the media, and literature. This class is practicing cultural studies.

Cultural studies approaches generally share four goals. First, cultural studies transcends the confines of a particular discipline such as literary criticism or history. Cultural studies involves scrutinizing the cultural phenomenon of a text—for example, Italian opera, a Latino telenovela, the architectural styles of prisons, body piercing—and drawing conclusions about the changes in textual phenomena over time. Cultural studies is not necessarily about literature in the traditional sense or even about art. Henry Giroux and others write in their *Dalhousie Review* manifesto that cultural studies practitioners are "resisting intellectuals" who see what they do as "an emancipatory project" because it erodes the traditional disciplinary divisions in most institutions of higher education. For students, this sometimes means that a professor might make his or her own political views part of the instruction, which, of course, can lead to problems. But this kind of criticism, like feminism, is an engaged rather than a detached activity.

Second, cultural studies is politically engaged. Cultural critics see themselves as "oppositional," not only within their own disciplines but to many of the power structures of society at large. They question inequalities within power structures and seek to discover models for restructuring relationships among dominant and "minority" or "subaltern" discourses. Because meaning and individual subjectivity are culturally constructed they can thus be reconstructed. Such a notion, taken to a philosophical extreme, denies the autonomy of the individual, whether an actual person or a character in literature, a rebuttal of the traditional humanistic "Great Man" or "Great Book" theory, and a relocation of aesthetics and culture from the ideal realms of taste and sensibility, into the arena of a whole society's everyday life as it is constructed.

Third, cultural studies denies the separation of "high" and "low" or elite and popular culture. You might hear someone remark at the symphony or at an art museum: "I came here to get a little culture." Being a "cultured" person used to mean being acquainted with "highbrow" art and intellectual pursuits. But isn't *culture* also to be found with a pair of tickets to a rock concert? Cultural critics today work to transfer the term *culture* to include *mass culture*, whether popular, folk, or urban. Transgressing of boundaries among disciplines high and low can make cultural studies just plain fun. Think, for example, of a possible cultural studies research paper with the following title: "The Birth of Captain Jack Sparrow: An Analysis." For sources of Johnny Depp's funky performance in Disney's *Pirates of the Caribbean* movies, you could research cultural topics ranging from the trade economies of the sea two hundred years ago, to real pirates of the Caribbean such as Blackbeard and Henry Morgan, then on to memorable screen pirates, John Cleese's rendition of Long John Silver on *Monty Python's Flying Circus*, and, of course, Keith Richards's eye makeup.

Finally, cultural studies analyzes not only the cultural work, but the means of production. Marxist critics have long recognized the importance of such paraliterary questions as, Who supports a given artist? Who publishes his or her books, and how are these books distributed? Who buys books? For that matter, who is literate and who is not? These studies help us recognize that literature does not occur in a space separate from other concerns of our lives. Cultural studies thus joins *subjectivity*— that is, culture in relation to individual lives—with *engagement*, a direct approach to attacking social ills. Though cultural studies practitioners deny "humanism" of "the humanities" as universal categories, they strive for what they might call "social reason," which often (closely) resembles the goals and values of humanistic and democratic ideals.

Material used in this particular passage has been adapted from the following source:

W. Guerin et al, *A Handbook of Critical Approaches to Literature.* © 2005 by Oxford University Press.

[handwritten: henry resisting intele rock concert]

1. Which of the following would be LEAST consistent with the author's description of cultural studies?

    A) An analysis of Missourian Mark Twain's *A Connecticut Yankee in King Arthur's Court* that examined questions regarding the oppressive inequality embodied in monarchical social etiquette and regional class structures
    B) A discussion of female image and intelligence as presented by reality TV dating shows such as VH1's *Rock of Love* with rock star Bret Michaels
    C) An exploration of whether Steven Spielberg's absent father characters in *E.T.*, *Catch Me If You Can*, and *Indiana Jones and the Last Crusade* are a response to his own father being absent in his childhood
    D) An examination of the influence of gospel hymns on the speechwriting of civil rights leaders such as Rev. Dr. Martin Luther King, Jr., and Medgar Evers

    [handwritten: new info—]

2. If a hard-line cultural studies practitioner were to conclude, after researching the text, that white supremacist Asa Earl Carter's novel *The Education of Little Tree* about the traditional upbringing of a Native American boy was written free of his opinions about non-Caucasian peoples, it would most *undermine* the author's assertion that:

    A) cultural studies is not exclusively about literature or even art.
    B) the oppositional nature of cultural studies, carried to an extreme, denies the sovereignty of individual will.
    C) analyzing the means of production is one of the important goals of cultural studies.
    D) cultural studies is politically engaged.

3. When the author quotes Henry Giroux's description of cultural studies practitioners as "resisting intellectuals" (paragraph 2), he most nearly means that:

    A) professors approaching literature this way reject an overly academic approach.
    B) the cultural studies movement began as an underground movement.
    C) professors reveal their own opinions in class in order to provoke disagreement and discussion from students.
    D) such academics take a multifarious approach to analyzing phenomena in a text.

*[handwritten notes:
#1: cultural studies discussion of A.w. the color purple
#2: cultural studies 1— cultural + not literal
P3: critics to power + inequalities due to constructivism ^subjec
P4: culture → mass culture not just high brow]*

4. The author's reference to a rock concert serves to indicate that:

    A) rock music combines both highbrow and lowbrow culture.
    B) music can serve political purposes.
    C) culture includes musical expression.
    D) popular artistic forms have not always been considered to be highly sophisticated.

5. Elsewhere the author writes, "Images of India circulated during the colonial rule of the British raj by writers like Rudyard Kipling seem innocent, but reveal an entrenched argument for white superiority and worldwide domination of other races." This, if taken as an example of cultural studies, illustrates the author's belief that such studies:

    A) deny the separation between lowbrow culture like Kipling's innocent stories and highbrow culture like discussions of political power.
    B) examine questions of power and influence, such as the structure of colonial society in India, and raise questions about who was circulating Kipling's writing.
    C) include mass culture such as Kipling's stories "The Jungle Book" and "Rikki-Tikki-Tavi."
    D) transcend historical analysis.

6. In the context of the passage as a whole, "emancipatory" (paragraph 2) most nearly means:

    A) excusing from an obligation.
    B) freeing from service.
    C) endorsing a wider perspective.
    D) promoting equality.

7. Suppose a critic were to propose a comparative analysis between Shakespeare's 16th-century play *Romeo and Juliet* and Tennessee Williams's 20th-century play *A Streetcar Named Desire*, focusing entirely on how the number of acts in each play affects the development of the main female character. Which of the following statements best represents how the author of the passage would most likely view this study and/or its author?

    A) This critic is not a cultural studies practitioner because she limits her investigations to questions internal to the plays.
    B) The critic is resisting historical disciplines by cutting across several centuries in her analysis.
    C) The critic should include an analysis of Shakespeare's and Williams's lives and the impact of personal events on their writing.
    D) Questions of who supported Shakespeare and Williams financially are irrelevant.

*[handwritten notes:
#5: cu. studies concerns itself w economics
P5: cul.st ⊕]*

SOLUTIONS TO CHAPTER 3 PRACTICE PASSAGE 1

1. **C**   This is a Tone/Attitude question.

    A: No. While the author does state in paragraph 2 that Harvard was a good school, the passage has a largely negative tone about Adam's experience. For example, the author states that Adams "got little more from his masters" than from his peers (paragraph 2), that in mathematics "his education failed lamentably" (paragraph 2), and that Adams got little out of his study of ancient languages, political economy, and chemistry (paragraph 3). The author also criticizes Adams' professors in paragraph 2.

    B: No. While the tone is largely negative, the author states in paragraph 4 that "Harvard College was a negative force, and negative forces have value. Slowly it weakened the violent political bias of childhood, not by putting interests in its place, but by mental habits which had no bias at all." Therefore, "complete waste" is too strong.

    C: Yes. While the author describes the failings of Adams' education in paragraphs 2 and 3, the author also states that there was some value to the experience: "Harvard College was a negative force, and negative forces have value. Slowly it weakened the violent political bias of childhood, not by putting interests in its place, but by mental habits which had no bias at all" (paragraph 4).

    D: No. While the passage does suggest Adams' opinion, it also clearly indicates the author's opinion of Adams as a student ("a partial [failure]" (paragraph 1)), of the professors at Harvard ("In the one branch he most needed—mathematics—barring the few first scholars, failure was so nearly universal that no attempt at grading could have had value, and whether he stood fortieth or ninetieth must have been an accident or the personal favor of the professor" (paragraph 2)), and of Adams' education as a whole, including the value Adams did get out of the experience ("Harvard College was a negative force, and negative forces have value." (paragraph 4)).

2. **A**   This is a Structure question.

    Note: The correct answer will be the statement made elsewhere in the passage that most contradicts the statement cited in the question stem. If a statement in an answer choice is on a different issue, it will not be inconsistent (that is, the two statements would be consistent in that they could both be true).

    A: Yes. Following the statement that grading could have had little value, the author states: "whether he stood fortieth or ninetieth must have been an accident or the personal favor of the professor" (paragraph 2). This suggests that grades or rankings did not in fact reflect the skill or accomplishment of the student. This would be inconsistent with the claim cited in choice A (from paragraph 4) that instructors accurately evaluate their students.

    B: No. The claim that the four years were wasted is consistent with the author's critique of how professors graded.

    C: No. The quote in this choice is on a different issue: that Adams was interested in only a small portion of his course material (paragraph 3). Therefore the two claims are not inconsistent with each other.

    D: No. This refers to a somewhat different issue (Adams' self-centeredness (paragraph 2)), rather than the value or accuracy of the grading. Furthermore, to the extent that this statement relates to the existence of other students (who were also graded by the same standards), it is consistent (not inconsistent) with the claim in the question stem.

3. **B** This is an Inference/Roman numeral question.

    I: False. This statement is not supported by the passage. While Adams' vanity is mentioned in the first paragraph, there was no mention of Adams being vain specifically about his appearance.

    II: False. While it is correct that Adams did teach, the passage states that Adams went "back to teach in his turn what no student naturally cared or needed to know" (paragraph 2). Therefore the claim that Adams was "motivated by instilling a new generation with useful information that was well received by his students" is inconsistent with the text.

    III: True. By stating that the Harvard experience "weakened the violent political bias of childhood" (paragraph 4), the author suggests that Adams did have an interest in, or predilection towards, politics in the first place. The author also mentions in paragraph 1 that because of Lee's request, "The diplomat felt his profession." As for literature, in paragraph 4 the author states: "Rather by instinct than by guidance, he turned to writing," suggesting that Adams had some interest himself in literature.

4. **D** This is an Inference/EXCEPT question.

    A: No. Paragraph 2 states: "Long afterwards, when the devious path of life led him back to teach in his turn what no student naturally cared or needed to know, he diverted some dreary hours of faculty-meetings by looking up his record in the class-lists, and found himself graded precisely in the middle." This suggests that Adams returned to Harvard as a professor.

    B: No. Paragraph 3 states: "The only teaching that appealed to his imagination was a course of lectures by Louis Agassiz on the Glacial Period and Paleontology, which had more influence on his curiosity than the rest of the college instruction altogether." This suggests Adams had an interest in paleontology.

    C: No. Paragraph 3 states: "The bit of practical teaching he afterwards reviewed with most curiosity was the course in Chemistry, which taught him a number of theories that befogged his mind for a lifetime." Even if Adams was confused by chemistry, the passage suggests that he did have some interest in or "curiosity" about it.

    D: Yes. There is no mention of Adams having any interest in military affairs. The passage does talk of Lee accepting a military commission (paragraph 1), but not of Adams doing the same or having any interest in military affairs.

5. **C** This is a Main Point/Primary Purpose question.

    A: No. While the passage does provide some details about Adams' education, it does not explicitly lobby for, or make suggestions concerning, education.

    B: No. There is no mention of preparing well-educated citizens.

    C: Yes. The author casts a critical eye on Adams' college experiences by speaking throughout the passage in largely negative terms; the value gained in lessening Adams' political biases (paragraph 4) still came out of the negative nature of the experiences themselves.

    D: No. While one could infer that some of the experiences described applied to other students as well (e.g., how they were evaluated), the main focus of the passage is on Adams himself. Furthermore, the emphasis is on the negative experiences; even the positive outcome mentioned in the beginning of the last paragraph came out of *negative experiences*.

SOLUTIONS TO CHAPTER 3 PRACTICE PASSAGE 2

1. **C** This is an Inference/LEAST question.

    A: No. This is consistent with the author's description of cultural studies in paragraph 2, where the author states that cultural studies transcends traditional boundaries between academic disciplines. It is also consistent with the author's discussion in paragraph 3: "Cultural critics see themselves as 'oppositional,'…to many of the power structures on society at large. They question inequalities within power structures…"

    B: No. This examination of gender depictions is consistent with the discussion of gender depictions in paragraph 1's example of cultural studies.

    C: Yes. This analysis is not consistent with any description of cultural studies laid out in the passage because it limits its scope to the artist's own life rather than the culture within which he or she created his or her movie.

    D: No. This is consistent with paragraph 2's assertion that "Cultural studies involves scrutinizing the cultural phenomenon of a text—for example, Italian opera," as well as with paragraph 4's examples of the types of cultural phenomena, including "mass culture," examined by cultural studies practitioners.

2. **B** This is a New Information question.

    A: No. The analysis of Carter's book would be consistent with the idea that history and traditional customs are also a part of cultural studies.

    B: Yes. Someone who is extremely committed to a cultural studies approach, according to the author, would be unlikely to assert that an artist could create a text in which he or she effectively and consciously omitted all trace or influence of his or her cultural context. According to the passage, an individual author would not be seen by this type of cultural critic as having this kind of autonomy (paragraph 3).

    C: No. There is no indication, either way, whether the critic examined questions of the means of production. Thus, the new information neither strengthens nor weakens this claim of the author.

    D: No. There is no reason, based on the passage, to believe that political engagement in this case would require a hard-line cultural critic to identify racist themes within the novel itself.

3. **D** This is an Inference question.

    A: No. While these practitioners are resisting traditional divisions in academia between disciplines (e.g., between literary criticism and history), being "academic" is not identified in the passage with respecting these divisions. Therefore, there is no evidence to support the idea that what they are rejecting is an "overly academic" approach.

    B: No. There is no evidence that cultural studies began as a secretive movement. This is taking the word "resisting" out of the context of the passage.

    C: No. This choice is wrong first because there is no evidence that professors introduce their own viewpoints *in order to* provoke disagreement, only that introduction of the professor's own political views may be part of instruction. Second, introduction of the professor's own views is given as perhaps one aspect of the "emancipatory project," but not as part of a definition of what the term "resisting intellectuals" itself means.

D: Yes. The author states that these intellectuals "see what they do as 'an emancipatory project' because it erodes the traditional disciplinary divisions" by "scrutinizing the cultural phenomenon of a text" (paragraph 2). This means that rather than studying only the text itself (or other aspects traditionally seen as "literary" issues related to it) cultural critics bring in other issues relating to the culture within which the text appears. This aligns with what the author said earlier in the paragraph, that "cultural studies transcends the confines of a particular discipline." Therefore, these academics take a multifarious or diverse approach to a text.

4. **D** This is an Inference question.
    A: No. There is no indication rock music is *both* highbrow and lowbrow—on the contrary, the passage indicates that rock music has traditionally been considered lowbrow instead of highbrow.
    B: No. Politics is not an issue in this paragraph. In addition, to the extent that the author discusses political motivations elsewhere in the passage, the issue is the political engagement of cultural critics, not of culture itself.
    C: No. The point of the reference is not to show that culture includes music; an earlier reference to the symphony suggests that at least some forms of music are already seen as cultural expression. Furthermore, the point being made is that cultural critics deny the distinction between high (the symphony) and low (the rock concert) culture.
    D: **Yes. In paragraph 4, the author writes that "cultural studies denies the separation of 'high' and 'low' or elite and popular culture...Being a 'cultured' person used to mean being acquainted with 'highbrow' art and intellectual pursuits. But isn't *culture* also to be found with a pair of tickets to a rock concert?" The change cultural studies has created from what culture "used to mean" has been to include forms (such as the rock concert) that were once considered not to be elite, intellectual, highbrow, or highly sophisticated.**

5. **B** This is a New Information question.
    A: No. Nothing indicates that Kipling's stories are or would have been considered lowbrow.
    B: **Yes. This is consistent with the author's description of the second major goal of cultural studies ("They question inequalities within power structures"), as detailed in paragraph 3; it is also consistent with the author's description of the fourth major goal of cultural studies ("Marxist critics have long recognized the importance of such paraliterary questions as, Who supports a given artist? Who publishes his or her books, and how are these books distributed?") as described in paragraph 5. (Note: Marxist critics are referred to as part of the description of cultural critics.)**
    C: No. Nothing indicates that Kipling's stories constitute mass culture. Note that A and C are saying basically the same thing, and they have the same problem—so you can cross them both out.
    D: No. This perspective is rooted in history, so it doesn't illustrate how cultural studies transcends, or goes beyond, history.

6. **C**   This is an Inference question.
    A: No. There is no indication of obligation in the passage. This choice takes the meaning of the word out of context.
    B: No. There is no indication of service in the passage. As in choice A, this answer represents a common definition of emancipation, but one that does not fit in the context of the passage.
    C: **Yes. Paragraph 2 says cultural studies practitioners see their field "as 'an emancipatory project' because it erodes the traditional disciplinary divisions." Eroding divisions would produce a "wider perspective;" that is, one not limited by the practices or assumptions of a particular academic field.**
    D: No. While the author indicates in paragraph 3 that cultural critics "question inequalities," this is not the context in which the word "emancipatory" appears in paragraph 2. This choice then has two problems: it uses a common definition of the word that does not fit in the context of the relevant part of the passage, and it refers to an issue that arises elsewhere in the passage but not in this paragraph.

7. **A**   This is a New Information question.
    A: **Yes. Because the question the critic asks is limited to the form of the plays and the development of characters within that structure, and because it does not address culture or any of the goals of cultural studies as they are outlined in the passage, the author is most likely to argue that the critic is not practicing cultural studies.**
    B: No. If anything, comparing texts from two different periods in history would be embracing a historical approach, not resisting it.
    C: No. Examining the text in terms of the events of the author's life is not one of the goals of cultural studies.
    D: No. We have no evidence the author disagrees with the fourth goal of cultural studies, as he described it in paragraph 5, which asserts the relevance of questions of finance and production.

Individual Passage Log

Passage # _____

Q#	Q type	Attractors	What did you do wrong?

Revised Strategy _____

Passage # _____

Q#	Q type	Attractors	What did you do wrong?

Revised Strategy _____

Think Like a Test-Writer: Exercise 1

MCAT CRITICAL ANALYSIS AND
REASONING SKILLS REVIEW

THINK LIKE A TEST-WRITER: EXERCISE 1

The AAMC gives this section the fancy name "Critical Analysis and Reasoning Skills" (instead of simply calling it "Reading Comprehension") to emphasize that the CARS section tests a variety of skills that go beyond simply understanding the information in the passage text. One of those skills is the ability to follow the logical structure of the passage. One of the most effective ways to track that structure is to ask questions of the text as you read, questions such as "What new idea is being introduced here?" or "How does this statement or paragraph relate to previous statements or paragraphs?" or "Has the author made their own position on this issue clear?" or "Why is the author making this claim?" or even "What might be coming next?"

The test-writers have these same questions in mind when they create the test questions. When you ask and answer these questions, you are getting into the minds of the test-writers; you are picking up on the aspects of the passage they will use to create the questions, the right answers, and those attractive wrong answers that are sometimes so tempting. To help you develop this way of reading and thinking, we have provided you with three "Think Like a Test-Writer" Exercises.

This first exercise focuses on asking questions as you read in order to effectively track the logical structure of the passage. The second (after Chapter 4) asks you to think about what kinds of questions a test-writer might create based on that logical structure. The third exercise (after Chapter 5) adds in the challenge of thinking about not only possible passage questions but types of attractive wrong answers they might create.

For this first exercise, read the following text, tracking the author's tone and purpose in each paragraph. Pay attention to key words that indicate transitions, emphasis, and tone.

As you read, you will see questions inserted into the text [in red and in brackets] to help you focus on defining the purpose of statements within the passage, the purpose of each paragraph, and the purpose of the passage as a whole. Some of these questions can be answered at that point in the text, while others are questions that will be answered later in the passage. Jot down your response to those questions as you read; answers are provided after the passage.

Note: This text is longer than a CARS passage in order to give you practice with tracking logical structure across multiple paragraphs.

EXERCISE 1

Three circumstances have seemed to liars to provide the strongest excuse for their behavior—a crisis where over-whelming harm can be averted only through deceit; complete harmlessness and triviality to the point where it seems absurd to quibble about whether a lie has been told; and the duty to particular individuals to protect their secrets. [**Q1:** Does the author agree that these are legitimate excuses?] I have shown how lies in times of crisis can expand into vast practices where the harm to be averted is less obvious and the crisis less and less immediate; how white lies can shade into equally vast practices no longer so harmless, with immense cumulative costs; and how lies to protect individuals and to cover up their secrets can be told for increasingly dubious purposes to the detriment of all. [**Q2:** Now do we know if the author agrees? **Q3:** Why is the author referring to her previous statements?]

_____

_____

_____

When these three expanding streams [**Q4:** What "three expanding streams" is the author referring to?] flow together and mingle with yet another—a desire to advance the public good—they form the most dangerous body of deceit of all. These lies may not be justified by immediate crisis nor by complete triviality nor by duty to any one person; rather, liars tend to consider them as right and unavoidable because of the altruism that motivates them….

_____

_____

_____

Naturally, there will be large areas of overlap between these lies and those considered earlier. But the most character-istic defense for these lies is a separate one, based on the benefits they may confer and the long range harm they can avoid. The intention may be broadly paternalistic, as when citizens are deceived "for their own good," or only a few may be lied to for the benefit of the community at large. Error and self-deception mingle with these altruistic pur-poses and blur them; the filters through which we must try to peer at lying are thicker and more distorting than ever in these practices. But I shall try to single out, among these lies, the elements that are consciously and purposefully intended to benefit society. [**Q5:** What new idea is introduced, starting with the word "But," in this paragraph?]

_____

_____

_____

A long tradition in political philosophy endorses some lies for the sake of the public. Plato…first used the expression "noble lie" for the fanciful story that might be told to people in order to persuade them to accept class distinctions and thereby safeguard social harmony. According to this story, God himself mingled gold, silver, iron, and brass in fash-ioning rulers, auxiliaries, farmers, and craftsmen, intending these groups for separate tasks in a harmonious hierarchy. … [**Q6:** What is the purpose of this discussion of Plato?]

_____

_____

_____

Rulers, both temporal and spiritual, have seen their deceits in the benign light of such social purposes. They have propagated and maintained myths played on the gullibility of the ignorant, and sought stability in shared beliefs. They have seen themselves as high minded and well bred—whether by birth or by training—and as superior to those they deceive. Some have gone so far as to claim that those who govern have a *right* to lie. The powerful tell lies believing that they have greater than ordinary understanding of what is at stake; very often, they regard their dupes as having inadequate judgment, or as likely to respond in the wrong way to truthful information. [**Q7:** Is the point of view described in this paragraph consistent or inconsistent with that of Plato?]

_____

_____

_____

At times, those who govern also regard particular circumstances as too uncomfortable, too painful, for most people to be able to cope with rationally. They may believe, for instance, that their country must prepare for long-term challenges of great importance, such as a war, an epidemic, or a belt-tightening in the face of future shortages. Yet they may fear that citizens will be able to respond only to short-range dangers. Deception at such times may seem to the government leaders as the only means of attaining the necessary results. [**Q8:** Is the author discussing a point of view shared by Plato, or is this a contrasting position?]

_____

_____

_____

The perspective of the liar is paramount in all such decisions to tell "noble" lies. If the liar considers the responses of the deceived at all, he assumes that they will, once the deceit comes to light and its benefits are understood, be uncomplaining if not positively grateful. The lies are often seen as necessary merely at one stage in the education of the public. …[**Q9:** Is there a new idea in this paragraph, or, is it simply further elaboration on the idea that some justify lying for the good of the public?]

_____

_____

_____

Some experienced public officials are impatient with any effort to question the ethics of such deceptive practices (except actions obviously taken for private ends). They argue that vital objectives in the national interest require a measure of deception to succeed in the face of powerful obstacles. Negotiations must be carried on that are best left hidden from public view; bargains must be struck that simply cannot be comprehended by a politically unsophisticated electorate. A certain amount of illusion is needed in order for public servants to be effective. Every government, therefore, has to deceive people to some extent in order to lead them. [**Q10:** Is this the author's point of view, or is she still describing someone else's argument?]

_____

_____

_____

If we assume the perspective of the deceived—those who experienced the consequences of government deception—such arguments are not persuasive. [**Q11:** What has changed in the nature of the author's argument in this part of the passage?] We cannot take for granted either the altruism or the good judgment of those who lie to us, no matter how much they intend to benefit us. We have learned that much deceit for private gain masquerades as being in the public interest. We know how deception, even for the most unselfish motive, corrupts and spreads. And we have lived through the consequences of lies told for what were believed to be noble purposes. Equally unpersuasive is the argument that there always has been government deception, and always will be, and that efforts to draw lines and set standards are therefore useless annoyances. It is certainly true that deception can never be completely absent from most human practices. But there are great differences among societies in the kinds of deceit that exist and the extent to which they are practiced, differences also among individuals in the same government and among successive governments within the same society. This strongly suggests that it is worthwhile trying to discover why such differences exist and to seek ways of raising the standards of truthfulness. ...[**Q12:** What is the purpose of the second part of this paragraph?]

_____

_____

_____

Can there be exceptions to the well-founded distrust of deception in public life? Are there times when the public itself might truly not care about possible lies, or might even prefer to be deceived? Are some white lies so trivial or so transparent that they can be ignored? And can we envisage public discussion of more seriously misleading government statements such that reasonable persons could consent to them in advance? [**Q13:** What is the author's purpose in asking this series of questions?]

_____

_____

_____

White lies, first of all, are as common to political and diplomatic affairs as they are to the private lives of most people. [**Q14:** What does the phrase "first of all" indicate about what may follow this discussion of one aspect of "white lies"?] Feigning enjoyment of an embassy gathering or a political rally, toasting the longevity of a dubious regime or an unimpressive candidate for office—these are forms of politeness that mislead few. It is difficult to regard them as threats to either individuals or communities. As with all white lies, however, the problem is that they spread so easily, and that lines are very hard to draw. Is it still a white lie for a Secretary of State to announce that he is going to one country when in reality he travels to another? Or for a president to issue a "cover story" to the effect that a cold is forcing him to return to the White House, when in reality an international crisis made him cancel the rest of his campaign trip? Is it a white lie to issue a letter of praise for a public servant one has just fired? Given the vulnerability of public trust, it is never more important than in public life to keep the deceptive element of white lies to an absolute minimum, and to hold down the danger of their turning into more widespread deceitful practices. ...[**Q15:** How does this paragraph about "white lies" answer the questions raised in the previous paragraph?]

_____

_____

_____

Another form of deception takes place when the government regards the public as frightened, or hostile, and highly volatile. In order not to create a panic, information about early signs of an epidemic may be suppressed or distorted. And the lie to a mob seeking its victim is like lying to the murderer asking where the person he is pursuing has gone. It can be acknowledged and defended as soon as the threat is over. In such cases, one may at times be justified in withholding information; perhaps, on rare occasions, even in lying. But such cases are so rare that they hardly exist for practical purposes. …[**Q16:** How does this paragraph about "another form of deception" relate to the questions raised in the earlier paragraph? Is the author going back on her argument against lying?]

_____

_____

_____

Whenever lies to the public become routine, then, very special safeguards should be required. The test of public justification of deceptive practices is more needed than ever. It will be a hard test to satisfy, the more so the more trust is invested in those who lie and the more power they wield. Those in government and other positions of trust should be held to the highest standard. Their lies are not ennobled by their positions; quite the contrary. Some lies—notably minor white lies and emergency lies rapidly acknowledged—may be more _excusable_ than others, but only those deceptive practices which can be openly debated and consented to in advance are _justifiable_ in a democracy. [**Q17:** What is the purpose of the last paragraph of this passage? Does it add anything new, or is it simply a summation of points already made?]

_____

_____

_____

[**Q18:** What is the author's overall purpose in writing this passage?]

_____

_____

_____

—Text adapted from S. Bok, _Lying: Moral Choice in Public and Private Life._ © 1978 by Sissela Bok.

SOLUTIONS TO EXERCISE 1

1. We don't know yet if the author agrees. The phrase "have seemed to liars," however, should make you wonder if the author may in fact disagree.

2. We still do not know, although the negative tone of this portion of the passage suggests that the author may not agree. However, you need more evidence to conclusively infer that the author believes that these particular lies are illegitimate.

3. The purpose is to set the stage for her judgment regarding the three excuses for lying listed at the beginning of the passage, and to suggest that at least some kinds of lies may be hard to justify.

4. This refers to the three expanding streams listed at the end of the previous paragraph; the theme of that list is that lies may have cumulative negative effects that go beyond any harm done by the initial lie, and that altruistic motives may not be enough to justify a lie.

5. This paragraph introduces the new idea that some lies are meant to benefit society, and that it is difficult to know if they are justified. Given the negative tone of the passage so far regarding lying, it is possible that the author will eventually claim that they are not in fact justified, but you need to read further before you can make that assessment.

6. The purpose of the reference to Plato is to give an example of a justification of lying for the public good. You don't know yet, however, if the author agrees or disagrees with Plato.

7. The point of view in this paragraph is consistent with that of Plato; the purpose of the paragraph is to further elaborate on the idea that some justify lying to the public for the public's own good. Note wording such as "myths played on the gullibility of the ignorant," and "dupes." This negative language suggests that the author of the passage may reject this justification, but we still don't know for sure what the author's own position is.

8. This paragraph is discussing, and elaborating on, the point of view shared by Plato: lying to the public may be necessary to protect the public interest.

9. While this paragraph is still discussing the claim that lying to the public may be in the public's own interest, it is introducing a new idea: the liars are not seriously considering the perspective of those being lied to.

10. The author is still describing someone else's argument in this paragraph. Note the wording in the beginning of the paragraph: "Some experienced public officials are impatient with any effort to question the ethics of such deceptive practices (except actions obviously taken for private ends). They argue…" Taken in that context, the statements at the end of the paragraph are still attributed to others.

11. Here the author is finally telling us what she thinks, and that she rejects the claim that lies for the public's own good are legitimate. Now it becomes clear why the author introduced, in the previous paragraph, the idea of the perspective of the deceived. When she says "If we assume the perspective of the deceived—those who experienced the consequences of government deception—such arguments are not persuasive" she is definitively saying that this perspective must be considered, and that that it invalidates the arguments made in defense of these kinds of lies.

12. The purpose of the rest of the paragraph is to elaborate on the claim made in the beginning, and to discount a series of possible justifications for lying in the public good, At the end of the paragraph the author also calls for investigation into differences in lies and into justifications for those lies between different societies.

13. Authors usually ask rhetorical questions (questions the reader is not expected to answer for themselves) to set up the next point. Here, the author is asking if the kind of lying she has criticized in the previous paragraph might ever be justified. As the reader, you should be looking out for a potential twist: is the author going to take this in an unexpected direction and actually justify certain types of lies, or is she using these questions to further elaborate on her rejection of such justifications?

14. "First of all" indicates that there will be multiple aspects of white lies discussed, not just how common they are in public life. Noting this phrase alerts you to the need to track where each different aspect is discussed.

15. The discussion of white lies in this paragraph constitutes a rejection of one possible justification for lying raised in the previous paragraph: "Are some white lies so trivial or so transparent that they can be ignored?" The author says no.

16. Here the author is conceding that in some cases lying can be justified, especially if the lie is soon exposed. But, she goes on to say that these cases are very rare. Therefore even though the author is conceding that some lies may be justified, she is still making her case against lying overall.

17. While this last paragraph does solidify the author's position against lying, it also introduces a new idea: lying may be *excusable* in rare cases after the fact, but it is only *justifiable* in a democracy when they are consented to in advance by the public.

18. The author's purpose in the passage as a whole is to address a variety of possible justifications for lying in public life and to warn us that even seemingly innocuous or well-motivated lies may have significant negative consequences.

Chapter 4
Question Types
and Strategies

GOALS

1) To learn the types of questions that are likely to be asked and strategies for attacking them
2) To refine the use of Process of Elimination (POE)

4.1 REVIEW: THE SIX STEPS

Here, one last time, is a brief outline of the six basic steps to approaching the MCAT CARS section:

▬ STEP 1: RANK AND ORDER THE PASSAGES

Decide whether to do the passage Now, Later, or Never (Killer) based on the difficulty level of the passage text.

▬ STEP 2: PREVIEW THE QUESTIONS

Read through the question stems (not the answer choices) before you read the passage. Look for and highlight words and phrases that indicate important passage content. Do not worry at this stage about identifying the question type.

▬ STEP 3: WORK THE PASSAGE

As you read through the passage, use the highlighting function (sparingly) to annotate the most important references in the passage, especially words that indicate the logical structure of the author's argument and references that appeared in your preview of the questions. Notice topic sentences that help you to identify conclusions made by the author. Articulate the Main Point of each chunk of information (usually, each paragraph). Use your noteboard, especially on difficult passages, to jot down these main points. As you read, think about how these chunks relate to each other, and identify the structure of the passage.

▬ STEP 4: BOTTOM LINE

After you have read the passage, sum up the Bottom Line: the Main Point and tone of the entire passage.

▬ STEP 5: ATTACK THE QUESTIONS

Read the question word for word, identifying the question type and translating the question task into your own words. Go back to the passage before reading the answer choices and find the relevant information (reading at least five lines above and below the reference). Think about what the correct answer will need to do, and generate an answer to the question in your own words. Use POE actively. Select the "least wrong" answer.

▬ STEP 6: INSPECT THE SECTION

At or before the 5-minute mark (ideally before you begin your last passage), double-check to make sure that you haven't left anything blank. You can use the Review function at this stage. Do NOT rethink questions you have already completed.

In the rest of this chapter, we'll focus on **Step Five: Attack the Questions.**

4.2 ATTACKING THE QUESTIONS

In order to continue to improve your CARS skills, you will need to refine your approach to the questions. In this chapter we will discuss the five basic steps you should take in answering any question, and the specific tactics appropriate to each question type.

Five Steps For Answering Questions

1) Read the question word for word and identify the question type.
2) Translate the question into your own words: identify what the question task is asking you to do with the information in the passage.
3) Identify any key words that refer to specific parts of the passage. If key words are provided, *go back to the passage* to locate that information.
4) Answer in your own words: articulate what the correct answer will need to do based on the question type and the information in the passage.
5) Use Process of Elimination (POE), and choose the *least wrong* answer choice.

Let's look at each step in more detail.

1) **Read the question word for word; identify the question type.**
   WHY?
   - If you misread or misinterpret the question now, you may never catch your mistake. Now is not the time to skim, or to get only a vague impression of what the question is asking.
   - No matter how good your annotation and mapping of the passage, if you're headed to the wrong destination, those signposts do you no good. You could have an excellent map of the United States, but if you're supposed to get to Boston and you think your destination is Biloxi, you are in big trouble. Know your destination!
   - The MCAT writers are highly skilled at predicting likely misinterpretations and at giving you wrong answers with which you could be perfectly happy. If you've ever completed a passage, pleased with how quickly and smoothly it went, only to realize upon checking your answers that you got many questions wrong, you may be reading the questions too carelessly.
   - Different kinds of questions ask for different kinds of information. Most importantly, General questions require general answers and can usually be answered with your own statement of the Bottom Line. Specific answer choices can be very narrow and always require going back to the passage. Reasoning and Application questions will usually also require you to go back to the passage, but they also ask you to either describe the logic or structure of the author's argument, or to apply new information to it. Identifying the question type is important because that will guide the rest of the process.
   HOW?
   - Read the question as if you have never seen it before. Focus on each word rather than taking it in as a chunk.
   - Think of the question as assigning you a task: what mission do you need to accomplish in answering the question? Do you need to find information that matches the passage? Describe the author's argument in the passage (in part or the whole)? Strengthen or weaken the author's argument? Apply new information from the question stem?

4.2

2) **Translate the question into your own words; identify what the question task is asking you to do.**
    WHY?
    - You may have noticed by now that questions are not always phrased in an easily comprehensible way. The test-writers do this on purpose to see if you can understand difficult, complex writing and ideas.

    HOW?
    - When you come across a long, complex, and convoluted question, take it out of MCAT-speak and put it into your own words. You may find it useful to jot down a few words on your noteboard.
    - The benefits of translation are two-fold. First, it helps you to clarify exactly what the question is asking. Second, it will enable you to remember exactly what you're looking for when you go back to the passage.

    For example, a question for a passage on Abstract Expressionism may ask

    1. Which of the following would be most inconsistent with Brown's claim that Jackson Pollock did not lack influence within the movement called Abstract Expressionism, as that movement and its subsequent offshoots and internal divisions are described in the passage?

    When you cut away the extraneous stuff and clarify the convoluted wording, all this question is asking is

    1. Which of the following answer choices indicates that Pollock had little or no influence on Abstract Expressionism?

3) **Identify any key words that refer to specific parts of the passage. If key words are provided, go back to the passage to locate that information.**
    WHY?
    - Going back to the passage to answer questions with specific lead words is fundamental. You simply don't have time to memorize the details. Relying on your ability to recall facts under time pressure will only get you into trouble.
    - If you don't check your answers against the text, you are likely to pick a choice that contains words from the passage taken out of context, or one that is true in the real world, but not supported by the passage.
    - Going back to the passage before you read the answer choices will not only increase your accuracy, but will also increase your overall speed. If you already have a solid grounding in the passage, you will more quickly recognize the correct choice, and you are much less likely to get stuck between two answers.

HOW?

- A key word or phrase is something in the question that appears only a few times in the passage, and it guides you toward the relevant sections in the passage that you'll need to reread.

- Looking again at the sample question above, the phrase "Abstract Expressionism" would not make a good key phrase if the whole passage is about Abstract Expressionism; it's likely to appear many times throughout the passage. The name Jackson Pollock, however, is likely to lead you right to the relevant sections for that particular question.

- Once you've identified the key words, *scan* the passage (using your annotations) until you locate those words, and then read a few sentences above and below until you find what you need. "Five lines above and five lines below" is a good guide. However, you should start reading where the relevant information begins, and keep reading until the passage moves on to another issue.

- Pay attention to the logical structure of the author's argument. For example, if the sixth line below begins with a word like *yet* or *additionally*, you need to keep reading. Pivotal and transitional words indicate that the author may be qualifying what he or she has just said, or adding an additional point that you need to take into account.

- Some Specific (such as, "With which of the following statements would the author be most likely to agree?") and Application questions do not give you lead words as clues. For these questions, eliminate the choices that are inconsistent with the Bottom Line (or, for a Weaken question, that are consistent with the passage), and then go back to the passage to check each of the remaining possibilities.

- For General questions, you can usually use your own articulation of the Bottom Line. You may, however, still need to go back to the passage when you are down to two choices.

4) **Answer in your own words; articulate what the correct answer will need to do, based on the question type and the information in the passage.**
WHY?

- Think of the answer choices as a minefield, full of potentially fatal missteps and pitfalls. Before you enter that minefield, you should have a detailed map of what a strong answer choice will accomplish.

- The wording of the credited response may be quite different from what you expect, but with your own answer as a guide, you will recognize it while avoiding the traps.

HOW?

- Once you've located the relevant information—and not before—articulate your own answer to the question. For particularly difficult questions, you may wish to jot this down on your noteboard.

- This does not mean, however, that you should try to predict the exact wording of the credited response. Instead, come up with a guide to what the correct answer needs to *do* (such as, in the sample question above, to show that Jackson Pollock had little or no influence).

4.3

5) **Use Process of Elimination (POE) to choose the *least wrong* answer choice.**
WHY?

- POE is the best friend of every strategic test-taker. Very often on the MCAT, there is no perfectly correct answer among the given choices, only better and worse choices. On particularly difficult passages, the credited response can even be a pretty bad answer. However, it will be *less bad* than the other three.
- There are a number of standard ways in which the MCAT writers make loser choices look like winners. The answer that at first glance "looks good" may in fact be a trap. See the rest of this chapter and Chapter 5 for more information on types of wrong answers.

HOW?

- Use your own understanding of the question task and of what the correct choice needs to do in order to eliminate the most clearly wrong answers. This will usually take you down to two choices.
- Reread the question and compare the choices you have left to each other. Identify what is wrong, if anything, with each choice. The winner is the choice that has the *least wrong* with it. You may not like that winner very much, but you score a point, which is all that matters in this game.
- When you are down to two choices, actively look for the types of Attractors that commonly appear for that question type.

4.3 QUESTION TYPES AND FORMATS

There are ten basic questions types that you will encounter in an MCAT CARS section. These ten types of questions fall into four categories.

Specific
1) Retrieval
2) Inference

General
3) Main Idea/Primary Purpose
4) Tone/Attitude

Reasoning
5) Structure
6) Evaluate

Application
7) Strengthen
8) Weaken
9) New Information
10) Analogy

Specific questions ask you for the answer that is best supported by a particular part of the author's argument. General questions ask you what is true of the passage as a whole. Reasoning questions ask you to describe some aspect of the logical structure of the author's argument. Finally, Application questions require you to apply new information (provided either in the question stem or in the answer choices) to the passage.

Occasionally, there can be a variation within a category. For example, a Tone/Attitude question could refer to a particular part of the passage rather than the passage as a whole, and so qualify as a Specific question. Or, a Structure question could ask for the overall organization of the passage, which would make it a General Reasoning question.

These ten types can appear in one of three formats.

1) **Standard:** The question task is direct.
2) **EXCEPT/LEAST/NOT:** The question asks you to find the exception.
   That is, the choice that does NOT address, or that LEAST addresses, the question task (e.g., the statement that is *not* supported by the passage). The three wrong answers will in fact address the task (e.g., *will be* supported by the passage).
3) **Roman numeral:** The question offers you three items. The correct answer will include all of the items that do appropriately address the question task and none of the items that do not.

A firm knowledge of all of these types and of the common trap answers that appear in each is necessary for dealing with the questions quickly and accurately. Before you take the MCAT, you will be able to easily identify each question and know immediately what strategy you will need to employ.

As you move through the set of questions for a passage, use your understanding of question types to attack the questions in the order that works best for you. If you hit a particularly difficult question, skip over it for the moment, and continue answering the easier questions on that passage. Then click back through the set of questions one more time, answering the harder questions. Here is the most efficient approach.

1) Preview the questions from first to last.
2) Work the passage from the screen containing the last question for that passage (remember—your highlighting will not disappear).
3) Then work backwards through the questions, answering the easier ones and skipping harder ones as you go.
4) Finally, click forward through the set of questions, answering the ones you left blank the first time through.
5) Click "Next" from the last question to move on to the next passage.

In the next part of this chapter, we will go through each question type in the Standard format, as well as the EXCEPT/LEAST/NOT and Roman numeral formats. After a discussion of the basic approach to the type, you will find a sample question and a description of how to apply the Five Steps to that question. The sample questions are attached to the passage on criminal procedure that you annotated for an Active Reading Exercise in Chapter 3. The passage is reproduced here; first rework the passage so that it is fresh in your mind.

4.4   QUESTION TYPES: SAMPLE PASSAGE AND QUESTIONS

There are two major systems of criminal procedure in the modern world—the adversarial and the inquisitorial. The former is associated with common law tradition and the latter with civil law tradition. Both systems were historically preceded by the system of private vengeance in which the victim of a crime fashioned his own remedy and administered it privately, either personally or through an agent. The vengeance system was a system of self-help, the essence of which was captured in the slogan "an eye for an eye, a tooth for a tooth." The modern adversarial system is only one historical step removed from the private vengeance system and still retains some of its characteristic features. Thus, for example, even though the right to institute criminal action has now been extended to all members of society, and even though the police department has taken over the pretrial investigative functions on behalf of the prosecution, the adversarial system still leaves the defendant to conduct his own pretrial investigation. The trial is still viewed as a duel between two adversaries, refereed by a judge who, at the beginning of the trial, has no knowledge of the investigative background of the case. In the final analysis the adversarial system of criminal procedure symbolizes and regularizes punitive combat.

By contrast, the inquisitorial system begins historically where the adversarial system stopped its development. It is two historical steps removed from the system of private vengeance. Therefore, from the standpoint of legal anthropology, it is historically superior to the adversarial system. Under the inquisitorial system the public investigator has the duty to investigate not just on behalf of the prosecutor but also on behalf of the defendant. Additionally, the public prosecutor has the duty to present to the court not only evidence that may lead to the conviction of the defendant but also evidence that may lead to his exoneration. This system mandates that both parties permit full pretrial discovery of the evidence in their possession. Finally, in an effort to make the trial less like a duel between two adversaries, the inquisitorial system mandates that the judge take an active part in the conduct of the trial, with a role that is both directive and protective.

Fact-finding is at the heart of the inquisitorial system. This system operates on the philosophical premise that in a criminal case the crucial factor is not the legal rule but the facts of the case and that the goal of the entire procedure is to experimentally recreate for the court the commission of the alleged crime.

Material used in this particular passage has been adapted from the following source:

M. A. Glendon, *Comparative Legal Traditions in a Nutshell.* © 1982 by West Academic Publishing.

Type 1: Specific—Retrieval Questions

Retrieval questions test your ability to locate information in the passage. They may also involve simple paraphrasing and summarizing, but they do not require any substantial analysis or interpretation. They will include some reference to a detail in the passage (a person's name, a theory, a time period, etc.).

Retrieval questions may be phrased in the following ways:

- "According to the passage, the three components of Brown's theory are..."
- "The passage states that Brown's theory is rejected by..."
- "Which of the following statements is *not* mentioned as a characteristic of Brown's theory?" (EXCEPT/LEAST/NOT format)

Sample Question 1:

1. According to the author, the inquisitorial system is two steps removed from:

   A) the adversarial system.
   B) the system of punitive vengeance.
   C) pretrial discovery.
   D) regularized punitive combat.

1) **Read the question word for word and identify the question type.**
   The words "according to the passage" tell you that this is a Retrieval question.

2) **Translate the question into your own words: identify what the question task is asking you to do with the information in the passage.**
   Retrieval questions tend to be fairly straightforward. Here, the question is asking you to locate information in the passage about the inquisitorial system, and to find an answer choice that is best supported by that information.

3) **Identify any key words that refer to specific parts of the passage. If key words are provided, go back to the passage to locate that information.**
   The word "inquisitorial" appears in all three paragraphs. However, "two historical steps" is found only in the beginning of paragraph 2. That is where you will find the answer to this question.

4) **Answer in your own words: articulate what the correct answer will need to do, based on the question type and the information in the passage.**
   The correct answer will state what the "inquisitorial system" is two steps removed from. If you start at the beginning of paragraph 2 and read five lines down, you will see that it is "two historical steps removed from the system of private vengeance." The correct answer needs to state or paraphrase this. Also note that paragraph 1 describes the two systems that preceded the inquisitorial system; any choice that mixes up the three systems will be incorrect.

5) **Use Process of Elimination (POE) to choose the *least wrong* answer choice.**
   As we indicated earlier, each question usually has at least one trap or Attractor answer; that is, a choice that "sounds good" but in fact has some significant flaw. (See Chapter 5 for further discussion of Attractors.) Because Retrieval questions tend to be relatively easy, the MCAT writers often try to distract you from the credited response by pairing it with an answer choice that sounds very similar to the passage but *is not* directly supported by it. These Attractors

often copy words and phrases directly from the passage text, but don't capture the meaning of those words in the passage. The test-writers may also give you an answer choice that *is* directly supported by the text, but that is not an appropriate answer to that particular question. They may also change or reverse a relationship (for example, the passage says A leads to B, and the wrong answer says that B leads to A). The only way to spot and avoid these traps is to go back to the passage and reread the relevant sections.

Let's take a look at each answer choice for our sample question.

A: No. The first sentence of paragraph 2 states that "the inquisitorial system begins historically where the adversarial system stopped its development." You also know from paragraph 1 that the adversarial system followed "the system of private vengeance." Therefore, the inquisitorial system is one step, not two steps, removed from the adversarial system. This is a classic trap answer on a Retrieval question; it gives you something that is discussed in the same part of the passage, but that doesn't match the specific reference in the question task.

B: **Yes. Notice that that the author uses "punitive combat" at the end of paragraph 1 to describe what came before the adversarial system (the adversarial system regularized that punitive combat). Thus "punitive vengeance" is another way of saying "private vengeance." Therefore, this choice is directly supported by the relevant part of the passage.**

C: No. This choice takes words from the passage out of context and doesn't directly address the question task. Pretrial discovery is part of the inquisitorial system; it isn't something that the inquisitorial system is removed from.

D: No. This choice is tricky because it sounds a lot like choice B. But when you compare the two, you will see that choice D mentions *regularized* punitive combat. The end of paragraph 1 states that "the adversarial system…symbolizes and regularizes punitive combat." "Punitive combat" itself describes the system of private vengeance. So, this is just another way of saying "the adversarial system," and, just like choice A, it is incorrect.

Type 2: Specific—Inference Questions

Inference questions are the most common question type in the CARS section. They require you to choose the answer that is best supported by the passage. They may ask you what can be inferred or concluded, what the author would agree with, what is implied or suggested by the author, what the author assumes to be true, or what the author means by a particular word or phrase. They may also ask which answer choice would be an example of something described in the passage.

There is no such thing as being "too close" to the passage to qualify as a correct answer to an Inference question. An answer that directly paraphrases the passage may in fact be the credited response. On the other hand, the correct answer may seem debatable (that is, you could argue that it isn't literally deducible from the passage information), but it will still be better supported by the passage text than the other three choices.

To approach an Inference question, find the relevant section or sections of the passage. Check each answer choice against that information, choosing the one that has the most support. The credited response may seem like a stretch (for example, something that you think is not particularly "reasonable" to conclude), but it will be the best supported of the four. Be flexible; the correct answer may be something that you would never have come up with on your own, but there will be some solid evidence for it in the passage.

There are a variety of ways in which Inference questions can be phrased. Some of the most common phrasings are:

- "It can be inferred from the passage that..."
- "An assumption underlying the author's discussion of Brown's theory is that..."
- "The author implies that Brown's theory is most closely linked to..."
- "Implicit in the passage is the contention that Brown's theory is..."
- "By *only dimly perceived*, the author most likely means:"
- "The author suggests that..."
- "Based on information in the passage, it can be most reasonably concluded that..."
- "With which of the following statements would the author be most likely to agree?"
- "Which of the following statements is best supported by the passage?"
- "Which of the following would be an example of Surrealism, as it is described in the passage?"

Sample Question 2:

[handwritten: find how IS diff A.S.]

2. The passage suggests that the inquisitorial system differs from the adversarial system in that: *[handwritten: (specific inference)   3)]*

A) it provides the judge with information about the findings of the pretrial investigation.

B) it makes the defendant solely responsible for gathering evidence.

C) it guarantees that all defendants get a fair trial.

D) a defendant who is innocent would prefer to be tried under the inquisitorial system.

1) **·Read the question word for word and identify the question type.**
The words "The passage suggests that" identify this as an Inference question.

2) **Translate the question into your own words: identify what the question task is asking you to do with the information in the passage.**
This question is asking you how the author contrasts the inquisitorial with the adversarial system.

3) **Identify any key words that refer to specific parts of the passage. If key words are provided, *go back to the passage* to locate that information.**
This is where many students falter, thinking that they don't need to go back to the passage because the question is asking us to infer something (or, in this case, what is suggested). The correct answer still must be closely based on the passage text, not on your own ideas or deductions.

The words "inquisitorial" and "adversarial" appear in multiple places. However, the words "in contrast" at the beginning of paragraph 2 indicate that this is the beginning of the author's discussion of the differences between the two systems. Your annotation should alert you to the fact that there are a variety of differences listed in this paragraph. Don't reread the whole paragraph at this point, but you will need to check the answer choices against it.

4) **Answer in your own words: articulate what the correct answer will need to do, based on the question type and the information in the passage.**

The credited response will need to not only match the description of the two systems, but will also need to correctly describe a difference between them.

5) **Use Process of Elimination (POE) to choose the *least wrong* answer choice.**

A wide variety of Attractors appear in Inference answer choices. One of the most common is a statement that puts information from the passage into overly absolutist or extreme language. For example, the passage may say that something *often* occurs, while the trap answer will say that same thing *always* occurs.

Do not, however, eliminate a choice for an Inference question only because it is narrower or more moderate than the scope or wording of the passage.

Be careful to eliminate answer choices that are out of scope; that is, answer choices which refer to issues that could be tangentially related but that are never discussed in the passage.

Just like for Retrieval questions, look out for Attractors that take words out of context, or that are supported by the passage but not relevant to the question.

Let's take a look at each answer choice from our sample question.

A: **Yes. At the end of paragraph 2, the author states (in the context of differences between the two systems) that "the judge takes an active part in the conduct of the trial that is both directive and protective." Earlier in that same paragraph, the author also states that the inquisitorial system requires "full pretrial discovery." From this you can infer that in the inquisitorial system the judge would have access to information uncovered in the pretrial investigation or discovery.**

B: No. The passage suggests that this is true of the adversarial, not the inquisitorial system.

C: No. This choice is too extreme. The passage suggests that the inquisitorial system may lead to increased fairness, but not that fairness is guaranteed.

D: No. Although many of these words appear in the passage, there is nothing to suggest which system an innocent person would prefer. While this choice makes common sense, it is too much of a stretch, especially when compared with choice A, which is directly supported by the passage text.

Type 3: General—Main Idea/Primary Purpose Questions

These questions require you to summarize claims and implications made throughout the passage in order to formulate a general statement of the central point or primary activity of the passage. Think of the passage as an argument. The Main Idea is the overall claim, supported by specific evidence in the various paragraphs, which the author wants to convince you to accept as true. The Primary Purpose is then very closely related; it will express what the author *does* in order to convey the Main Idea.

Good active reading is the key to these questions; don't wait until you encounter a Main Idea question to think about the Main Point or Bottom Line of the passage. Synthesize the major themes as you read the passage. Distill these themes into a summary of the content and tone of the author's argument or

Type 3 → general: main idea & primary purpose

presentation. Don't ignore the author's attitude as expressed in the passage. An answer may have the correct content and scope, but if the tone or attitude doesn't match the passage, the choice is incorrect.

Main Idea questions are often phrased in the following ways:

- "The main idea of the passage is that…"
- "The central thesis of this passage is…"

Primary Purpose questions are often phrased as follows:

- "The author's primary purpose is to explain that…"

Sample Question 3:

3. The primary purpose of the passage is to: *(General – main idea)*

   A) explain why the inquisitorial system is the best system of criminal justice. *(too extreme)*
   B) explain how the adversarial and the inquisitorial systems of criminal justice both evolved from the system of private vengeance. *(too narrow)*
   C) show how the adversarial and inquisitorial systems of criminal justice can both complement and hinder each other's development.
   D) analyze two systems of criminal justice and deduce which one is more advanced.

1) **Read the question word for word and identify the question type.**
   General questions are generally very easy to identify. Here, the words "primary purpose" tip you off.

2) **Translate the question into your own words: identify what the question task is asking you to do with the information in the passage.**
   The question is asking you to summarize the author's overall goal in writing this passage. A good translation of this question would be: "Why did the author describe the two modern criminal procedure systems, as well as the pre-modern system of private vengeance?"

3) **Identify any key words that refer to specific parts of the passage. If key words are provided, *go back to the passage* to locate that information.**
   On Main Idea and Primary Purpose questions you will not usually need to go back to the passage before reading the choices. Use your original articulation of the Bottom Line to take a first pass or cut through the choices. You may, however, need to go back to the passage when you are down to two or three choices.

4) **Answer in your own words: articulate what the correct answer will need to do, based on the question type and the information in the passage.**
   For this type, the correct answer needs to include (explicitly or implicitly) all of the major themes of the passage, without going beyond the scope of the author's argument. Your own answer to this question would be something like: "The author describes the pre-modern system of private vengeance in order to set up contrast between the adversarial and inquisitorial systems; the adversarial system is closer to the system of private vengeance, and the inquisitorial system is more highly evolved."

4.4

5) **Use Process of Elimination (POE) to choose the *least wrong* answer choice.**
Common Attractors for Main Idea and Primary Purpose questions will understate or overstate the author's point. Choices that summarize the main idea of a paragraph or two but which leave out other major themes are too narrow. Vague or overly inclusive choices that go beyond the scope of the passage are too broad. Take the "Goldilocks approach": eliminate what is too big or too small, and find the one that is the best fit.

For Primary Purpose questions, focus in part on the verb in each answer choice, and eliminate the ones that are inappropriate; that is, too opinionated, too neutral, or that go in the opposite direction from the passage.

Eliminate choices that are too extreme. Is the author really *proving* or *disproving* a claim, or just *supporting* or *challenging* that claim? Eliminate any verb that expresses an opinion (*criticizing*, *propounding*, etc.) on a neutral passage (*explaining*, *describing*, etc.) and vice versa.

Be very careful to read and evaluate all parts of each answer choice. An answer choice may begin beautifully, but change halfway through to bring in something inconsistent with or irrelevant to the author's argument. If any part of the choice is wrong, the whole thing is wrong.

Let's take a look at the choices for this question.

A: No. This choice is too extreme ("the best") and too broad in scope. The passage only compares the inquisitorial system to the adversarial and private vengeance systems, not to all other systems of criminal justice.

B: No. This choice is too narrow in scope. The author not only explains this evolutionary connection, but explicitly contrasts the inquisitorial with the adversarial system in order to judge the former to be "historically superior."

C: No. This choice is out of scope. The passage never suggests that these two systems coexist, or that one would either contribute to, or get in the way of, the other.

D: **Yes. While this choice does not explicitly mention the system of private vengeance, it doesn't need to; the author discusses the pre-modern system of private vengeance in order to argue that the inquisitorial system is historically superior to the adversarial system (because the adversarial system is closer to the system of private vengeance).**

Type 4: General—Tone/Attitude Questions

Tone and Attitude questions ask you to evaluate whether or not the author expresses an opinion regarding the material in the passage, and if so, to judge how strongly positive or negative that opinion is. Or, the question may ask you who or what the author is most likely to be. Pure Tone or Attitude questions are fairly rare (however, Main Idea and Primary Purpose questions always involve assessing the tone of the passage).

Just as for Main Idea and Primary Purpose questions, you must identify the tone of the author through active reading before you begin any of the questions.

type 4: general - tone / attitue

When pure Tone/Attitude questions do appear, they are usually general questions, as in the following:

- "In this passage, the author's tone is one of…"
- "The author's attitude can best be described as…"   *general*
- "The passage makes it clear that the author is…"

However, Tone/Attitude questions may also appear in Specific form, asking about the author's attitude towards a particular part of the passage (in which case they are Specific Tone/Attitude question), as in:

- "The author's attitude toward Brown's claim can best be described as…"
- "What is the tone of the author's response to Brown's critics?"   *specific*
- "The author's attitude towards the controversy surrounding Brown's theory can best be char-acterized as exhibiting…"

Sample Question 4:

4. The author's attitude regarding the evolution of criminal *general tone - specific*
   procedure systems can best be characterized as:

   A) condemnatory. *(tov –)*
   B) instructive.
   C) admiring. *(tov +)*
   D) ambivalent. *(neutral*

1) **Read the question word for word and identify the question type.**
   The word "attitude" is a pretty clear indication of a tone question. Because the passage as a whole is about the evolution of criminal procedure systems, this is a General Attitude question.

2) **Translate the question into your own words: identify what the question task is asking you to do with the information in the passage.**
   This question is asking you what the author thinks about how criminal procedures have changed over time.

3) **Identify any key words that refer to specific parts of the passage. If key words are pro-vided, *go back to the passage* to locate that information.**
   As with most General questions, you already have an answer, based on the passage, in mind. Therefore you may not need to go back to the passage before you begin evaluating the answer choices. However, you may well need to refer back to the passage during POE.

4) **Answer in your own words: articulate what the correct answer will need to do, based on the question type and the information in the passage.**
   The correct answer must be fairly neutral in tone. The author is describing how criminal procedure has evolved, not condemning or advocating any particular system. The author does state that the inquisitorial system is superior, but in the context of being "historically supe-rior;" that is, more highly evolved.

5) **Use Process of Elimination (POE) to choose the *least wrong* answer choice.**

Common Attractors on Attitude and Tone questions are choices that take the author's opinion to extremes. If the passage expresses qualified or moderate admiration, for example, an Attractor may incorrectly describe the author as "enthusiastic." If the author expresses both positive and negative thoughts about a subject, incorrect answer choices may leave out the positive or ignore the negative. Also, positive and negative comments don't cancel each other out to create a neutral tone. If the passage is neutral, any choice that expresses an opinion one way or the other is incorrect.

Beware of choices that express strange attitudes rarely seen in MCAT passages. For example, if you see a choice like "obtuse ambiguity," you should be highly suspicious of it.

Let's apply POE to our sample question.

A: No. This choice is too strong—and too negative. The author does not condemn earlier criminal procedure systems; the passage only labels them as less highly evolved. The author definitely does not condemn "the evolution of criminal procedure systems" as a whole; the author says nothing negative about the inquisitorial system, which is the most highly evolved version.

B: **Yes. The author is describing this evolution in a fairly neutral tone. Thus you can say that the tone of the passage is instructive; its goal is to teach us about the evolution of criminal procedure.**

C: No. This choice is too strong and too positive. It is tempting, given that reference to "historically superior." However, the passage isn't praising the inquisitorial system, but just describing it as the most recent system. Even if you speculate that the author may have positive feelings about the inquisitorial system, this would be only speculation; "instructive," based only on passage information, is the least wrong choice.

D: No. "Ambivalent" means uncertain, or torn between multiple options. Nothing in the passage suggests that the author is torn between different opinions regarding the evolution of criminal procedure systems.

Type 5: Reasoning—Structure Questions

Structure questions ask you to describe how the author makes his or her argument. They differ from other questions in that they address the passage's construction or logical structure along with its content. This is what puts them into the category of Reasoning Questions, even though they almost always relate to one specific area of the passage. Structure questions may ask you for the purpose of a particular reference within the passage. That reference could be to an example, a conclusion, a contrasting point of view, etc. For example, the question stem may cite evidence from the passage and ask you to find the answer that describes the claim or larger point being supported by that evidence. This version of a Structure question often includes the wording "in order to," as in: "The author states X in order to...."

Alternatively, a Structure question might cite a claim from the passage and ask you how, or if, that claim is supported by the author. Similarly, the question may ask what kinds of support are not used in the passage, or what claims are not supported in a particular way; for example: "Which of the following statements is NOT supported by an example or explanation?"

To answer these questions, it is crucial to identify the Main Point of the paragraph or chunk of information in which a reference cited in the question appears, and to separate the claims made by the author

type 5- reasoning structure how the author makes his or her argument

from the evidence (if any is given) supporting those claims. Look for words—like *for example* or *for instance*—that indicate that what comes next is the support or evidence, and conclusion words—like *therefore, thus, so,* or *hence*—that indicate that what comes next is the claim being supported.

It is also possible for Structure questions to appear in General form, asking you to describe the organization of the passage as a whole. When answering a General Structure question, separate the choices into pieces and check for pieces that are out of order, that have an inappropriate tone, or that describe things that never happened in the passage.

Specific Structure questions may be worded as follows:

- "The author probably mentions the controversy surrounding Brown's ideas in order to…"
- "The three experiments carried out by Brown are cited in the passage as evidence that…"
- "The author describes Brown's unique methodology in order to make the point that…"

or

- "Which of the following items of information presented in the passage provides the most support for the author's claim that Brown's methodology is unique?"
- "The author's claim that Brown's methodology is unique is supported by…"
- "Which of the following claims made by the author regarding Brown's methodology is NOT supported by example or reference to authority?"

General structure questions can be phrased as:

- "Which of the following best describes the overall organization of the passage?"
- "Which of the following statements best describes the logical progression of the author's argument?"

Sample Question 5:

5. The author cites the slogan "an eye for an eye and a tooth for a tooth" (paragraph 1) in order to:

A) show how aspects of the private vengeance system persist in today's legal system.

B) criticize pre-modern systems of justice as overly violent.

C) characterize private vengeance as a system that required the victim himself to seek justice.

D) demonstrate how the legal rule rather than the facts of the case provided the foundation of the system of private vengeance.

1) **Read the question word for word and identify the question type.**
   The words "in order to" tell you that this is a Structure question.

2) **Translate the question into your own words: identify what the question task is asking you to do with the information in the passage.**
   The question is asking you to describe why the author used this phrase at this point in the passage.

4.4

3) **Identify any key words that refer to specific parts of the passage. If key words are pro-vided,** *go back to the passage* **to locate that information.**

The quote "An eye for an eye..." appears in paragraph 1. The author argues that it "captures the essence" of the private vengeance system, in which "the victim of a crime fashioned his own remedy and administered it privately...."

4) **Answer in your own words: articulate what the correct answer will need to do, based on the question type and the information in the passage.**

The correct answer must connect the quote to the system of private vengeance, and describe it as part of the author's explanation of how victims themselves had to administer punishments to those who had wronged them.

5) **Use Process of Elimination (POE) to choose the** *least wrong* **answer choice.**

For Structure questions, beware of Attractors that describe claims that are made in the passage but that are not relevant to or directly supported by the reference given in the question. Also beware of half right, half wrong choices. All parts of the correct answer choice must check out.

The correct choice must be consistent with the Main Point and tone of the relevant chunk of passage, as well as with the Bottom Line of the passage as a whole.

Let's evaluate the answer choices for our sample question.

A: No. The author argues that while the adversarial system does share some aspects with private vengeance, we have moved on to a system based on "fact-finding" where the judge directs the proceedings. Our modern inquisitorial system is "two historical steps removed from the system of private vengeance" (paragraph 2). Therefore, today's legal system is shown to be very different from the system of private vengeance.

B: No. The tone of this choice does not match the passage. While you might think of "an eye for an eye" as a violent way to mete out justice, the author does not describe it that way, or criticize it as such.

C: **Yes. The quote appears in a sentence describing private vengeance as "a system of self-help." The preceding sentence also discusses how "the victim had to fashion his own remedy and administer it privately...." This choice fits with both the content and tone of the passage and with the specific reference in the question.**

D: No. This choice takes words from the end of the passage out of context. There is no direct connection made by the author between basing a system on a legal rule, and the "eye for an eye" approach to justice.

Type 6: Reasoning—Evaluate Questions

Evaluate questions are similar to Structure questions in that you need to identify the logical structure of the author's argument. Evaluate questions, however, go a step further by asking either how well an author supports their claims *(Type 1: "Claims and Evidence")* or for a logical error or contradiction in the passage *(Type 2: "Flaw")*. That is, the question asks you to evaluate whether or not the author does a good job justifying his or her conclusions.

Type 1—"Claims and Evidence": The answers for these questions often come in two parts. One part will be some version of "strongly" or "weakly" supported. The other part will be the explanation or justification *reasoning evaluate*

for that evaluation (for example, that it is weakly supported *because* no examples are given, or, strongly supported *because* relevant examples are provided). When choosing an answer, make sure to check that both parts of the choice are supported by the text; that is, both the judgment itself (strongly or weakly) and the justification for that judgment.

These questions may be phrased as follows:

- "The author asserts that Brown's theoretical model is 'dangerously incomplete.' The support offered for this conclusion is…"
- "Is Brown's analysis of the implications of Herrera's theoretical model well supported?"
- "The author's assertion that Brown's model is incomplete is…"

Type 2—"Flaw": This version of an Evaluate question asks you for an error or self-contradiction in the passage. Unless the question stem references a particular part of the passage, go straight into POE rather than trying to answer in your own words first. That is, use the answer choices to go back and locate the relevant parts of the passage, and then decide if that part of the author's argument is logically flawed.

These questions may be phrased as follows:

- "Which of the following represents a logical error in the passage?"
- "The author's claim regarding Brown's model is flawed in which of the following ways?"
- "Which of the following pairs of statements from the passage represent a logical contradiction?"

Sample Question 6:

reasoning- evaluate

6. How well supported is the author's claim that the adversarial system still retains some features of private vengeance?

    A) Strongly, because the claim is inherent in the meaning of the word "adversarial"
    B) Strongly, because examples of similarities between the two are provided by the author
    C) Weakly, because the claim is logically inconsistent with the author's description of the inquisitorial system
    D) Weakly, because no evidence is cited to bolster the claim

1) **Read the question word for word and identify the question type.**
    The question asks *how well* supported the author's claim is, which makes it an Evaluate question. Notice that it doesn't just ask *what* the author's claim is (this would be a Retrieval or Inference question).
2) **Translate the question into your own words: identify what the question task is asking you to do with the information in the passage.**
    The question is asking if there are any significant flaws or weaknesses in the author's argument about the relationship between private vengeance and the adversarial system. If so, what are those flaws? If not, why is it a strong argument?

4.4

3) **Identify any key words that refer to specific parts of the passage. If key words are provided, *go back to the passage* to locate that information.**

This question sends you back to paragraph 1. The claim cited in the question comes in the middle of the paragraph. Immediately after the claim, the author discusses particular similarities (as well as some differences) between private vengeance and the adversarial system.

4) **Answer in your own words: articulate what the correct answer will need to do, based on the question type and the information in the passage.**

Read through the examples supporting the claim: the defendant must conduct "his own pretrial investigation," and "the trial is still viewed as a duel between two adversaries." This leads the author to the conclusion that the adversarial system "symbolizes and regularizes punitive combat;" punitive combat characterizes private vengeance. Because the author gives relevant examples, and draws reasonably well-supported conclusions based on those examples, you can say that the claim is strongly supported.

5) **Use Process of Elimination (POE) to choose the *least wrong* answer choice.**

Answer choices that mischaracterize the strength of the argument are incorrect.

Once you have narrowed it down to the choices that fall on the correct side (in this case, "strongly" or "weakly") narrow it down further by analyzing precisely what is either good or bad about the author's logic.

Let's go through the answer choices for our sample question.

A: No. While the claim is in fact supported strongly, it is not because of the definition of "adversarial." Instead, it is because the author provides relevant examples.

B: **Yes. The fact that the defendant must carry out his own pretrial investigation; and that the trial is still seen as a duel, show that the adversarial system retains aspects of private vengeance, even if they are in a somewhat more symbolic or institutionalized form.**

C: No. There is no inconsistency in the logic of the author's argument (which claims that the adversarial and inquisitorial systems are in fact quite different).

D: No. Direct, relevant evidence is in fact given (note the phrase "for example" in the passage, directly following the claim cited in the question).

Type 7: Application—Strengthen Questions

A Strengthen question asks you to find the answer that most supports the passage (as opposed to Structure and Evaluate questions, which ask how, if, or how well the author has supported his or her own argument). That is, the correct answer will make the author's argument more convincing than it already was.

Notice that Strengthen questions often use the phrase, "which of the following, if true…." Take those words *if true*—whether implied or explicitly stated—seriously. Do not try to find the answer choices *in* the passage. Take each statement as if it were true and find the one that does what it needs to do *to* the relevant part of the passage. These questions are quite different from Specific, General, and Reasoning questions in that they give you new information in the answer choices; the correct answer will change (for the better), not just describe or reflect, the passage. These questions are also distinct from other question types (except for Weaken questions) in that it is impossible for an answer to be "too extreme" to be correct. You want the answer that goes the farthest in the correct direction.

Strengthen questions may be phrased as follows:

- "Which of the following, if valid, would provide the best support for the author's conclusion in the last paragraph?"
- "Which of the following, if true, would most strengthen the author's claims?"

Strengthen EXCEPT/LEAST/NOT

Strengthen questions sometimes appear in the EXCEPT/LEAST/NOT format. EXCEPT/LEAST/NOT Strengthen questions have a bit of a twist, compared to most other questions in this format; the correct answer may do the opposite (in this case, Weaken), but they may also just do nothing (have no effect or be irrelevant), or not go as far in the strengthening direction as the three wrong answers (that is, barely strengthen the passage, but less so than the other choices). It is especially crucial to compare choices to each other and pick the one that is the farthest away from strengthening as possible.

The correct answer is the one that goes the farthest to the left along this spectrum.

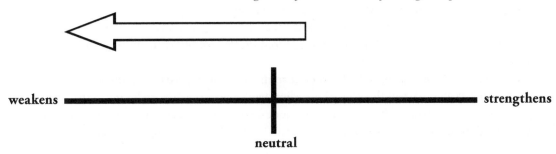

Sample Question 7:

7. Which of the following, if true, would most strengthen the author's claim that the inquisitorial system is historically superior to the adversarial system of justice?

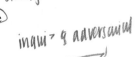

app- strengthen

inqui > g adversarial

A) Judges within the inquisitorial system are expected to be familiar with the facts of the case before a trial begins.

B) The justice systems currently used in some countries still treat a trial as a duel between two adversaries.

C) While the inquisitorial system in theory is based on fact-finding, in practice it often takes on the form of a private contest between victim and defendant.

D) In some cases tried under the adversarial system, the judge is biased towards either the defendant or the victim.

4.4

1) **Read the question word for word and identify the question type.**

   The words "most strengthen" tell you that this is a Strengthen question.

2) **Translate the question into your own words: identify what the question task is asking you to do with the information in the passage.**

   You will need to take each choice as true, rather than looking for support for the right answer in the passage. You will still need to go back to the passage, however, to pin down what is being strengthened. The question is asking you to find new evidence in the passage that makes the author's claim that the inquisitorial system is more historically developed than the adversarial system (that is, that it is even further away from the system of private vengeance) even more compelling.

3) **Identify any key words that refer to specific parts of the passage. If key words are provided, *go back to the passage* to locate that information.**

   The passage as a whole is making the argument that the inquisitorial system is more historically developed. Therefore, you can take the Bottom Line into the answer choices and look for the one that most supports this overall claim. You may, however, need to go back to the passage as you go through POE to pin down the relevance of details included in the answer choices.

4) **Answer in your own words: articulate what the correct answer will need to do, based on the question type and the information in the passage.**

   The correct answer will provide new evidence that the inquisitorial system is in fact different, along the lines discussed in the passage, from the system of private vengeance, from the adversarial system, or from both.

5) **Use Process of Elimination (POE) to choose the *least wrong* answer choice.**

   When using POE on Strengthen questions, eliminate choices that are irrelevant to the cited part or issue in the passage (that is, that are out of scope). Remember, however, that the correct answer will bring in new information: "irrelevant" is not the same thing as "never mentioned."

Do *not* eliminate choices on the basis of absolute or extreme wording. It is impossible on these questions (in contrast to Specific, General, and Reasoning questions) for an answer to be wrong solely on the basis of being too strong. The more it strengthens the passage, the better. In fact, choices on this question type may be wrong because they don't go far enough to have a significant impact on the author's argument. Also, make sure to look out for wrong answers that weaken instead of strengthen by suggesting that the inquisitorial system is less historically superior than the author claims.

Let's use POE on our sample question.

A: Yes. The author states in the first paragraph that one reason that the adversarial system is "only one historical step removed from the private vengeance system" is that the judge has no knowledge of the background of the case as the trial begins. While the author does state in the second paragraph that "the inquisitorial system mandates that the judge take an active part in the conduct of the trial, with a role that is both directive and protective," the passage never indicates that this also means that the judge is familiar before the trial with the facts of the case. Therefore, this answer choice strengthens the author's claim by providing one more relevant way in which the inquisitorial system has evolved even further from private vengeance than the adversarial system.

B: No. This choice has no impact on the author's argument. While the author does suggest that the adversarial system still exists in the world, this isn't relevant to his or her claim that the *qualities* of the inquisitorial system make it historically superior.

C: No. This choice does the opposite of what the question requires. It weakens, not strengthens, the author's claim by suggesting that the inquisitorial system is not as different from the adversarial system (or from the system of private vengeance) as the author claims.

D: No. While this choice is consistent with the author's argument, it doesn't go far enough to actually strengthen it, especially when compared to choice A. The author does imply that the judge plays a neutral role in the inquisitorial system. However, the fact in *some* (which could be one or two) adversarial justice systems the judge plays a biased role doesn't strongly support the author's claim that *in general* the inquisitorial system is more distinct than the adversarial system from private vengeance.

4.4

Type 8: Application—Weaken Questions

A Weaken question requires you to find the answer choice that most undermines or calls into question the claim or claims made by the author.

Notice that just like Strengthen questions, Weaken questions often use the phrase, "which of the following, if true…." Take those words *if true*—whether implied or explicitly stated—seriously. Do not try to find the answer choices *in* the passage. Take each statement as if it were true and find the one that is most *inconsistent* with the relevant part of the passage. These questions are quite different from Specific, General, and Reasoning questions in that they give you new information in the answer choices; the correct answer will change the passage by making the author's argument less convincing than it originally was. These questions are also distinct from other question types (except for Strengthen questions) in that it is impossible for an answer to be "too extreme" to be correct. You want the answer that goes the farthest in the correct direction.

Weaken questions are often phrased as follows:

* "Which of the following, if valid, would most *weaken* the author's point?"
* "Which of the following, if true, would most *undermine* the author's claims?"
* "Which of the following results, if proven to be valid, would most call into question the author's conclusion regarding Brown's methodology?"

You might also see a variation on Weaken questions that cites a statement from the passage, and asks you to decide which *answer choice* would be most weakened by that statement. For example:

* "The claims made by Brown, if true, would cast the most *doubt* on which of the following statements?"

Regardless of the wording, you are doing the same thing in answering any Weaken question in the Standard format: finding the answer choice that is *most inconsistent* with the cited part of the passage.

4.4

Weaken EXCEPT/LEAST/NOT

As with Strengthen questions, Weaken questions sometimes appear in the EXCEPT/LEAST/NOT format, as in, "Which of the following would LEAST weaken the claims made by the author?" EXCEPT/LEAST/NOT Weaken questions have the same twist as Strengthen questions in this format; the correct answer may do the opposite (Strengthen), but they may also just do nothing (have no effect or be irrelevant), or not go as far in weakening as the three wrong answers (i.e., weaken a little bit but less than the other choices). It is especially crucial to compare choices to each other and pick the one furthest along the spectrum we discussed for Strengthen EXCEPT/LEAST/NOT questions, but in this case in the opposite direction.

The correct answer is the one that goes the farthest to the right along this spectrum.

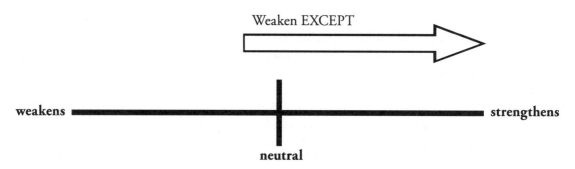

Sample Question 8:

inqui > adversar

8. Which of the following, if true, would most *undermine* the author's *main argument* in the passage?

A) The vengeance system did not precede all systems of criminal procedure in the world. *RAWD*

B) The inquisitorial and adversarial systems have many things in common.

C) The adversarial system is a system of self-help. *(RAWD)*

D) Personal vengeance is at the heart of the inquisitorial system. ✓

1) **Read the question word for word and identify the question type.**
   The words "most undermine" identify this as a Weaken question. The question is asking you to undermine the author's central argument.

2) **Translate the question into your own words: identify what the question task is asking you to do with the information in the passage.**
   You will need to take each choice as true, rather than looking for support for the right answer in the passage. You will still need to go back to the passage, however, to pin down the credited response. You need the response that most undermines the author's argument as a whole.

3) **Identify any key words that refer to specific parts of the passage. If key words are provided, *go back to the passage* to locate that information.**
   Because the question asks you to weaken the author's main argument, you can use your own articulation of the Bottom Line of the passage. With that already clearly defined, you don't need to go back to the passage before you start evaluating the choices. If the question stem had asked you to weaken a particular claim within the passage, you would need to first go back and find and paraphrase that part of the author's argument.

4.4

4) **Answer in your own words: articulate what the correct answer will need to do, based on the question type and the information in the passage.**

The correct answer will suggest that the adversarial and inquisitorial systems are more similar than the author claims, and/or that the inquisitorial system is not in fact historically superior.

5) **Use Process of Elimination (POE) to choose the *least wrong* answer choice.**

For a Weaken question, the best answer will go the furthest toward making it impossible for the claim made in the passage to be true. Look for the answer choice that is most inconsistent with the relevant part of the passage.

When using POE on Weaken questions, eliminate choices that are irrelevant to the cited part or issue in the passage (that is, that are out of scope). Remember, however, that the correct answer will bring in new information: "irrelevant" is not the same thing as "never mentioned."

Do *not* eliminate choices on the basis of absolute or extreme wording. It is impossible on these questions (in contrast to all other question types except for Strengthen questions) for an answer to be wrong solely on the basis of being too strong. The more it weakens the passage, the better.

In fact, choices on this question type may be wrong because they don't go far enough to have a significant impact on the author's argument.

Finally, look out for Attractors that strengthen instead of weaken.

Let's use POE on our sample question.

A: No. The author does not claim that private vengeance was the very first system used to punish criminals. For all you know, there could have been other pre-modern systems that preceded private vengeance. This choice attacks a claim that is never made by the author; it is therefore out of scope.

B: No. The passage itself suggests some similarities: e.g., there is a judge, and there is a private investigator searching for evidence to support the prosecution (the inquisitorial system just broadens those duties to include finding evidence for the defense as well). Because the author's main argument is not founded on the assumption that there are few or no similarities between the two, this choice does not go far enough to weaken the passage.

C: No. This choice is entirely consistent with the author's depiction of the adversarial system in paragraph 1. This choice strengthens, not weakens, the author's contrast between the adversarial and inquisitorial systems.

D: **Yes. The author argues that the inquisitorial system is historically superior because it is "two historical steps removed from the system of private vengeance" (paragraph 2) and because it is based on "the facts of the case" (paragraph 3). The adversarial system, in contrast, "is only one historical step removed from the private vengeance system and still retains some of its characteristic features" (paragraph 1). If private vengeance was in fact at the heart of the inquisitorial system, this would undermine the author's argument about the historical character and evolutionary place of the inquisitorial system. Thus, choice D is the best answer.**

Type 9: Application—New Information Questions

All New Information questions have one thing in common: they provide new facts or scenarios in the question stem that are never mentioned in the passage. That said, the question may require you to do a variety of things with that new information. New Information questions break down into two general types.

4.4

Type 1: New Information/Inference questions

These questions give you new facts that are in the same general issue area of the passage and then ask what, according to the passage, is likely to be true. In essence, you're inserting the new facts into the existing passage, and then drawing an inference from both the new and the old information. Before you read the answer choices, answer the question in your own words, based on the information already in the passage and on the new facts in the question stem.

For example, the question might ask the following:

- "If China experienced an unusually rainy winter, what would also be true, based on the passage?"
- "According to the passage, what would likely happen if China experienced an unusually rainy winter?"
- "What would the author recommend as the best way to predict whether China is likely to experience an unusually rainy winter next year?"
- "If a meteorologist were to claim that China's climate can be studied in isolation, how would the author respond?"

Type 2: New Information/Strengthen/Weaken questions

These questions provide you with new facts in the question stem (as opposed to pure Strengthen or Weaken questions that give the new information only in the answer choices). They then ask you to evaluate what effect those new facts would have on the author's argument as a whole, or on one specific claim made or described in the passage.

Use the passage much like you do Strengthen, Weaken, and Structure questions. Identify the issue of the question, and go back to the passage to find the relevant sections. Pay close attention to the logical structure of the author's argument. Define what the correct answer needs to do based on the passage, the information in the question stem, and the direction (strengthen or weaken) the correct choice must take.

This type of New Information question may be phrased as follows:

- "Suppose it was shown to be true that when winters in China are unusually rainy, summers in Latin America are unusually dry. What effect would this have on the author's argument as it is described in the passage?"
- "Which of the following claims made in the passage would be most strengthened by data showing that industrialization has affected global weather patterns?"
- "Recent studies have shown that the jet stream has shifted 10 degrees in latitude over the past five years. This fact tends to *undermine* the author's claim that…"
- "El Niño has been proven to be a recurring and invariant pattern. This fact tends to support the author's claims in paragraph 2 because…"

type 9 - application - new information question

The following sample question falls into the *Type 1* category.

Sample Question 9:

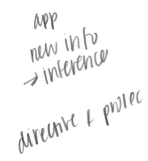

*app
new info
→ inference*

directive + protec

4.4

9. Suppose that in an inquisitorial system of justice a judge perceives that the prosecution is misdirecting the trial by introducing irrelevant evidence. The author would most likely advise the judge to:

   A) protect the prosecution by turning a blind eye to the proceedings.
   B) admonish the prosecution and get the trial back to the issues at hand.
   C) call a mistrial and free the defendant.
   D) refuse to participate in the trial.

1) **Read the question word for word and identify the question type.**

   The word "suppose" is our first indication that this is a New Information question. What follows is a scenario that does not already appear in the passage. The question asks you what the author of the passage would advise, making this a *Type 1* question.

2) **Translate the question into your own words: identify what the question task is asking you to do with the information in the passage.**

   The question is asking you to find an answer choice that is consistent both with the passage and with the new situation in the question stem; in this new scenario, the judge discovers that the prosecution is breaking the rules.

3) **Identify any key words that refer to specific parts of the passage. If key words are provided, *go back to the passage* to locate that information.**

   The role of the judge in the inquisitorial system is described at the end of paragraph 2. The judge must "take an active part in the conduct of the trial, with a role that is both directive and protective."

4) **Answer in your own words: articulate what the correct answer will need to do, based on the question type and the information in the passage.**

   Based on the passage, the judge in this situation must take action to protect the defense from the unfair tactics used by the prosecution, and must direct the trial in a way consistent with the system's rules.

5) **Use Process of Elimination (POE) to choose the *least wrong* answer choice.**

   A common Attractor for any New Information question is an answer choice that focuses on the wrong part of the passage. Also beware of answer choices that are inconsistent with the passage (for all but the Weaken version of this question type), or that deal with irrelevant issues. This means choices that do not connect to the passage, or that are not relevant to the theme of the new information in the question.

   For *Type 1* questions, beware of extreme language. The correct answer can't go too far beyond the scope and tone of the passage.

   For *Type 2* questions, beware of choices that go in the opposite direction (e.g., that strengthen instead of weaken or vice versa).

4.4

Let's go through POE on our sample question.

A: No. This is inconsistent with the author's claim that in the inquisitorial system, the interests of the defense as well as of the prosecution should be protected. This is also inconsistent with the author's claim that the judge must take an active role to direct the proceedings.

B: Yes. This is consistent with the author's claim that the judge has a protective role (protecting the rights of the defense by admonishing the prosecution) and a directive role (getting the trial back on track). This choice is relevant to the theme of the new information and is consistent with the passage (as required by the question task). Thus, it is the "least wrong" of the four choices.

C: No. This choice is too extreme; the passage does not indicate that prosecutorial misbehavior would invalidate the trial as a whole. This choice is also out of scope; the issue of calling a mistrial arises in neither the passage nor the question stem.

D: No. As in choice A, this is inconsistent with the author's claim that judges in the inquisitorial system must play an active role.

Type 10: Application—Analogy Questions

These questions ask you to take something described in the passage, abstract or generalize it, and then apply it to an entirely new situation. They differ from New Information questions in that the new information is in the answer choices, not in the question stem. They differ from Strengthen questions in that the new information in the correct choice will not make the original argument stronger than it already was. It will be similar to it in logic, but is likely to be on a different issue or subject matter.

These questions can be tricky, as all the answers at first glance may seem to have nothing to do with the passage. However, you are matching the logic or purpose of the author's argument, not the informational content of the passage. Therefore, the correct answer can match the logic of the passage (or relevant part of the passage) while still bringing in entirely new content.

Take, for example, a passage in which the author argues the following: "Weather is the result of a global interactive system. Therefore, to understand and predict the weather in a particular region, you must analyze how the climates of all regions interact with each other, and not limit your focus to the weather patterns in that region alone."

The question might ask:

- "Which of the following approaches to educational reform would most likely be advocated by a school board member following the same logic as the author of the passage?"

To answer this question, you must *first* generalize the author's own claims to create an abstracted model that could be applied to other situations. For example, you might say, "Large interactive systems cannot be understood by looking at the parts in isolation from the whole; you must understand how those parts relate to and affect each other," or, more simply, "the whole is more than the sum of its parts."

Now, take this generalized version into the answer choices, and look for a choice that has the same theme. The school board member might place the school system within the context of larger socioeconomic forces that also affect educational performance. Or, she might argue that the school itself is a large interactive system, and that you can't improve education by addressing only one piece of the puzzle (standardized testing, for example). As you can see, a wide variety of answer choices are possible. Don't waste time coming up with specific scenarios; generalize the passage's argument as much as possible, and then match each answer choice against that abstracted model.

Remember that the correct answer must depend solely on the content of the passage, not on outside information or your own opinion!

Sample Question 10:

application – analogy

10. The author's discussion of the history of systems of criminal procedure is most similar to which of the following?

(neg tone)

A) A study of the transmission of infectious diseases
B) A proposal for civil rights reforms
C) An evolutionary biologist's study of plant species
D) An architect's blueprint

*primitive
↓
secondary
↓
tertiary
} change over time*

*difference &
contrast*

1) **Read the question word for word and identify the question type.**
   The phrase "most similar to" tells you that this is an Analogy question.
2) **Translate the question into your own words: identify what the question task is asking you to do with the information in the passage.**
   The question is asking you to describe the overall logic and purpose of the passage in order to match it to a similar logic and purpose (but, in a different subject area) in the correct answer.
3) **Identify any key words that refer to specific parts of the passage. If key words are provided, *go back to the passage* to locate that information.**
   Because this question asks you to make an analogy to the author's overall logic and purpose in the passage as a whole, you don't necessarily need to go back the passage at this point; use your own articulation of the Bottom Line and your understanding of the logical structure of the passage as a guide.
4) **Answer in your own words: articulate what the correct answer will need to do, based on the question type and the information in the passage.**
   The passage describes the historical evolution of criminal procedure: how private vengeance evolved into the adversarial system, which then evolved into the inquisitorial system. Therefore, you need an answer that has this theme of evolution or change over time.
5) **Use Process of Elimination (POE) to choose the *least wrong* answer choice.**
   Keep in mind that all of the answer choices may be on different topics (i.e., not on criminal procedure). The correct choice will be the one that is most similar in logic to the author's overall argument in the passage. Be careful to eliminate choices that have the wrong tone (compared to the passage).

   When you are down to two, pick the choice that has the most similarities to the passage. If one of the two remaining choices has one similarity, but the other remaining choice is similar in two ways, the latter choice will be the credited response.

4.4

Let's use POE on our sample answer choices.

A: No. First of all, this choice has a negative tone that does not match the passage. While the passage does describe how the adversarial system maintained some of the characteristics of private vengeance, the author doesn't use language suggesting it was "infected" (which has an overly negative tone) by the earlier system. Furthermore, this theme of transmission of a disease from one thing to another doesn't fit with the passage's theme of difference and contrast (between the adversarial and inquisitorial systems).

B: No. The tone of this choice does not match the tone and purpose of the passage. The author describes change over time, but does not recommend further change.

C: Yes. An evolutionary biologist studying plant species would look at change over time through the succession of species. This choice is most similar to the logic and purpose of the passage, and matches the tone reasonably well.

D: No. Compare this choice to choice C. While there are some aspects of a blueprint (describing the structure a system), there is no theme in this choice of change over time. Also, the author of the passage is describing structures themselves (that already exist) not plans for structures.

Now that we have looked at the ten question types in the Standard format, let's look at examples of the other two formats: EXCEPT/LEAST/NOT and Roman numeral questions.

EXCEPT/LEAST/NOT Questions

This question type can appear in combination with most of the question tasks described above. Because of its potentially confusing structure (looking for the worst instead of the best), students often misread or misapply the question. In fact, the correct answer to this question type can be the wacky or totally irrelevant answer choice that you are used to eliminating first.

To avoid making a mistake, use your noteboard. Write down the passage number (if you haven't already) and the number of the question. Next to the question number jot down a translation of the question, including what kind of choices you will be eliminating. Do this before looking at the answer choices. For example, in a Weaken EXCEPT question, write down

eliminate what weakens, pick what strengthens or does nothing.

Also jot down the four letters. As you assess each answer choice write "W" (for "yes this weakens") next to each choice that definitely weakens, cross it off on your noteboard, and then strike it out on the screen. If an answer does not appear to weaken, either leave it as is, or give it an "N" for "No, it does not weaken." At the end, you should have three "W"s and one "N" (or one with nothing written next to it). That is, it should look something like this:

1 A̶ W
   Ⓑ N
   C̶ W
   D̶ W

Use notation for the wrong answers that is specific to the question type; for example "S" for "Strengthen" or "T" (for true) or "I" (for inference) for Inference questions.

Sample Question 11:

4.4

11. The author would be most likely to agree with all of the following statements EXCEPT

A) the judge actively participates in the inquisitorial system. T
B) the prosecutor in the adversarial system need not disclose evidence to the defense.
C) the inquisitorial system regularizes punitive combat. F
D) the vengeance system was a system of self-help. T

1) **Read the question word for word and identify the question type.**
EXCEPT/LEAST/NOT questions are quite easy to recognize. Here, the key word is "EXCEPT." This is an Inference question ("The author would be most likely to agree") in EXCEPT/LEAST/ NOT format.

2) **Translate the question into your own words: identify what the question task is asking you to do with the information in the passage.**
This question is asking you to eliminate the choices that are supported by the passage (that is, statements that the author of the passage would accept as true), and to pick the one that is most inconsistent with the author's argument.

3) **Identify any key words that refer to specific parts of the passage. If key words are provided, *go back to the passage* to locate that information.**
In this question, there is no specific reference to the passage. You will need, however, to go back to the passage as you work through the answer choices. If the question had given you a specific reference (e.g., to "the police department"), you would go back to the passage and read above and below that reference before moving on to the next step.

4) **Answer in your own words: articulate what the correct answer will need to do, based on the question type and the information in the passage.**
The correct choice will contradict the passage in some way. The incorrect answers will be consistent with the passage information as well as consistent with the author's tone and purpose.

5) **Use Process of Elimination (POE) to choose the *least wrong* answer choice.**
As you might predict, the most common Attractor is the opposite: a choice that would be the correct answer to a Standard Format question. Approach EXCEPT/LEAST/NOT questions carefully and methodically to avoid falling into this (very annoying) trap. Keep in mind that your reasons for eliminating choices on a Standard question (e.g., language that is too extreme, or a statement that mixes up two different things in the passage) now become your reasons for keeping, and perhaps selecting, an answer.

4.4

Let's take a look at our answer choices.

A: No. This choice is directly supported by the end of paragraph 1.

B: No. This choice is supported by the discussion of pretrial discovery in paragraph 2. If the inquisitorial system is different in that it does require the prosecutor to disclose its evidence to the court (and so to the defense), the author would agree that the prosecutor need not disclose it under the adversarial system.

C: **Yes. This is true of the adversarial, not the inquisitorial system (see the end of paragraph 1). This choice contradicts the passage; therefore, it is the credited response.**

D: No. This choice is supported by the middle of paragraph 1.

Roman Numeral Questions

Like EXCEPT/LEAST/NOT questions, Roman numeral questions can appear in combination with a variety of question tasks.

To approach these questions, evaluate numeral I (unless it appears in all four choices, in which case it must be true). If it is not an appropriate answer to the question, strike out all of the choices that include it. If it *is* appropriate, eliminate the choices that do *not* include it. (If you are not sure about a numeral, leave it and look at the next numeral before eliminating any more answer choices.) Compare the choices you have left to each other. If numeral II or III appears in all of them, read it but don't overthink it. Unless there is something terribly wrong with it, it must also be true based on the combinations you have.

Sample Question 12:

12. According to the passage, which of the following is a duty of the prosecutor in the inquisitorial system?

   I. To present evidence that may lead to the defendant's exoneration ✓
   II. To disclose all evidence in his/her possession ✓
   III. To assume a role that is both protective and directive

   evidence for depth

   A) II only
   B) III only
   C) I and II only
   D) I and III only

1) **Read the question word for word and identify the question type.**
   This is a Retrieval question ("According to the passage") in Roman numeral format.

2) **Translate the question into your own words: identify what the question task is asking you to do with the information in the passage.**
   The question is asking which of the three statements accurately represent things that are required of a prosecutor within the inquisitorial system.

3) **Identify any key words that refer to specific parts of the passage. If key words are provided,** *go back to the passage* **to locate that information.**

The inquisitorial system is described in paragraphs 2 and 3. Prosecutor's duties are specifically mentioned in the context of pretrial discovery, in the second half of paragraph 2 (after the word "additionally," and before the word "finally").

4) **Answer in your own words: articulate what the correct answer will need to do, based on the question type and the information in the passage.**

Prosecutors in the inquisitorial system must permit full disclosure of all evidence they have uncovered, even if that evidence would help the defense. They must also comply with all of the other rules of the inquisitorial system.

5) **Use Process of Elimination (POE) to choose the** *least wrong* **answer choice.**

In some ways, you are approaching the choices just as you would for a Standard question (in our Sample, a Retrieval task). For each numeral, ask yourself if this statement accomplishes the question task (here, if it describes a prosecutor's duty in the inquisitorial system).

However, you can also often use the combinations in the answer choices to your advantage. If, for example, you are sure that numeral I is supported, and unsure about numeral III, but no choice includes both I and III, you know that numeral III is in fact not supported (as it doesn't appear in any of the possible correct answer choices).

If you tend to miss Roman numeral questions, diagnose the most common reasons for your mistakes. If you tend to pick incomplete answers that are missing one or two numerals, you may be reading the numerals too quickly, picking only the ones that are the most obvious, and missing the more subtly supported statements. If you tend to pick choices that include too many, you may not be going back to the passage enough to check your answers carefully against the text.

Let's go through POE on our sample question item by item.

I: **True. This statement is supported by the author's discussion of pretrial discovery in paragraph 2. Therefore, you can eliminate choices A and B, because neither includes Roman numeral I. You are now down to choices C and D. The difference between them is that choice C includes II but not III, and choice D includes III but not II. It is now a battle between choices II and III—only one of them can be correct!**

II: **True. This is also supported by the author's description of pretrial discovery. Note that you essentially have the correct answer at this stage, as there is no answer that includes all three numerals.**

III: False. This is the role of the judge, not of the prosecutor (see the end of paragraph 2, after the word "finally").

So, your credited response is **choice C: I and II only**.

4.4

MCAT CRITICAL ANALYSIS AND REASONING SKILLS: QUESTION TYPES			
QUESTION TYPES AND STRATEGIES			
Question	Sample Wording	Strategy Tips	Common Types of Wrong Answers
1. Specific: Retrieval	"According to the passage, what is true of 'X'?" "The author states that 'X' is:"	• Go back to the passage before POE: find and paraphrase the relevant information. • Answer in your own words.	• uses similar language as passage but changes meaning • good answer to a question on a different passage topic or to a different question type • too strong to be supported by passage • relies too much on speculation or outside knowledge
2. Specific: Inference	"The passage implies/ suggests/assumes that…" "Based on the passage, it is reasonable to conclude/infer which of the following regarding 'X'?" "With which of the following statements would the author be most likely to agree?"	• Go back to passage as soon as possible to find and paraphrase relevant information. • Answer in your own words.	
3. General: Main Point/ Primary Purpose	"Which of the following best expresses the main point of the passage?" "The author's primary purpose in the passage is to:"	• Use your Bottom Line, including author's tone.	• too narrow to represent the passage as a whole • too broad/goes beyond scope of the passage • too extreme • wrong tone • part right, part wrong
4. General: Overall Tone/ Attitude	"The author's apparent attitude toward 'X' can best be described as…"	• Use your Bottom Line. • Look for tone indicators you have highlighted in passage.	• positive or negative tone for a neutral passage • opposite tone (e.g., negative instead of positive) • too strong/extreme
5. Reasoning: Structure	"The author of the passage states 'X' in order to…" "The author's claim 'X' is based on evidence that:"	• Go back to the passage before POE. • Determine if the statement is a conclusion or evidence for a conclusion. • Pay attention to context of the cited statement.	• references wrong part of the author's argument • can be inferred from the passage, but doesn't describe logical structure

MCAT CRITICAL ANALYSIS AND REASONING SKILLS: QUESTION TYPES			
QUESTION TYPES AND STRATEGIES			
Question	Sample Wording	Strategy Tips	Common Types of Wrong Answers
6. Reasoning: Evaluate	"How well supported is the author's claim that 'X'?" "Which of the following represents a logical error in the passage?"	• Go back to the passage and find the cited claim. • Use your highlighting to help locate the support, if any, given for claim. • If question asks for an error or contradiction, go straight to POE and then back to the passage as needed.	• incorrectly describes logical structure of argument • opposite evaluation (e.g., strongly rather than weakly supported) • Part of the passage that is NOT flawed or self-contradictory (for question asking for a flaw)
7. Application: Strengthen	"Which of the following, if true, most strengthens/supports the passage author's argument?"	• Go back to the passage; find and paraphrase the relevant claim. • Define the necessary issue and direction (consistent or inconsistent with passage) of the correct choice.	• opposite • not relevant to cited claim • not strong enough to have a significant impact
8. Application: Weaken	"Which of the following statements, if true, most *weakens/ undermines/calls into question* the author's argument in the passage?"		
9. Application: New Information	"Elsewhere, the author of the passage states 'X.' Given the information in the passage, this is most likely due to:"	• Summarize theme of new info. • Define the relationship of new info to relevant parts of the passage/Bottom Line.	• not relevant to new info and/or the passage • relevant only to wrong part of passage • incorrectly describes the new information's impact on or relevance to the passage.
10. Application: Analogy	"Which of the following relationships is most similar to 'X' as it is described in the passage?"	• Go back to passage; define the theme or logic of the relevant part of the passage.	• similar content but different logic • incomplete match compared to other choices • reversal or opposite of passage logic

4.4

4.5 EXERCISE 1: IDENTIFYING QUESTION TYPES

Here are 10 sample questions. Read each question carefully, and identify the question type and format. Also think about what this question type is asking you to do.

1. The author lists the duties of City Council representatives in order to:

   reasoning: structure

2. If it is shown to be true that only two species of egg-laying mammals exist, the author would most likely conclude that the platypus:

   new info: inference

3. The passage suggests which of the following to be true of the Treaty of Versailles?

   reasoning: specific

4. According to passage information, the Sahara Desert:

   specific retrieval

5. Which of the following claims, if true, would most *undermine* the author's contention that most environmental regulation is counterproductive?

   app: weaken

6. Which of the following is most similar to Professor Bybee's experimental methodology?

   app: analogy

7. By "quarantine" the author most likely means:

   a retrieval inference

8. All of the following strengthen the author's claim that caps on jury awards should be lifted EXCEPT:

   strengthen except

9. How well is the author's criticism of deconstructionist literary theory supported?

   specific evaluate   reasoning/app/evaluate

10. Which of the following claims is NOT supported by the author's argument in the passage?

    weaken

Answers for CARS Exercise 1: Identifying Question Types

1. **Structure:** What role does this list play in the author's argument?
2. **New Information *Type 1*:** What would the author say is true about the platypus, based both on the new information and on the existing information in the passage?
3. **Inference:** Which statement about the Treaty of Versailles is best supported by information in the passage?
4. **Retrieval:** Which statement about the Sahara Desert is best supported by information in the passage?
5. **Weaken:** Which answer choice goes farthest to suggest that environmental regulation *is* productive?
6. **Analogy:** Which choice most describes the same kind of methodology or process as that used, according to the passage, by Bybee?
7. **Inference:** Which definition of quarantine best fits with the author's use of that word in the passage?
8. **Strengthen EXCEPT:** Which choice either weakens that claim (by indicating caps should not be lifted) or has no effect on that claim? *Eliminate* the choices that do suggest that caps should be lifted.
9. **Evaluate:** Is the author's criticism of deconstructionist literary theory strongly or weakly supported? If strongly, then how? If weakly, then what are the flaws in the argument?
10. **Inference/NOT:** Look for the answer that is least supported by the passage. *Eliminate* the choices that are most supported by the information presented in the passage.

4.6 EXERCISE 2: FOCUS ON QUESTION TYPES— PRACTICE PASSAGES

Once you have learned the basic approach to each question type, it is time to dig in and solidify your understanding of type-specific logic and approach. The passages in this exercise will help you to accomplish this as they are specialized to include only one or two questions types. On the real MCAT, passages will include a mix of different question types. However, practicing the different types in isolation is a useful exercise; as you work each passage below, keep your focus on the logic of each type. Don't rely on the heading to tell you the type; still read the question stem word for word, and think about what type corresponds to that wording and why. Translate the question, thinking about what it is really asking you to do. As you do POE, keep your focus on predicting Attractors, and on identifying them as they come up.

Do not do these passages timed. However, do work the passage efficiently, just as you would on a test, and focus on taking the most efficient route to the correct answer.

There are six passages in this exercise, followed by explanations for each one.

PASSAGE I: SPECIFIC—RETRIEVAL QUESTIONS

4.6

For as long as they have been inhabited, Shenandoah National Park lands have been subject to direct human change. Homesteads, farms, cattle pastures, and orchards dotted the slopes of the Blue Ridge until the National Park Service took possession of the lands in 1936, and, to use the landscape architect's term, obliterated almost all traces of human history. In recent decades, the official story of Shenandoah has been one of "re-creation," of a wilderness lost to human exploitation and then restored by natural processes. But nature alone did not re-create a lost wilderness. The National Park Service and the Civilian Conservation Corps created a landscape never before seen on the Blue Ridge, through fire suppression, road construction, wildlife protection, human removal, landscaping, and engineering. Through the various stages of acquiring park lands, establishing Shenandoah, and re-creating the landscape, park officials and supporters told a variety of stories that justified both the "preservation" and the transformation of the Blue Ridge Mountains. Throughout Shenandoah's history, stories and landscapes have re-created each other.

This history of storytelling and land management in Shenandoah National Park attempts to make a contribution to the broader study of environmental history. In unveiling evidence of significant human influence in Shenandoah, it suggests that the historiography of the national parks, while focusing on how parks preserve landscapes, continues to underemphasize how these places create new landscapes. This history highlights the dynamic relationship between stories about nature and the landscapes of a national park.

Shenandoah National Park has occupied an uncomfortable position in the history of the National Park Service. The master narrative of this history, exemplified by Alfred Runte's National Parks: The American Experience, describes a progression from parks designed to preserve natural wonders and scenic grandeur to ones designed to preserve representative environments from around the country. Runte treats Shenandoah as a "transition" between the two types of preservation in the park system. He argues Shenandoah "anticipated the ecological standards of the later twentieth century" but could only "approximate the visual standards of the national park idea as originally conceived." He defines Shenandoah as a marginalized follower to the "crown jewels" of the West.

The management of landscapes and the management of stories can be woven into a single history of Shenandoah. Land management in Shenandoah has been deeply influenced by the stories that park officials have told about nature and about appropriate human relations with the environment. At the same time, the official park narrative has always reflected the contemporary condition of the environment on the Blue Ridge. Stories about Shenandoah's nature lead to management practices that in turn lead to new stories. For the last seventy-five years, Shenandoah's landscape and story have changed and have changed each other.

Every park faces a tension between what it is and what it is supposed to be; otherwise management would be unnecessary. Parks can resolve this tension in two ways: rhetorically or materially. Supporters and officials can either argue that the park meets the relevant standards or that those standards ought to be changed to include the park. Or, park managers can materially change parklands so they approach the ideal landscape. This tension between ideal and reality has motivated the evolution of stories and land management in Shenandoah.

The history of Shenandoah began when the National Park Service first proposed a park in the Southern Appalachians in 1924. To those who suggested that no place in the East could meet standards for western parks, boosters retorted that eastern scenery had its own virtues. In 1936, the Virginia lobby celebrated their success at the dedication of Shenandoah National Park. In the decade that followed, Shenandoah attempted to transform the landscape into a model of Southern Appalachian wilderness. So successful were landscape architects in both executing and veiling their efforts that the following generation of park managers described Shenandoah's re-creation entirely in terms of natural processes. This re-creation narrative is the one that presently dominates the signs, guides, and histories of Shenandoah National Park. Only recently, as Shenandoah officials have found a renewed interest in the cultural history of their park, has the narrative of Shenandoah begun to again recognize the park's landscape as a collaboration between human and natural actors.

Material used in this particular passage has been adapted from the following source:

J. Reich, *"Re-Creating the Wilderness: Shaping Narratives and Land-scapes in Shenandoah National Park"* © 2001 by Forest History Society and American Society for Environmental History.

1. According to the passage, why is park management necessary?

(A) To navigate the tension between what a park is and what it should be
B) To protect and preserve that natural environment
C) To manage the re-creation processes
D) To prevent human destruction and encroachment

specific retrieval

2. According to the author, what contribution can an understanding of land management at Shenandoah National Park make to a broader study of environmental history?

A) Emphasizing the importance of preservation in national parks *no too narrow*
(B) Drawing attention to the idea that national parks create new landscapes
C) Demonstrating that eastern parks can be just as beautiful as western parks *too extreme*
D) Encouraging more communities to engage with wildlife

3. According to the passage: *specific retrieval*

A) because of model preservation practices, Shenandoah National Park has remained a near-pristine monument to nature in Appalachia.
B) Shenandoah National Park serves as an excellent example of how stories about nature usurp the actual natural resources the stories were originally created about in the first place.
C) Shenandoah National Park is considered by many to be the crown jewel of the East.
(D) there is a cyclical relationship between Shenandoah's lore and management practices.

(specific retrieval)

4. The author mentions all of the following EXCEPT:

A) the acknowledgment of human as well as natural forces in shaping Shenandoah National Park is a more recent phenomenon.
B) fire prevention played an important role in shaping Shenandoah National Park.
C) land management of Shenandoah National Park has evolved over the decades.
(D) Shenandoah National Park was preserved (merely) as a representative of Appalachian wilderness.

5. According to Alfred Runte, Shenandoah is:
(specific retrieval)

A) a marginalized victim in the competition for the best representative landscape.
(B) a transition between national parks intended to protect the wilderness, and parks designed as a paradigm.
C) an important contribution to the broader study of environmental land management. *RAWO*
D) an example of the relationship between stories about landscapes and the actual landscapes themselves. *(RAWO)*

natural wonder /scenic
→ rep environ from
around country
anticipation

4.6

PASSAGE II: SPECIFIC—INFERENCE QUESTIONS

The Migratory Bird Treaty Act (MBTA) is a strict liability statute that makes it "unlawful, at any time, by any means or in any manner, to pursue, hunt, take, capture, kill, attempt to take or capture any migratory bird, or any part, nest, or egg of any such bird." The Fish and Wildlife Service (FWS) has defined the scope of the term "take" to encompass "to pursue, hunt, shoot, wound, kill, trap, capture, or collect, or attempt to pursue, hunt, shoot, wound, kill, trap, capture, or collect." Unlike the Endangered Species Act, the MBTA does not provide for "incidental take" permits. Thus, the United States may prosecute for death or other "take" of migratory birds under the MBTA even if the take occurred as part of an activity conducted under a federal permit.

Courts in the Ninth Circuit have confirmed that the MBTA does not require an intent to kill, capture, or wound a bird; the fact of killing, wounding, or capturing by the defendant would suffice. As with other similar regulatory acts, where the penalties are small and there is no "grave harm to an offender's reputation," the Supreme Court has long recognized that a different standard applies to those federal criminal statutes that are essentially regulatory. Therefore, there is no requirement that proof be offered that a defendant specifically intended to violate the MBTA, or that the defendant was aware of the violation. Accordingly, the courts have upheld convictions under the MBTA for the deaths of birds caused by electric power line, pesticide application, oil sump pumps, and oil drilling equipment.

The scope of strict liability is not unlimited, but neither is it well-defined. The Ninth Circuit and the District of California courts have found that the reach of the MBTA is limited by the overlapping requirements for the government to prove causation in fact, proximate causation, and that the defendant had some reasonable knowledge of the potential for danger. Questions abound regarding what types of predicate acts—acts which lead to the MBTA's specifically prohibited acts—can constitute a crime. Conceptually, the constitutional challenge to the criminalization of these predicate acts can be placed under a rubric of notice or causation. The inquiries regarding whether a defendant was on notice that an innocuous predicate act would lead to a crime, and whether a defendant caused a crime in a legally meaningful sense, are analytically indistinct and go to the heart of due process constraints on criminal statutes. The Ninth Circuit noted and approved the attempts of one district court to limit the MBTA's reach by holding that the defendants must "proximately cause" the MBTA violation in order to be found guilty. Specifically, the court focused on whether the government had demonstrated "proximate causation" or "legal causation beyond a reasonable doubt" by showing that trapped birds are a reasonably anticipated or foreseeable consequence

of failing to cap an exhaust stack and cover access holes to the heater. Unfortunately, the courts have not fully defined how the concept of proximate cause would limit the scope of MBTA liability in the real world. Courts have speculated in dicta that some everyday activities like driving cars or piloting aircraft would not reasonably be linked to bird death, while other (more industrial or hazardous) activities like operating power lines or oil drilling equipment would. "Because the death of a protected bird is generally not a probable consequence of driving an automobile, piloting an aircraft, maintaining an office building, or living in a residential dwelling with a picture window, such activities would not normally result in liability under the provisions of proximate cause, even if such activities would/could cause the death of protected birds. Proper application of the law to an MBTA prosecution should not lead to absurd results." When the MBTA is stretched to criminalize predicate acts that could not have been reasonably foreseen to result in a proscribed effect on birds, the statute reaches its constitutional breaking point.

Recently, a case was brought to the Ninth Circuit court regarding an environmental project entitled "Borderlands" erected near the U.S./Mexico border in California. The U.S. Attorney is bringing suit under the provisions of the MBTA on the basis that the project, consisting of a high net fence (meant to dramatize the environmental and cultural effects of the border), both blocks the migration path of various bird species and presents a clear danger to the lives of the birds that might fly into the fence.

Material used in this particular passage has been adapted from the following source:
L. Standers, "*Liability and Causation in the Migratory Bird Treaty Act*" © 2011

specific - inference

1. The passage indicates that the MBTA:

A) entails harsher penalties for those who violate its
    provisions than does the Endangered Species Act.
B) is in some ways stricter than the Endangered Species Act
    in regard to the activities that are allowed or disallowed
    under its provisions.
C) was enacted in part because it was felt that the
    Endangered Species Act was not strict enough in its
    provisions.
D) controls the hunting, capturing, wounding, or killing of
    endangered bird species.

2. Which of the following best represents the relationship
    between a predicate act and a proximate cause, in the
    context of the author's discussion of the MBTA?

A) A predicate act is defined by the motives of the
    actors, while a proximate cause directly results in
    the relevant effects.
B) A predicate act is behavior that precedes the harm, while
    proximate causation is legal responsibility for the harmful
    act.
C) A predicate act is innocuous, while a proximate cause is
    harmful.
D) A predicate act, unlike a proximate cause, does not have
    a foreseeable negative effect.

reasonable knowledge

3. The U.S. Attorney's suit against the "Borderlands"
    project would be least likely to succeed if:

A) it can be shown that it is probable that migratory birds
    would become trapped in the net and be harmed and/or
    die as a result. S
B) it can be shown that the project was undertaken with
    the intent of mitigating the negative effects of industrial
    activity on the health of migratory birds. (Kno
C) it can be shown that the motion of the net in the high
    winds that predictably occur in the area of the project can
    reasonably be anticipated to break the eggs of migratory
    birds nesting nearby. S
D) it can be shown that there was no foreseeable negative
    effect of the project on migratory birds.

4. The passage most supports which of the following
    conclusions?

A) Criminalizing predicate acts that cannot reasonably
    be predicted to result in harm to migratory birds has
    a negative effect on the legitimacy of other important
    regulatory measures.
B) Causation is more important in determining liability than
    whether or not an act is a proximate cause.
C) An activity that does cause the death of migratory birds
    but that can be considered a normal activity that does not
    normally pose a threat to birds should not be prosecuted.
D) An activity undertaken without the express intent of
    harming migratory birds should not be prosecuted.

4.6

5. The author indicates that which of the following would
    qualify as "taking" a migratory bird under the provisions
    of the MBTA?

I.   Damaging its eggs
II. Wounding its leg
III. Capturing it with a net

A) I only
B) III only
C) II and III only
D) I, II, and III

6. It can be most reasonably concluded, based on the passage,
    that prosecution for breaking a regulatory statute:

penalties are small

A) is likely to occur even if permission for the action has
    been granted under an "incidental take" permit.
B) is unlikely, even if successful, to cause significant harm to
    the reputation of the offender.
C) can result in the offender being charged with a felony
    rather than a misdemeanor if the offense is serious
    enough.
D) is carried out by the Fish and Wildlife Service.

7. The passage suggests that the author most likely
    believes that:

A) the role of proximate causes in defining strict liability
    under a statute should be clearly defined.
B) the severity of punishment for violating a regulatory
    statute should take the level of intent to cause harm into
    account as a mitigating factor.
C) the MBTA should not be used to prosecute harmful
    actions that are not related to industrial activity.
D) the notion of strict liability is inappropriately applied
    within the provisions of the MBTA.

PASSAGE III: GENERAL—MAIN POINT, PRIMARY PURPOSE, AND TONE QUESTIONS

4.6

A child and a man were one day walking on the seashore when the child found a little shell and held it to his ear. Suddenly he heard sounds—strange, low, melodious sounds, as if the shell were remembering and repeating to itself the murmurs of its ocean home. The child's face filled with wonder as he listened. Then came the man, explaining that the pearly curves of the shell simply caught a multitude of sounds too faint for human ears, and filled the glimmering hollows with the murmur of innumerable echoes. It was not a new world, but only the unnoticed harmony of the old that had aroused the child's wonder.

Some such experience as this awaits us when we begin the study of literature, which has always two aspects, one of simple enjoyment and appreciation, the other of analysis and exact description. Let a little song appeal to the ear, or a noble book to the heart, and for the moment, at least, we discover a new world, a world so different from our own that it seems a place of dreams and magic. To enter and enjoy this new world, to love good books for their own sake, is the chief thing; to analyze and explain them is a less joyous but still an important matter.... We have now reached a point where we wish to understand as well as to enjoy literature; and the first step, since exact definition is impossible, is to determine some of its essential qualities.

The first significant thing is the essentially artistic quality of all literature. All art is the expression of life in forms of truth and beauty; or rather, it is the reflection of some truth and beauty which are in the world, but which remain unnoticed until brought to our attention by some sensitive human soul, just as the delicate curves of the shell reflect sounds and harmonies too faint to be otherwise noticed. A hundred men may pass a hayfield and see only the sweaty toil and the windrows of dried grass, but there is one who pauses by a meadow, where girls are making hay and singing as they work. He looks deeper, sees truth and beauty where we see only dead grass, and reflects what he sees in a little poem in which the hay tells its own story.

The second quality of literature is its suggestiveness, its appeal to our emotions and imagination rather than to our intellect. It is not so much what it says as what it awakens in us that constitutes its charm.... When Faustus in the presence of Helen asks, "Was this the face that launched a thousand ships?" he does not state a fact or expect an answer. He opens a door through which our imagination enters a new world, a world of music, love, beauty, heroism—the whole splendid world of Greek literature. Such magic is in words.... The province of all art is not to instruct but to delight.

The third characteristic of literature, arising directly from the other two, is its permanence. The world does not willingly let any beautiful thing perish. History records deeds, outward acts largely, but every great act springs from an ideal, and to understand this we must read literature, where we find ideals recorded. When we read a history of the Anglo-Saxons, for instance, we learn that they were sea rovers, pirates, explorers, great eaters and drinkers; and we know something of their hovels and habits, and the lands which they harried and plundered. All that is interesting, but it does not tell us what most we want to know about these old ancestors of ours—not only what they did, but what they thought and felt; how they looked on life and death; what they loved, what they feared, and what they reverenced. Then we turn from history to the literature which they themselves produced, and instantly we become acquainted. These hardy people were not simply fighters and freebooters; they were people like ourselves. Their emotions awaken instant response in the souls of their descendants.

It is so with any age or people. To understand them, we must read not simply their history, which records their deeds, but their literature, which records the dreams that made their deeds possible. So Aristotle was profoundly right when he said that "poetry is more serious and philosophical than history"; and Goethe, when he explained literature as "the humanization of the whole world."

Material used in this particular passage has been adapted from the following source:
W. Long, *English Literature: Its History and Its Significance for the Life of the English-Speaking World,* 1909.

1. What is the main idea of the passage?

A) Literature's permanence allows us to better understand our ancestors. (narrow)
B) Literature has three fundamental qualities that must be debated by serious students of literature.
C) Literature, in the recording of ideals rather than deeds, tells us more about the past than history can. ✓
D) Literature calls attention to aspects of the world that would otherwise escape our notice; it appeals to emotion above reason, and it enriches our understanding of the past.

2. Which of the following statements best describes the author's tone in the passage?

A) He is enthusiastic about literature and disparaging about history.
B) He expresses his belief in the superiority of English literature over that in other languages.
C) He believes that reading literature is not only pleasurable, but fundamentally important to culture.
D) He considers contemporary literature inferior to that of the past.

3. What is the purpose of the first paragraph of the passage?

A) To illustrate that, like literature, nature can appear mysterious to a person who has not learned how to "read" it
B) To provide an analogy introducing literature's ability to delight its reader through the discovery of subtle beauty in the world
C) To introduce the author's discussion of how literature teaches us about the lives of those who produced that literature
D) To illustrate, through a narrative, the appeal of narrative literature

4. The author most likely intended this passage to be read by: Did not go back

A) literary critics. ✓ ?
B) students.
C) historians.
D) writers.

5. What is the central theme of the passage's third paragraph?

A) Literature renders nature capable of telling its own story.
B) It takes a true artist to be able to see beauty in quotidian work.
C) Literature does not just create truth and beauty, but exposes their presence in the world.
D) All art is ostensibly based on the natural world, whose beauty transcends what the average person sees in a cursory glance.   ↑ too narrow

6. Which of the following statements best describes the author's feelings about the analysis of literature?

A) He believes that it is of equal importance to the pure enjoyment of literature.
B) He feels it diminishes the joy one experiences immediately when reading a work of literature.
C) He acknowledges that while it is not the primary aspect of the experience of reading literature, it is nonetheless important.
D) He feels that those who do not wish to analyze literature beyond the simple pleasure it induces are missing out on a fundamental purpose of reading.

4.6

PASSAGE IV: REASONING—STRUCTURE AND EVALUATE QUESTIONS

4.6

If you were writing a morality play about class privilege, you couldn't do better than to dream up a glamorous ship of fools and load it with everyone from the A-list to immigrants coming to America for a better life. The class issue is one major reason the Titanic disaster has always been so ripe for dramatization…. If the indignant depictions of the class system in so many Titanic dramas coexist uneasily with their adoring depictions of upper-crust privilege, that, too, is part of the appeal: it allows us to demonstrate our liberalism even as we indulge our consumerism. In [James] Cameron's movie, you root for the steerage passenger who improbably pauses, during a last dash for a boat, to make a sardonic comment about the band as it famously played on…but you're also happy to lounge with Kate Winslet on a sunbathed private promenade deck while a uniformed maid cleans up on her hands and knees after breakfast.

Like all ships, the Titanic was a "she," and Cameron went to some lengths to push the identification between the ship and the young woman. Both are, to all appearances, "maidens" who are en route to losing their virginity; both are presented as the beautiful objects of men's possessive adoration. "She's the largest moving object ever made by the hand of man in all of history," a smug Ismay boasts to some appreciative tablemates at lunch. Later, as Rose goes in to dinner, one of Cal's fat-cat friends commends him on his fiancée as if she, too, were a prized object: "Congratulations, Hockley—she's splendid!"

All the energy spent on the mechanics, the romance, the construction, the passenger list, the endless debates about what the Californian might have done and just how many people perished…has distracted from what may, in the end, be the most obvious thing about the Titanic's story: it uncannily replicates the structure and the themes of our most fundamental myths and oldest tragedies…. The forty-six-thousand-ton liner is just the latest in a long line of lovely girl victims, an archetype of vulnerable femininity that stands at the core of the Western literary tradition.

But the Titanic embodies another strain of tragedy. This is the drama of a flawed and self-destructive hero…. The ship starts out like Oedipus: admired, idolized, hailed as different, special, exalted. Sophocles' play [*Oedipus Rex*] derives its horrible excitement from a relentless exposition of its protagonist's fall from grace. Cameron… knew that there is an ancient theatrical pleasure… in watching something beautiful fall apart.

All this is why we keep watching Cameron's movie, and why we can't stop thinking about the Titanic. The tale irresistibly conflates two of the oldest archetypes in literature…. Perhaps the most unsettling item in the immense inventory of Titanic trivia is a novel called *Futility*, by an American writer named

Morgan Robertson…. As the title suggests, the themes of this work of fiction are the old ones: the vanity of human striving, divine punishment for overweening confidence in our technological achievement, the futility of human effort in a world ruled by indifferent nature. But the writing comes to life only when Robertson focuses on the mechanical details, as in the scene of the aftermath of the collision.

> Seventy-five thousand tons—dead-weight—rushing through the fog at the rate of fifty feet per second, had hurled itself at an iceberg…. She rose out of the sea, higher and higher—until the propellers in the stern were half exposed…. The holding-down bolts of twelve boilers and three triple-expansion engines, unintended to hold such weights from a perpendicular flooring, snapped, and down through a maze of ladders, gratings, and fore-and-after bulkheads came these giant masses of steel and iron, puncturing the sides of the ship….

Down to the most idiosyncratic detail, all this is familiar…. And yet it couldn't be. Robertson published his book in 1898, fourteen years before the Titanic sailed. If she continues to haunt our imagination, it's because we were dreaming her long before the fresh spring afternoon when she turned her bows westward and, for the first time, headed toward the open sea.

Material used in this particular passage has been adapted from the following source:

D. Mendelsohn, "*Unsinkable: Why we can't let go of the Titanic,*" *The New Yorker,* April 16, 2012. © 2012 by Condé Nast.

1. Which of the following best describes the progression of ideas in this passage?

A) The author presents some reasons why the story of the Titanic is so compelling, and then argues that these reasons obscure the real meaning of the 1912 disaster.

B) The author discusses several interpretations of the Titanic story, and then suggests that Cameron's is the most compelling.

C) The author notes that the Titanic is a story of class privilege as well as that of an archetypal feminine vulnerability; he then moves on to suggest that it is compelling because the story has tragic themes that are among the oldest in Western literature.

D) The author notes several historical interpretations of the Titanic, and then suggests they are all undermined by Robertson's anticipation of the tragedy in his novel.

2. The author provides two quotations from Cameron's film in paragraph 2 in order to:

A) indicate that women should not be considered property.
B) express views, common at the time of the Titanic but out of fashion now, that women were little more than objects to be adored and possessed by men.
C) illustrate the similar terms by which the ship and Rose are defined.
D) give an example of Cameron's genius in film direction.

3. The author's claim that the Titanic "is the drama of a flawed and self-destructive hero" is:

A) undermined by the comparison with Oedipus.
B) not supported by any evidence in the passage.
C) supported by his claim that the ship is "an archetype of vulnerable femininity that stands at the core of the Western literary tradition."
D) supported with a reference to a play.

4. The author provides a passage from Robertson's novel primarily in order to:

A) demonstrate Robertson's skill at rendering a depiction of the fateful events leading to the Titanic's sinking.
B) note the uncanny resemblance of Robertson's prose to the story of the Titanic.
C) indicate some of the themes of Robertson's text.
D) give an example of the pleasure found in watching something beautiful fall apart.

5. The author's claim in paragraph 1 that the Titanic story "allows us to demonstrate our liberalism even as we indulge our consumerism" is best supported in the passage by:

A) the preponderance of sardonic treatments of the class issue in many interpretations of the story.
B) reference to conflicting responses the viewer of Cameron's film experiences.
C) the discussion in paragraph 2 about the parallels between the ship and Rose.
D) nothing; this is a claim made without evidence.

6. The author's claim that the story of the Titanic "conflates two of the oldest archetypes in literature" is:

A) weak: he does not indicate what either of these archetypes are.
B) strong: the paragraphs preceding this claim provide evidence supporting it.
C) weak: the author cannot claim to know what the oldest archetypes in Western literature are.
D) strong: the author supports this claim through his discussion of consumerism.

7. The author's claim that the Titanic was "admired, idolized, hailed as different, special, [and] exalted" in its time (paragraph 4) is supported by evidence in the passage about the ship's:

A) unique mechanical system.
B) absence of lower-class passengers.
C) size.
D) elaborate décor.

8. The author suggests that the viewer of Cameron's film is "happy to lounge with Kate Winslet on a sunbathed private promenade deck" in order to:

A) highlight an instance when we are tempted to indulge in upper-class fantasy even while we otherwise scorn the unfairness of the class system.
B) indicate the universal allure of Cameron's film's female protagonist.
C) criticize our hypocrisy in both appreciating and denouncing privilege.
D) express his approval of Cameron's directorial choices.

9. The author notes that the Titanic was a "she" in order to:

A) remark upon this eccentricity of assigning a gender to inanimate objects, unique to Cameron's interpretation.
B) question why all ships are assigned the feminine pronoun.
C) set up another argument for why the Titanic endures in our collective imagination.
D) indicate the sexism pervasive in the era in which the Titanic sailed.

4.6

PASSAGE V: APPLICATION—STRENGTHEN AND WEAKEN QUESTIONS

4.6

In ordinary community life, in which individuals depend on one another and yet remain divided by different interests and passions, courtesy creates possibilities for cooperation by offering an artificial code of behavior. Genuine respect and mutual affection are not required for the "false friendships" of polite society to form; courtesy offers social coordination and civil peace so long as everyone simply agrees to be well-mannered. This offer is widely accepted, in part, because most individuals are capable of only appearing to live up to community ideals. The opportunity for polite pretense is valuable in a world where people strive to keep up appearances because it permits everyone "to be better than they might be" by giving them a chance to pretend to be better than they are.

Courtesy and law are often connected in terms of symbiosis: manners mavens and legal professionals alike both argue that courtesy and law work together to maintain communal harmony. In this vein, for example, Justice Ruth Bader Ginsburg has called on fellow Supreme Court judges to avoid intemperate and abrasive language in their opinions (and especially in their dissents) in order to promote the judiciary's capacity and standing as an authoritative, dispute-resolving institution. It is by speaking in a polite "judicial voice" that courts may become more effective at performing their official duties.

Although the symbiotic view has its merits, my approach to the relationship between courtesy and law is somewhat different. Rather than examining how courtesy and law may work in combination, I wish to explore what the functioning of courtesy can tell us about the function of law. Unlike Justice Ginsburg, I do not intend to consider how the judicial voice can be made more decorous; instead, I plan to assess the ways in which judicial action may itself be a form of decorum.

To see how the dynamics that drive courtesy may also be at work in the judicial process, we should first, for the sake of analysis, accede to the proposition that the same understanding of human nature out of which courtesy grows also provides the context in which law must function. That is, we should accept, as a working premise, that differences between individuals are significant and irreducible; thus we should view disagreements as an obstinate fact of community life, never to be fully overcome but only to be more or less successfully managed. Moreover, we should accept that humans are governed by an inextricable mix of high principle and low passion. As a result, we should stipulate that most people take public moral standards seriously yet remain too filled with ambition and vanity to actually practice what they preach.

I recommend this somewhat pessimistic view of human nature, along with the understanding of courtesy that flows from it, as a way of explaining how the American judicial process works. I do not claim that this view of human nature perfectly represents how people are, nor do I claim that courtesy and law are identical. My claim is instead that an analytical model built on these ideas serves the purpose of explanation by generating new insights into how the rule of law currently operates.

What, then, does courtesy tell us about law? To begin to develop an answer to this question, consider that law, like courtesy, has often been thought to fulfill a facilitating function. A number of scholars have argued that courts effectively manage disputes by pursuing acceptable settlements without altering the fundamental factors that generate the disputes in the first place. Law, on this understanding, is an artificial medium in which otherwise opposed parties may jointly find ways of moving on.

A leading example of such thinking can be found in the classic discussion of legal reasoning by Lief Carter and Thomas Burke. Carter and Burke argue that the rule of law, in its essence, is a matter of requiring people to "look outside [their] own will for criteria of judgment." Whatever the specific features of a given political order may be, the rule of law directs individuals to adopt independent, publicly shared principles outside the sphere of personal attachments and private beliefs. Highly charged conflicts will certainly tempt people to evaluate competing claims by their own feelings and convictions. But the rule of law asks us to push beyond individual preferences....

According to Carter and Burke, one great advantage of having such independent standards of governance is that they create a highly useful language of dispute management for the courts. The rule of law sets aside the "dramatic and emotional work of poetics and theatrics" and commits the judiciary to "the logic of ideas." Unlike the world of electoral politics, in which "smart participants know that they should obfuscate, change the subject, [and] hurl mud" to achieve their goals, the rule of law requires judges to work out their arguments openly and to furnish reasons for their rulings. It is a deliberate process that relies on "elaborate mechanisms for sequencing questions" and structured frameworks that dictate how each sequenced question is to be addressed. The payoff of such "slow and steady (and often boring)" legal procedures is that they help broker community peace, channeling hotly contested questions into a forum in which they can be more easily handled.

Material used in this particular passage has been adapted from the following source:

K. Bybee, *All Judges Are Political Except When They Are Not*
© 2010 by Stanford University Press.

1. Which of the following, if true, would most challenge Justice Ginsburg's argument that judges should "avoid intemperate and abrasive language in their opinions"?

A) Some legal experts argue that the fact that few, other than legal experts, are aware of the specific nature of judicial decisions suggests that the language used in those decisions has little effect on public perceptions regarding the judiciary.
B) Professionals are especially sensitive to criticism by others in their own field, which can lead to defensiveness and unwillingness to cooperate in the future.
C) Moderation is often perceived as an indication of weakness and indecision.
D) Courtesy and law function in qualitatively different ways in society, and no relevant analogy can be drawn between them.

2. Which of the following statements, if true, would go the furthest in validating the contrast drawn in the last paragraph between the rule of law and electoral politics?

A) Candidates for office often achieve success by sticking tightly to pre-scripted talking points and repeating them by rote rather than by engaging in authentic discussion and debate.
B) Laws requiring candidates to divulge all sources of campaign donations have contributed to a healthy transparency and openness in the electoral process.
C) The level of public interest in an electoral campaign often turns on how many hotly contested issues are matters of public debate at the time.
D) Candidates for office who project a friendly and accessible image are often the most successful.

3. Which of the following, if true, would most undermine the author's suggestion that courtesy is valuable largely because it allows people to appear to be better than they really are?

A) Polite pretense, when obviously inauthentic to an extreme, can have the effect of increasing social tensions, but the effect is usually temporary.
B) The belief that aggression and dominance are prized over all other characteristics in a competitive, free-market economy is for the most part false.
C) When a person pretends for any length of time to live by certain values that he or she does not in fact hold, that person usually begins to actually believe in and live by those values.
D) Human beings do sometimes act selflessly, putting aside their own ambitions and vanity.

4. Which of the following statements, if true, would most weaken the author's central argument?

A) Human beings do sincerely value cooperation and wish, for the most part, to act in the interests of the community rather than for their own good alone.
B) Statistical studies show no correlation over the last 100 years between the level of open hostility and discourteous behavior amongst Supreme Court judges and those judges' capacity to effectively perform their judicial functions.
C) The structure provided by the rule of law allows people to compromise somewhat on their own goals and preferences without feeling that they are being taken advantage of by other individuals.
D) The facilitating function performed by the rule of law arises only when and because the existence of a stable legal structure allows community members to come to equate their own interests with those of the community; self-interest becomes one with group-interest.

5. Which of the following statements, if true, would most support the author's central argument?

A) Many studies of human decision-making have shown that fear of being taken advantage of often leads people to make choices that lead to a less-than-optimal outcome for all involved.
B) Many studies of human decision-making show that people are more highly motivated by the fear of losing than by the hope of winning.
C) Many studies in behavioral psychology show that the more time people have to consider a conflict, the more able they are to put aside emotion and consider perspectives other than their own.
D) Many psychological studies have shown that when people are bored and impatient, they often make choices based on emotion rather than on rational consideration of the pros and cons of different possible decision paths.

6. Which of the following, if true, would least weaken Carter and Burke's contention that the rule of law excludes "poetics and theatrics" from the business of the courts?

A) Legal language is often convoluted and dry due to the goal of removing any room for ambiguity, emotion, or unnecessary debate over semantics.
B) The power of the courtroom is based in large part on the ritualistic and performative aspects of a trial, rather than on the intellectual basis for those legal processes.
C) Jury members are much more likely to be swayed by appeals to the emotions of either sympathy or anger than by arguments based on the letter of the law.
D) The influence of television has led judges at all levels to base their rulings more on popular expectations of a shocking and dramatic outcome than on traditionally accepted legal rules and procedures.

PASSAGE VI: APPLICATION—NEW INFORMATION AND ANALOGY QUESTIONS

The historical roots of the civic community are astonishingly deep. Enduring traditions of civic involvement and social solidarity can be traced back nearly a millennium to the eleventh century, when communal republics were established in places like Florence, Bologna, and Genoa, exactly the communities that today enjoy civic engagement and successful government. At the core of this civic heritage are rich networks of organized reciprocity and civic solidarity—guilds, religious fraternities, and tower societies for self-defense in the medieval communes; cooperatives, mutual aid societies, neighborhood associations, and choral societies in the twentieth century.

These communities did not become civic simply because they were rich. The historical record strongly suggests precisely the opposite: They have become rich because they were civic. The social capital embodied in norms and networks of civic engagement seems to be a precondition for economic development, as well as for effective government. Development economists take note: Civics matters.

How does social capital undergird good government and economic progress? First, networks of civic engagement foster sturdy norms of generalized reciprocity: I'll do this for you now, in the expectation that down the road you or someone else will return the favor. "Social capital is akin to what Tom Wolfe called the 'favor bank' in his novel, *The Bonfire of the Vanities*, notes economist Robert Frank. A society that relies on generalized reciprocity is more efficient than a distrustful society.

Networks of civic engagement also facilitate coordination and communication and amplify information about the trustworthiness of other individuals. Students of prisoners' dilemmas and related games report that cooperation is most easily sustained through repeat play. When economic and political dealing is embedded in dense networks of social interaction, incentives for opportunism and malfeasance are reduced. This is why the diamond trade, with its extreme possibilities for fraud, is concentrated within close-knit ethnic enclaves. Dense social ties facilitate gossip and other valuable ways of cultivating reputation—an essential foundation for trust in a complex society.

Finally, networks of civic engagement embody past success at collaboration, which can serve as a cultural template for future collaboration. The civic traditions of north central Italy provide a historical repertoire of forms of cooperation that, having proved their worth in the past, are available to citizens for addressing new problems of collective action.

Sociologist James Coleman concludes, "Like other forms of capital, social capital is productive, making possible the achievement of certain ends that would not be attainable in its absence.... In a farming community...where one farmer gets his hay baled by another and where farm tools are extensively borrowed and lent, the social capital allows each farmer to get his work done with less physical capital in the form of tools and equipment." Social capital, in short, enables Hume's farmers to surmount their dilemma of collective action.

Stocks of social capital, such as trust, norms, and networks, tend to be self-reinforcing and cumulative. Successful collaboration in one endeavor builds connections and trust—social assets that facilitate future collaboration in other, unrelated tasks. As with conventional capital, those who have social capital tend to accumulate more: "them as has, gets." Social capital is what the social philosopher Albert O. Hirschman calls a "moral resource," that is, a resource whose supply increases rather than decreases through use and which (unlike physical capital) becomes depleted if not used.

Like other public goods, from clean air to safe streets, social capital tends to be underprovided by private agents. This means that social capital must often be a byproduct of other social activities. Social capital typically consists in ties, norms, and trust transferable from one social setting to another. Members of Florentine choral societies participate because they like to sing, not because their participation strengthens the Tuscan social fabric. But it does.

Material used in this particular passage has been adapted from the following source:
R. Putnam, *"The Prosperous Community"* © 1993 by *The American Prospect.*

1. Which of the following scenarios most closely demonstrates the logic of reciprocity, as described in the passage?

A) A diamond trader who pays fair prices for crude diamond ore
B) A free babysitting collective in which each parent participates in watching each other's children
C) A government that subsidizes health care and education using taxpayer money
D) A couple that signs a prenuptial agreement before their wedding

2. Which of the following is the most analogous to the relationship described by the author in the second paragraph?

A) Employees at small start-up companies often engage in after-hours collaborations and events outside of work in order to facilitate team-building and efficiency long before their companies become profitable.
B) Private universities with the largest endowments also boast the most student involvement in the academic community.
C) The wealthiest citizens are responsible for the largest private donations to charitable and community. organizations, especially to those involved in the arts.
D) Large stock market investments tend to make the most money, and, as this money is re-invested, it generates even more money.

3. Which of the following is most analogous to social capital, as it is described in the passage?

A) In long-term relationships, passionate love declines gradually as companionate love increases.
B) Positive reinforcement from peers is often more effective than parental punishment in moderating adolescent behavior.
C) Because heat is generated by electricity, electrical circuits will automatically shut down when the heat reaches a certain threshold.
D) As the temperature rises, permafrost begins to thaw, releasing carbon dioxide and methane gases into the atmosphere, which further increases the temperature.

4. Which of the following would be LEAST comparable to a network of civic engagement, as it is described in paragraph 4?

A) Businesses that are run entirely by family networks are most successful.
B) Olympic teams composed of individuals from all over the country who have not played together before tend to require much more practice than teams that have played together for years.
C) Individual consultants are routinely shuffled into new teams in order to maximize performance.
D) Prisoners tend do best when their cell mates and security personnel remain consistent.

4.6

5. Which of the following is most analogous to Florentine choral societies, as they are portrayed by the author?

A) Children who stay after school to receive tutoring in social studies, English, and math
B) Men drafted into military service during times of war
C) Community members forming a Neighborhood Watch group in an effort to reduce crime and make the neighborhood safer
D) People participating in amateur sports clubs in their free time

6. Which of the following claims made in the passage would be most strengthened by data showing a strong positive correlation between the number of Boy Scout and Girl Scout troops in a community and median income?

A) "The historical roots of the civic community are astonishingly deep."
B) "The social capital embodied in norms and networks of civic engagement seems to be a precondition for economic development."
C) "Networks of civic engagement also facilitate coordination and communication and amplify information about the trustworthiness of other individuals."
D) "Successful collaboration in one endeavor builds connections and trust—social assets that facilitate future collaboration in other, unrelated tasks."

7. Suppose that the gossip fostered by modern-day social media networks has been shown to cultivate more mistrust, bullying, and sullied reputations. Which of the following claims made in the passage is most undermined by this information?

A) Social networks are essential for effective democracy.
B) Distrustful societies are less efficient than societies built on trust.
C) Trust and repute are cultivated by gossip.
D) None; the information provided is not applicable to the information about civic engagement in the passage.

4.6

8. In the past three decades, the number of Americans who attend public meetings or political rallies has radically decreased, to less than ten percent of the total population. What might the author of this passage suggest as a possible outcome of this decline?

A) More organized protests
B) Slowing of economic progress
C) Heightened sociocultural awareness
D) Increased participation in other activities

9. If religion is the most common associational membership among people in various societies today, what is most likely true, based on the passage?

A) Government continues to rely on religion, and vice versa.
B) Active members of a religion have more social capital than those who are not religious.
C) Religious affiliation serves as a venue for modern-day civic engagement.
D) Places of worship enjoy an economic boost from high membership.

EXPLANATIONS

Passage I: Specific—Retrieval Questions

Question Type Strategies

Retrieval questions test your ability to locate and paraphrase information in the passage. Pick the answer that is best supported by the relevant part of the text. Look out for wrong answers that are supported by the passage but that are not relevant to the specific reference in the question stem, that use words from the passage out of context, or that rely on outside knowledge.

1. **A**   This is a Retrieval question.

   The term "land management" is used in several places in the passage, so it is important to narrow in on the place where the author also explains why it is necessary. In paragraph 5, the passage states: "Every park faces a tension between what it is and what it is supposed to be; otherwise management would be unnecessary…. This tension between ideal and reality has motivated the evolution of stories and land management in Shenandoah." Therefore, land management is necessary because of the tension between what a park is and what it should be.

   A: **Yes. This choice is most supported by the information in paragraph 5.**

   B: No. This is an "outside knowledge" Attractor; most people probably consider land management to serve this function for national parks, but this is not supported by the passage.

   C: No. The term "re-creation" is used frequently in the passage, but the author does not suggest that land management is specifically necessary for re-creation.

   D: No. This is an "outside knowledge" Attractor; most people probably consider land management to serve this function for national parks, but this is not supported by the passage.

2. **B**   This is a Retrieval question.

   In paragraph 2, the passage states: "This history of storytelling and land management in Shenandoah National Park attempts to make a contribution to the broader study of environmental history. In unveiling evidence of significant human influence in Shenandoah, it suggests that the historiography of the national parks, while focusing on how parks preserve landscapes, continues to underemphasize how these places create new landscapes. This history highlights the dynamic relationship between stories about nature and the landscapes of a national park."

   A: No. This is an "outside knowledge" Attractor; the importance of preservation is not the contribution to a broader study of environmental history.

   B: **Yes. This choice is most closely supported by the information in paragraph 2.**

   C: No. While this choice is supported in the final paragraph, it is not the contribution to a broader study of environmental history. This is the right answer to the wrong question.

   D: No. This choice is outside the scope of the passage and relies on outside knowledge.

3. **D**   This is a Retrieval question.

The question stem does not provide any useful information. Therefore, translate each answer choice and determine if it is supported by information in the passage.

A: No. The passage does not suggest that the preservation practices at Shenandoah National Park were "model," nor does it suggest that Shenandoah National Park is a "near-pristine monument to nature in Appalachia."

B: No. The passage does not suggest that the stories about nature usurp or surpass the actual natural resources. Instead, the passage states: "Shenandoah's landscape and story have changed and have changed each other" (paragraph 4).

C: No. This answer uses words taken out of context; the passage states: "He defines Shenandoah as a marginalized follower to the 'crown jewels' of the West" (paragraph 3). Therefore, this choice is not supported by the passage.

D: **Yes. The passage states: "Stories about Shenandoah's nature lead to management practices that in turn lead to new stories" (paragraph 4). Therefore this choice is most directly supported by the passage.**

4. **D**   This is a Retrieval question in EXCEPT/LEAST/NOT format.

The question stem does not provide much useful information. So, translate each answer choice and determine if it is mentioned in the passage.

A: No. The final paragraph states: "Only recently, as Shenandoah officials have found a renewed interest in the cultural history of their park, has the narrative of Shenandoah begun to again recognize the park's landscape as a collaboration between human and natural actors." The recent acknowledgment of human forces is mentioned in the passage, so this is not the correct choice.

B: No. The first paragraph states: "The National Park Service and the Civilian Conservation Corps created a landscape never before seen on the Blue Ridge, through fire suppression, road construction, wildlife protection, human removal, landscaping, and engineering." Therefore, fire prevention is mentioned as playing a role in shaping Shenandoah, and this is not the correct choice.

C: No. This passage describes how land management has evolved over the decades; therefore this is not the correct choice.

D: **Yes. The passage never mentions that Shenandoah was preserved merely as a representative of Appalachian wilderness. This, therefore, is the best choice for an EXCEPT/LEAST/NOT Retrieval question.**

5. **B**   This is a Retrieval question.

The question is asking you specifically about Alfred Runte's take on Shenandoah; the third paragraph of this passage contains all the information that you need in order to answer this question. In the paragraph, it states there is a: "…progression from parks designed to preserve natural wonders and scenic grandeur to ones designed to preserve representative environments from around the country. Runte treats Shenandoah as a 'transition' between the two types of preservation in the park system." The best answer choice should describe this idea of transition.

A: No. This choice is too extreme ("marginalized victim" is not in line with the passage's tone), and does not reflect Runte's description of Shenandoah; be careful not to seize on an answer simply because one word in it rings true with the passage: Runte says Shenandoah is "marginalized" but not that it is a "victim."

B: **Yes. This choice summarizes Runte's sentiment about Shenandoah; this choice is best supported by paragraph 3.**

C: No. The contribution to the broader study of land management is described in paragraph 2, not paragraph 3. This choice, while supported by the passage, does not answer the question being asked about Runte.

D: No. This is an example of a "right answer to the wrong question" response because the information in this choice appears in the passage, but not in paragraph 3. It is mentioned at the end of paragraph 2 in a different context: "This history highlights the dynamic relationship between stories about nature and the landscapes of a national park." This idea also appears at the ends of paragraphs 4 and 5, but again, not in the context of Runte's argument.

Passage II: Specific—Inference Questions

Question Type Strategies

When attacking Inference questions, choose the answer choice that is best supported by the passage. The correct answer may be more or less stated in the text (there is no such thing as being "too close to the passage" to qualify as a correct answer for this question type). More commonly, however, the answer is not directly stated, but there is direct evidence supporting it in the passage. Occasionally, it will seem like the correct answer is a bit too much of a stretch from the passage, but, if it is better supported than the other three choices, it is the "least wrong" answer (i.e., the credited response). In particular, look out for wrong answers that are too extreme, that take words from the passage out of context, or that are supported by the passage but do not respond to the specific issue cited in the question stem.

1.   **B**   This is an Inference question.

A: No. The only mention of the Endangered Species Act is in paragraph 1, and there is no direct discussion of what penalties it entails. Although the author's discussion in paragraph 2 of penalties for violations of regulatory measures may apply to the Endangered Species Act, there is no indication that those penalties are less severe than for violations of the MBTA.

B: **Yes. In the first paragraph the author writes: "Unlike the Endangered Species Act, the MBTA does not provide for 'incidental take' permits. Thus, the United States may prosecute for death or other 'take' of migratory birds under the MBTA even if the take occurred as part of an activity conducted under a federal permit." Therefore, you can infer that the Endangered Species Act, unlike the MBTA, does allow for "incidental take" permits, and that it is in at least that way less strict. Note the moderate wording of the choice ("in some ways").**

C: No. While the MBTA is in at least one way stricter than the Endangered Species Act (paragraph 1), the author never discusses the motivations for enacting the MBTA. This choice is out of scope and too extreme.

D: No. This choice is half-right but half-wrong. While those activities are in fact controlled, they are controlled specifically for migratory birds, and the passage does not suggest that migratory birds are endangered.

2. **B** This is an Inference question.

Predicate acts and proximate causes are discussed in paragraph 3. The author writes: "Questions abound regarding what types of predicate acts—acts which lead to the MBTA's specifically prohibited acts—can constitute a crime.… The Ninth Circuit noted and approved the attempts of one district court to limit the MBTA's reach by holding that the defendants must 'proximately cause' the MBTA violation in order to be found guilty. Specifically, the court focused on whether the government had demonstrated 'proximate causation' or 'legal causation beyond a reasonable doubt' by showing that trapped birds are a reasonably anticipated or foreseeable consequence of failing to cap an exhaust stack and cover access holes to the heater." By going back to this part of the passage before doing POE, you would know that predicate acts lead up to the harm, while proximate cause is legal responsibility for the harm.

A: No. This choice is half-right, half-wrong. There is no suggestion that the definition of predicate acts takes motivation into account. In fact, at least under the MBTA, motive is not a relevant factor in defining liability (paragraph 2).

B: **Yes. Both parts of this answer choice correspond to the author's discussion in the passage (see explanation in the note above).**

C: No. This choice takes words out of context, making the first half too extreme. For that reason the choice is half-right but half-wrong. While the author states in paragraph 3 that the "inquiries regarding whether a defendant was on notice that an innocuous predicate act would lead to a crime, and whether a defendant caused a crime in a legally meaningful sense, are analytically indistinct," she is not suggesting that all predicate acts are innocuous or harmless.

D: No. Neither term is defined by the predictability of harm. Rather, they are defined by their relative proximity to actual harm. This choice takes words out of the context of the passage.

3. **D** This is an Inference question.

A: No. The passage suggests just the opposite. The author writes in paragraph 3 that "The Ninth Circuit noted and approved the attempts of one district court to limit the MBTA's reach by holding that the defendants must '"proximately cause"' the MBTA violation in order to be found guilty. Specifically, the court focused on whether the government had demonstrated '"proximate causation"' or '"legal causation beyond a reasonable doubt"' by showing that trapped birds are a reasonably anticipated or foreseeable consequence of failing to cap an exhaust stack and cover access holes to the heater." This indicates that a case showing proximate causation would likely succeed in the Ninth Circuit court.

B: No. The passage suggests that motivation, good or bad, is not a relevant factor in proving liability under the MBTA (paragraph 2). Therefore, this would make it neither more nor less likely that the suit would succeed.

C: No. First, the effect on the eggs of migratory birds is a relevant factor (see the definition of "take" in paragraph 1). Second, if a negative result is foreseeable, this would make the suit more, not less, likely to succeed (paragraph 2).

D: **Yes. This choice is the opposite of choices A and C. According to paragraph 3, foreseeability of the harm is a major factor in the likely success of a suit under the provisions of the MBTA. If there is no predictable harm, the suit is not likely to succeed.**

4. **C** This is an Inference question.

A: No. While this choice would strengthen the author's argument at the end of paragraph 3, it cannot be inferred from the passage: it is too extreme and out of scope. Make sure to determine if the question is asking you to support the passage (a Strengthen question), or what is supported by the passage (an Inference question).

B: No. It is unclear in the passage what the relationship between "causation in fact" and "proximate" causation are. (The author writes in paragraph 3 that "the reach of the MBTA is limited by the overlapping requirements for the government to prove causation in fact, proximate causation, and that the defendant had some reasonable knowledge of the potential for danger.") There is no suggestion that one is or should be more important than the other in determining liability.

C: **Yes. At the end of paragraph 3, the author discusses activities that "would not normally result in liability under the provisions of proximate cause, even if such activities would/could cause the death of protected birds." The author goes on to argue that "proper application of the law to an MBTA prosecution should not lead to absurd results. When the MBTA is stretched to criminalize predicate acts that could not have been reasonably foreseen to result in a proscribed effect on birds, the statute reaches its constitutional breaking point."**

D: No. Paragraph 2 discusses how intent is not a relevant factor in determining liability under the MBTA; the author does not express any disagreement with this.

5. **D** This is an Inference question in the Roman numeral format.

The first step in answering this question should be to go back to paragraph 1, where the passage states that "The Migratory Bird Treaty Act (MBTA) is a strict liability statute that makes it 'unlawful, at any time, by any means or in any manner, to pursue, hunt, take, capture, kill, attempt to take or capture any migratory bird, or any part, nest, or egg of any such bird.' The Fish and Wildlife Service (FWS) has defined the scope of the term 'take' to encompass 'to pursue, hunt, shoot, wound, kill, trap, capture, or collect, or attempt to pursue, hunt, shoot, wound, kill, trap, capture, or collect.' Under this statute, any person, association, partnership, or corporation is guilty of a misdemeanor if they violate any provisions of the Act." Any item that would (1) be covered by the MBTA and (2) qualify as a "take" by this definition must be included in the correct answer.

Numeral I: True. The MBTA covers "any part, nest, or egg of any such bird," and damage to eggs could reasonably be considered a "wound." While this may not be an intuitively obvious definition of "take," it is supported by the passage.

Numeral II: True. The MBTA covers "any part, nest, or egg of any such bird," and "take" includes wounding. As with item I, while this may not be an intuitively obvious definition of "take," it is supported by the passage.

Numeral III: True. The MBTA covers capturing of birds, and so does the FWS definition of "take."

6. **B** This is an Inference question.

A: No. First, you know from paragraph 1 that the MBTA does not grant incidental take permits. Second, while the passage does indicate that other regulatory measures, including the Endangered Species Act, do grant such permits, the passage does not indicate that prosecution is likely to occur even if a permit has been granted. This choice is too extreme.

4.6

B: Yes. This choice more or less paraphrases a statement made in the passage. In the first paragraph the author writes: "As with other similar regulatory acts, where the penalties are small and there is no 'grave harm to an offender's reputation,' the Supreme Court has long recognized that a different standard applies to those federal criminal statutes that are essentially regulatory." From this you can reasonably infer that prosecution for breaking regulatory statutes is unlikely to damage the reputation of the offender. While it is a bit ambiguous in the passage whether or not this applies to all regulatory acts, this is still the "least wrong" answer.

C: No. The passage only mentions misdemeanors (paragraph 1). Being charged with a felony is out of the scope of the passage.

D: No. While the FWS definition of a "take" is relevant to prosecution under the MBTA (paragraph 1), the passage never suggests that the FWS itself carries out prosecutions. Only "the United States" (paragraph 1) and the U.S. Attorney (paragraph 4) are mentioned as actually bringing suit or prosecuting cases.

7.   **A**   This is an Inference question.

A: **Yes. In paragraph 3, the author states: "Unfortunately, the courts have not fully defined how the concept of proximate cause would limit the scope of MBTA liability in the real world." If the author believes that the lack of a clear definition is unfortunate in this case, you can infer that the author thinks that the role, in general, should be clearly defined.**

B: No. The author never expresses disapproval of the fact that the MBTA does not take intent into account.

C: No. This choice takes words out of context, and is also too extreme. While the author states in paragraph 3 that "Courts have speculated in dicta that some everyday activities like driving cars or piloting aircraft would not reasonably be linked to bird death, while other (more industrial or hazardous) activities like operating power lines or oil drilling equipment would," the passage does not suggest that the author believes that only industrial activity should be considered liable under the MBTA.

D: No. The author never indicates that she has a problem with the fact that the MBTA is "a strict liability statute" (paragraph 1).

Passage III: General—Main Point, Primary Purpose, and Tone Questions

Question Type Strategies

Main Point and Primary Purpose questions

These questions generally ask you about the Bottom Line of the passage as a whole. Make sure to choose answers that cover all of the major themes in the passage, without going beyond its scope. Also make sure that the answer you select matches the tone (positive, negative, or neutral) of the author. A similar type of question will ask you for the main point or purpose of a paragraph. Make sure to pick an answer specific to the content, tone, and scope of that paragraph.

Tone questions

These questions directly ask you about the author's attitude toward the overall subject being discussed (General Tone questions), or toward one particular aspect of it (Specific Tone questions). Be careful to choose answers that are supported by evidence in the passage (for example, by the tone indicators that you should be highlighting); don't speculate about what the author "might" think. Beware of choices that go in the right direction but that are too extreme.

1. **D** This is a Main Point question.

    A: No. This answer choice only addresses the second-to-last paragraph of the passage; it does not go far enough in encompassing the ideas of the passage as a whole.

    B: No. While the author does discuss three qualities of literature, he does not discuss the need for debate on the part of "serious students" or anyone else. This choice is half-right but half-wrong.

    C: No. This answer choice only addresses the final two paragraphs of the passage, and is therefore too limited in scope. A common trick of MCAT questions is to feature as an Attractor the part of the passage you most recently read; you can avoid this trick by ensuring that you summarize your own Bottom Line before starting the questions.

    D: Yes. This answer choice summarizes the three qualities of literature that the author discusses, making it the best answer choice among those listed.

2. **C** This is a Tone/Attitude question.

    A: No. While the first part of this answer is correct, the second part is too strong in tone, and too negative, making this a half-right/half-wrong Attractor. While the author notes that literature can tell us things that history cannot, he does not "disparage," or harshly criticize, history.

    B: No. There is nothing in the passage to indicate that the author thinks English literature is superior to any other sort of literature; in paragraph 4, in fact, he refers to "the whole splendid world of Greek literature."

    C: Yes. In the second paragraph, the author says "…to love good books for their own sake, is the chief thing; to analyze and explain them is a less joyous but still an important matter." In the passage's final paragraph he emphasizes the seriousness and importance of literature, agreeing with Goethe that literature is "the humanization of the world." This assertion supports the strong language in this answer choice; additionally, the other answer choices all have more discernible flaws.

    D: No. The author makes no claims about contemporary literature, and does not make any comparative statements regarding the literature of the present and that of the past.

3. **B** This is a "purpose of a paragraph" question.

    A: No. The author does not explain the story in the first paragraph in terms of people who have learned how to read nature or literature versus people who have not. The author does not suggest, either, that the mystery and delight inspired by good literature is something that goes away once someone knows how to "read" it.

    B: Yes. In the first paragraph, the author describes the man's explanation of the shell: "It was not a new world, but only the unnoticed harmony of the old that had aroused the child's wonder." This relationship between the apparent newness of the world and the fact that it is in fact something that has been there all along is addressed explicitly in the third paragraph with reference to literature and the shell: "All art is the expression of life in forms of truth and beauty; or rather, it is the reflection of some truth and beauty which are in the world, but which remain unnoticed until brought to our attention by some sensitive human soul, just as the delicate curves of the shell reflect

sounds and harmonies too faint to be otherwise noticed." **This explanation by the author in terms of his opening narrative is the most concrete evidence in the passage to explain the purpose of the first paragraph, making B the best answer choice.**

C: No. This is an appealing answer that addresses things that are discussed elsewhere in the passage, but it is not the point or purpose of this particular paragraph.

D: No. The author makes no statements about narrative literature in particular; this answer choice is beyond the scope of the passage.

4. **B** This is a variation on a Tone question.

This question requires you to take the scope, tone, and subject matter into account. Eliminate choices that are not appropriate to the focus and level of the passage, for example historians (for a passage that is largely about literature) or literary critics (for a passage that is not at all technical or academic).

A: No. This discussion of literature is too basic for literary critics themselves; presumably they would know the basic qualities of literature. This answer is not supported by the passage's tone.

B: **Yes. In the second paragraph, the author says, "We have now reached a point where we wish to understand as well as to enjoy literature; and the first step, since exact definition is impossible, is to determine some of its essential qualities." This talk of a "first step" in a "wish to understand" indicates an instructive tone, making students the most likely intended audience of this passage.**

C: No. While the author mentions the difference between literature and history, there is nothing in the passage to suggest that his intended audience consists of historians.

D: No. The passage is clearly addressed to readers of literature; there is no indication that the author is addressing writers themselves.

5. **C** This is a "point of the paragraph" question.

A: No. While the author says that the poem mentioned in paragraph 3 allows the hay to tell its story, this is merely an expression, and this answer choice is therefore a good example of an Attractor that uses a word or phrase out of context. This paragraph does not support the idea that literature renders nature capable of telling its own story, but rather that literature—written by someone who sees the beauty in the mundane—reflects the truth and beauty in the world.

B: No. The author does not discuss qualities of "true" artists versus presumably lesser artists, or fakes. He notes that, in this example, there is one man who takes notice of the meadow's beauty after a hundred men have merely noted its surface appearance, but there is nothing in this statement about the particular qualities of that man and whether or not he is a true artist; the author merely notes that it is a "sensitive human soul" who regards the meadow in a different light.

C: **Yes. Paragraph 3 follows up on the idea introduced by the opening narrative. Like the shell, literature does not only reveal a new world but reveals aspects of the world that often go unnoticed in daily life. The second sentence of the third paragraph nicely paraphrases this answer choice.**

D: No. This statement is too extreme. While the author makes statements about "all art," and refers in paragraph 3 to an example involving nature, he does not make the connection that all art is based on the natural world. For example, there is no suggestion that this is true of the literature of the Anglo-Saxons discussed in paragraph 5.

6. **C**   This is a Tone/Attitude question.

A: No. While the author indicates in the second paragraph that "To enter and enjoy this new world [of literature], to love good books for their own sake, is the chief thing; to analyze and explain them is a less joyous but still an important matter." To say that analysis is "still an important matter" is not the same as saying it is an "equally important matter." That he isolates enjoyment as the "chief" thing indicates that analysis must be ranked below enjoyment.

B: No. See paragraph 2. The author indicates that analyzing literature itself is "less joyous" than entering and loving good books, but does not say that analysis itself diminishes the immediate joy of reading.

C: **Yes. This answer choice best paraphrases the author's remark in paragraph 2 that "To enter and enjoy this new world [of literature], to love good books for their own sake, is the chief thing; to analyze and explain them is a less joyous but still an important matter."**

D: No. While the author says that analysis and explanation of literature is "an important matter," he does not make such extreme statements as to say that those who do not engage in analysis and explanation "are missing out on a fundamental purpose of reading." This answer is out of scope and too extreme in tone.

Passage IV: Reasoning—Structure and Evaluate Questions

Question Type Strategies

Structure questions

These questions ask you either for the purpose of a statement or paragraph within the passage, or how a particular statement is supported by the author. They are called Structure questions because they deal with not just the content, but also the logical structure of the passage. Therefore, in choosing an answer, make sure you select a choice that not only accurately represents the content of the passage, but also the purpose of the reference (that is, how it relates to other parts of the text) or the support given for the claim (that is, what evidence the author provides to explain or justify it). A rare version of this question type is the General Structure question, which asks you to find an answer that correctly describes the progression of claims or ideas in the passage. When evaluating the answers for these General Structure questions, make sure that the different parts of the answer choice match not only the content but the ordering of the referenced parts of the passage.

Evaluate questions

Evaluate questions ask you *how well* a claim is supported by the author within the passage. When answering these questions make sure that both the judgment (usually some form of "strongly" or "weakly") and the description (of why it is strongly or weakly supported) match the passage.

1. **C**   This is a General Structure question.

A: No. This answer choice gets the tone of the passage wrong by tweaking it a bit too far toward the negative. While the author does build up to his larger points, he discusses the earlier reasons "obscuring" the "real" reasons nowhere. In paragraph 3, he merely notes that some of the reasons "distract" from what may be the "most obvious" reason. "Obscure" and "distract" are not synonyms, nor are "obvious" and "real," so this choice is an inadequate paraphrasing of passage material.

B: No. While the author makes reference to Cameron's interpretation of the Titanic story, he nowhere privileges it as the "most compelling."

C: Yes. This answer comes the closest to following the trajectory of the passage, and does not feature any changes in tone from what is found in the passage. The ordering of ideas is exactly as it occurs in the passage.

D: No. While this one gets the ordering of the passage right, the author never suggests that the interpretations of the Titanic story are undermined by Robertson's novel.

2. **C** This is a Specific Structure question.

A: No. This is not the author's purpose in using these two quotes in paragraph 2; he does not offer an explicit value judgment on the parallel between Rose and the Titanic as both female entities.

B: No. The author does not contrast the attitudes of the Titanic's era with those held today.

C: Yes. In the sentences preceding the two quotations, one of which is about the ship and the other about Rose, the author says "Both…" and lists several factors that both the ship and Rose have in common.

D: No. While Cameron's film is quoted, the author is not singling out Cameron as a genius or noting anything exceptional about his direction. This is not the purpose of using the two quotes from Cameron's film in paragraph 2.

3. **D** This is an Evaluate question.

A: No. The discussion of Oedipus supports rather than undermines the author's claim. This is the opposite of the correct answer.

B: No. The author clearly backs up his claim with reference to Oedipus, a character from Sophocles' drama.

C: No. This is in fact a claim, not support, and comes in a different paragraph (paragraph 3) from the one referenced in the question stem (paragraph 4). The author begins paragraph 4 with "But the Titanic embodies another strain of tragedy": the words in quotations (here) are ones you should have highlighted to indicate that the author was making a separate point.

D: Yes. The author discusses Oedipus from Sophocles' *Oedipus Rex* to illustrate another drama that featured a "flawed and self-destructive hero." Notice that in classic MCAT form, the more moderate answer here is preferable—as is often the case—to the more extreme answer, which in this case is A.

4. **B** This is a Specific Structure question.

A: No. This answer does not go far enough and misses the point. As with the incorrect answer choices in other questions that emphasize Cameron's strength as a director, this answer is incorrect because it valorizes Robertson rather than positions him in the context of a larger discussion of our cultural fascination with the Titanic.

B: Yes. The author quotes Robertson to note the similarity of his account with the story of the Titanic: immediately following the quote, he says, "Down to the most idiosyncratic detail, all this is familiar," only to then surprise the reader by saying Robertson's novel preceded the Titanic disaster by 14 years. In the end, his point is that even before the Titanic, our imaginations were caught up in themes present in the story of the disaster.

C: No. While the author precedes the quotation by talking about the themes of Robertson's text, the quotation itself does not address themes as much as specific details of the scene of a sinking ship. And most importantly, the author uses the quotation primarily to draw a comparison between Robertson's story and that of the Titanic.

D: No. The author does not cite this explicitly in relation to the quotation from Robertson's book. He mentions this a few paragraphs earlier as part of the theatrical appeal of the Titanic disaster, but not as a direct reference to Robertson.

5. **B** This is a Specific Structure question.

A: No. The quotation given in the question stem notes a tension or an ambivalence: we "demonstrate liberalism even as we indulge our consumerism." This answer choice only deals with the "demonstrate liberalism" aspect of the question stem. The author does note that many versions of the Titanic story feature "indignant depictions of the class system" but these "coexist uneasily with their adoring depictions of upper-crust privilege": this latter quotation addresses the "indulge our consumerism" aspect of the question stem.

B: **Yes. See the explanation for choice A above. The quotation given in the question stem notes a tension in reactions of viewers/readers to class issues in the Titanic story. The author then provides specific moments from Cameron's film as evidence to support his claims about our reactions.**

C: No. This is not relevant to the question stem; it is part of a second argument made by the author, whereas the question stem refers to the first.

D: No. As choice B explains, the author supports his claim with specific references to Cameron's film.

6. **B** This is an Evaluate question.

A: No. The author does indicate that one archetype is of feminine vulnerability, so this answer choice directly contradicts information provided in the passage.

B: **Yes. In the paragraphs preceding the claim in the question stem, the author notes the archetype of female vulnerability, and then indicates another archetype by saying "But the Titanic embodies another strain of tragedy. This is the drama of a flawed and self-destructive hero." Admittedly, the author does not use the term "archetype" in the second case, but by the time he makes his claim that the Titanic "conflates two of the oldest archetypes in literature," we have a pretty good sense of what he means. If this feels like a stretch, it at least helps to definitively rule out choice D, which is much more definitive than the words "provide evidence supporting it" in this answer choice. Process of elimination leaves choice B as the "least wrong" answer.**

C: No. This answer choice extrapolates too much on the author's credentials and focuses on something that is not really the issue here: the age of the archetypes rather than the existence of them. There is no reason to doubt the author's knowledge about Western literature: his references to Sophocles' work and Robertson's novel, for instance, illustrate that he has knowledge about literature.

D: No. The discussion of consumerism in the first paragraph is not directly tied to the author's claim about archetypes. This is the right answer to the wrong question.

7. **C** This is a Specific Structure question.

A: No. The author never mentions anything unique about the ship's mechanical system.

B: No. This information is directly refuted by the passage's first paragraph, in which the author discusses the tension between classes present in the Titanic story.

4.6

C: Yes. In paragraph 2, the author quotes a character from Cameron's movie who says the Titanic is "the largest moving object ever made by the hand of man in all of history," and in paragraph 3 he refers to it as "the forty-six-thousand-ton liner."

D: No. The author does not mention the ship's décor.

8. **A** This is a Specific Structure question.

A: **Yes: This answer choice properly captures the tension that is the focus of the author in this paragraph: the tension between our liberalism and consumerism. The author provides the example of the sunbathed deck to illustrate that while we also identify with the scornful remark of the lower-class passenger to the music from the first-class section of the boat, we cannot help but enjoy the indulgence of seeing Winslet on the private deck.**

B: No. The allure, and the universal allure in particular, of the female protagonist is not something addressed in this paragraph. The allure of the sunbathed deck is more about the elitist indulgence than the attractiveness of the female enjoying it.

C: No. This choice is too extreme. The author does not suggest that this tension represents or indicates hypocrisy.

D: No: The point of this paragraph is not for the author to express his approval of Cameron's directorial choices; he does not explicitly express approval or disapproval at any point in the passage.

9. **C** This is a Specific Structure question.

A: No. The author never suggests that the Titanic's feminine status is unique to Cameron's interpretation, but merely that "the Titanic was a 'she'" and "Cameron went to some lengths to push the identification between the ship and the young woman."

B: No. The author does not question or investigate why ships are assigned the feminine pronoun; he merely states it as fact and then explores consequences for interpretation.

C: **Yes. The author notes that the feminine pronoun used for the ship creates room for an identification between the ship and the woman in Cameron's film; this parallel leads the author to comment on the story's archetype of feminine vulnerability, which is one of his arguments for the enduring appeal of the Titanic story in our imagination.**

D: No. The author does not contrast the Titanic's era with others, and the main point of paragraph 2 is not to discuss sexism, either at that time or at any time in history.

Passage V: Application—Strengthen and Weaken Questions

Question Type Strategies

Weaken questions

First, clearly define what you are weakening (the overall argument or some part of it in the passage) based on the question stem. Next, go back to the passage to clarify the logic of the argument. You can't literally answer these questions in your own words, as the correct answer will include new information. But you do want to create a guide for yourself regarding what the direction and issue of the correct answer needs to be. As you go through POE, make sure that the answer that you choose is relevant, that it weakens rather than strengthens, and that it is strong enough to have a real impact on the passage.

Strengthen questions

First, clearly define what you are strengthening (the overall argument or some part of it in the passage) based on the question stem. Next, go back to the passage to clarify the logic of the argument. As with Weaken questions, you can't come up with an exact answer in your own words, but do create a guide for yourself based on what the direction and issue of the correct answer needs to be. As you go through POE, make sure that the answer that you choose is relevant, that it strengthens rather than weakens, and that it is strong enough to have a significant impact on the passage.

1. **C**   This is a Weaken question.

   Look for the answer that provides the strongest reason to doubt Ginsburg's argument, described in paragraph 2, that judges should avoid discourteous language in order to preserve the status and effectiveness of the judiciary.

   A: No. While this answer goes in the right direction, it isn't strong enough to significantly weaken Ginsburg's claim. The fact that some (which could be only a few) experts believe something doesn't mean that it is actually true.

   B: No. This choice strengthens rather than weakens by suggesting that strong language in a dissent could undermine the functioning of the court. Note that Ginsburg states that courtesy is especially important in dissents.

   C: Yes. Ginsburg argues that it is by speaking in a "polite 'judicial voice' that courts may become more effective at performing their official duties" and preserving the status of the institution. If moderation is widely seen as a sign of weakness, however, then courteous language might undermine rather than promote the standing of the court.

   D: No. This choice is the right answer to the wrong question; it weakens the author's argument, but not Ginsburg's. Note that it is the author who argues that the law is itself a form of courtesy (see paragraph 3), whereas Ginsburg is simply calling for more courtesy within the legal system (paragraph 3).

2. **A**   This is a Strengthen question.

   In the last paragraph, the author offers (and agrees with) Carter and Burke's claim that "Unlike the world of electoral politics, in which 'smart participants know that they should obfuscate, change the subject, [and] hurl mud' to achieve their goals, the rule of law requires judges to work out their arguments openly and to furnish reasons for their rulings." Look for the answer that goes the furthest in suggesting that the rule of law and electoral politics are in fact different on this basis.

   A: Yes. Sticking to scripted responses and avoiding open debate would be the opposite of "work[ing] out arguments openly and furnish[ing] reasons for their rulings." Therefore this choice does support the author's contrast between the law and politics.

   B: No. This choice weakens rather than strengthens by suggesting that politics is becoming more open, with less obfuscation (i.e., hiding things).

   C: No. This choice takes words out of context from the passage. The fact that public interest is affected by how many controversial issues are involved in a campaign doesn't tell you anything about the openness of politics as compared to the law.

   D: No. Given that you don't know how authentic this image is, this choice has no impact on the author's claim.

3. **C**   This is a Weaken question.

The correct answer will either indicate that courtesy is not valuable, or that it is valuable largely for some reason other than that it allows people to "pretend to be better than they are."

A: No. This choice is not strong enough to most undermine the author's argument. It only indicates that courtesy can have the opposite effect in extreme cases, and for a limited amount of time.

B: No. This choice strengthens rather than weakens. If aggression and dominance are not in fact highly prized characteristics, it strengthens the claim that a "polite pretense" of cooperation and friendliness is valuable because it helps people to keep up the appearance of having good qualities ("pretend to be better than they are").

C: **Yes. The author's claim rests on the assumption that the value of courtesy lies in the fact that it hides reality, since "most individuals are capable only of appearing [emphasis added] to live up to community ideals." If pretending, through courtesy, to live up to those ideals made one able to actually do so, it would undermine the author's argument by giving an alternative explanation for the value of courtesy.**

D: No. The author does not claim that human beings never act selflessly; in fact, he says in paragraph 5: "I do not claim that this [pessimistic] view of human nature perfectly represents how people are...."

4. **D**   This is a Weaken question.

The author states in paragraph 3 that while he thinks that courtesy and the law may work in symbiosis, what he really wishes to talk about is how "judicial action may itself be a form of decorum." The rest of the passage discusses reasons for this claim. Therefore, the correct answer will be the one that most undermines this claim and/or the reasoning supporting the claim.

A: No. The author does not argue that people do not want to be selfless, but rather that they are for the most part unable to do so: "most people take public moral standards seriously, yet remain too filled with ambition and vanity to actually practice what they preach" (paragraph 4). Therefore, this answer choice weakens an argument more extreme than the one that the author actually makes.

B: No. The connection between civility and the functioning of the court is made by Ginsburg (paragraph 2). While the author does not disagree with her recommendation, it is not a central part of the author's own argument.

C: No. This would do the opposite; it strengthens the author's indication in the last paragraph that the structure of the rule of law contributes to cooperation and social peace.

D: **Yes. The author argues that the law, like courtesy, is an "artificial medium in which otherwise opposed parties may jointly find ways of moving on" without affecting "the fundamental factors that generate the disputes in the first place" (paragraph 3). When the author, through citation of Carter and Burke, states that the law helps us to "look outside [our] own will for criteria of judgment," he means that we act in spite of our individual preferences, not that we change those preferences. If the law acted to transform our perceptions in the way described in this answer choice, the author's argument that the law is a form of courtesy would fall apart.**

5. **C** This is a Strengthen question.

The author argues that law is a form of courtesy. Part of this argument is that the structure of the rule of law allows and directs people to look beyond their own perceptions and self-interest. The correct answer will either directly support the overall claim that one can see the law as itself a "form of decorum," or it will support the rationale given for the author's claim in the last two paragraphs.

A: No. There is no suggestion in this choice that the rule of law lessens this fear. Therefore, this choice is out of scope.

B: No. There is no suggestion in this choice of how the rule of law might relate either to this fear or to this hope. Therefore, this choice is out of scope.

C: **Yes. In the last paragraph, in the course of explaining and supporting his argument, the author cites Carter and Burke's claim that "The payoff of such 'slow and steady (and often boring)' legal procedures is that they help broker community peace." If it is the case that time is an issue, and if the more time people have to consider their options, the less likely they are to act purely on self-interest, this would support the author's argument.**

D: No. This would weaken the author's (and Carter and Burke's) argument in the last paragraph that "The payoff of such 'slow and steady (and often boring)' legal procedures is that they help broker community peace, channeling hotly contested questions into a forum in which they can be more easily handled."

6. **A** This is a LEAST Weaken question.

For a LEAST Weaken (or Weaken EXCEPT) question, eliminate the answers that most weaken the relevant claims in the passage. The correct answer may (1) strengthen, (2) have no impact, or (3) weaken less than the other three. (The last of these three is rarely seen.) For this question, you are eliminating answers that indicate that the rule of law does NOT "set aside the 'dramatic and emotional work of poetics and theatrics'" by "commit[ting] the judiciary to the logic of ideas" (paragraph 8).

A: **Yes. This answer strengthens the relevant claim by providing more evidence that the rule of law entails excluding emotion and drama from the court.**

B: No. This would weaken the argument by suggesting that the influence of the court comes more through drama and theater than through "the logic of ideas."

C: No. This would weaken the argument by suggesting that the rule of law is unsuccessful at excluding emotion from the work of the court.

D: No. This would weaken the argument by suggesting that the rule of law is unsuccessful at committing the judiciary to the "logic of ideas," and that drama and theatrics have come to play a major role in judges' decision-making.

Passage VI: Application—New Information and Analogy Questions

Question Type Strategies

New Information questions

First, identify the theme of the new information in the question stem. Next, define if it is a New Information-Inference (Type I) or New Information-Strengthen/Weaken (Type II) question. Then define the relationship of the new information to the passage, and answer the question in your own words as best you can. Be on the lookout for wrong answers that correspond to the passage but not the new information, or that are consistent with the new information but inconsistent with the passage.

Analogy questions

First, identify the theme of the relevant part of the passage. Your goal is to generalize at this point and to get away from the precise content of the passage in order to find the more general logical theme of structure. Your goal is to find the best match in the choices; beware of answers that match the content but not the logic of the passage, or that match one part of it but not another.

1. **B**   This is an Analogy question.
    Paragraph 2 describes the logic of reciprocity as a "favor bank." That is, one person does something for another with the expectation that the favor will be returned later. The correct answer will have this theme.

    A: No. This choice is tempting because diamond trading is mentioned in the passage. Do not be fooled, however—remember that the answer choices to analogy questions will often contain new information, and they only rarely will reproduce the actual content or subject matter of the passage. Furthermore, this does not demonstrate the concept of reciprocity as described in paragraph 3: "I'll do this for you now, in the expectation that down the road you or someone else will return the favor."

    B: Yes. This choice most closely demonstrates the concept of "I'll do this for you now, in the expectation that down the road you or someone else will return the favor" (paragraph 3). Each parent who participates watches someone else's children with the expectation that they will also have their own children watched, when needed.

    C: No. This choice involves the government implementing something for the people, using the money gathered from taxing them. It does not demonstrate "I'll do this for you now, in the expectation that down the road you or someone else will return the favor."

    D: No. This choice involves two people mutually agreeing about assets before entering into marriage; as written, it does not demonstrate one of them doing something for the other now, with the expectation of payback later on.

2. **A**   This is an Analogy question.
    This question asks you to find the choice with the most similar relationship to the one established in the second paragraph: "...communities did not become civic simply because they were rich. The historical record strongly suggests precisely the opposite: They have become rich because they were civic." In other words, the best answer will demonstrate that civic engagement results in (and precedes) prosperity.

A: Yes. This choice describes employees who were civically involved (by participating in "after-hours collaborations and events outside of work") before their companies become prosperous. Of the four choices, this is the one that comes closest to suggesting that civic engagement contributed to wealth and prosperity (through facilitating team building and efficiency).

B: No. There is no indication in this choice whether the prosperity (large endowment) preceded the students' involvement in the community or vice versa.

C: No. This choice states that wealthy individuals donate generously to organizations; it does not demonstrate the relationship between civic engagement and wealth, as described in the second paragraph of the passage.

D: No. This choice is analogous to the relationship the author establishes about social capital in the final paragraph, not to the relationship between civic engagement and wealth as described in the second paragraph of the passage. This is an example of a "right answer, wrong question" Attractor.

3. **D** This is an Analogy question.
In the seventh paragraph, the author describes the accumulation of social capital: "Stocks of social capital, such as trust, norms, and networks, tend to be self-reinforcing and cumulative. Successful collaboration in one endeavor builds connections and trust—social assets that facilitate future collaboration in other, unrelated tasks. As with conventional capital, those who have social capital tend to accumulate more—'them as has, gets.'" Therefore, the correct answer will be a positive feedback loop (the more social capital you have, the more you get, therefore the more you will have, and so on).

A: No. This choice describes the decline of one thing (passionate love) as something else increases (companionate love); this choice does not describe a positive feedback cycle.

B: No. This choice states that peer reinforcement and parental punishment have differential impacts on adolescent behavior; this choice does not describe a positive feedback cycle.

C: No. This choice describes a negative feedback cycle: electricity generates heat, and as heat increases, it shuts off the source of the electricity, thereby reducing heat.

D: Yes. This choice describes a positive feedback cycle: as temperature rises and permafrost thaws, carbon dioxide and methane gases are released into the atmosphere, which will further increase the temperature and increase the melting of the permafrost, releasing more gases, and so on.

4. **C** This is an Analogy question in an EXCEPT/LEAST/NOT format.
The question asks you to take information from the fourth paragraph about how networks of civic engagement best operate and apply it to the examples given in the answers. The best choice will be the one that is least consistent with the information in paragraph 4.

A: No. Paragraph 4 states: "This is why the diamond trade, with its extreme possibilities for fraud, is concentrated within close-knit ethnic enclaves." This choice is consistent with the description of a network of civic engagement.

B: No. Paragraph 4 states: "Students of prisoners' dilemmas and related games report that cooperation is most easily sustained through repeat play." If a team is composed of people that have not played together before, it is consistent with the information in paragraph 4 that they would need more practice.

C: Yes. Paragraph 4 suggests that repeated interaction with the same people fosters trust. However, this choice suggests the opposite—that teams of people that are frequently changed "maximizes performance." This choice is the most inconsistent with what the passage says about networks of civic engagement in paragraph 4.

D: No. Paragraph 4 suggests that repeated interaction with the same people fosters trust; this choice implies something similar.

4.6

5. **D**   This is an Analogy question.
        At the end of the last paragraph, the author states: "Members of Florentine choral societies participate because they like to sing, not because their participation strengthens the Tuscan social fabric." Therefore, the author states that people engage in "civic participation" because they want to, not because they are consciously trying to "strengthen the…social fabric."
    A: No. There is no indication that this after-school study involves group or social activities, or that the students participate because they want to.
    B: No. This choice describes a situation wherein men join the military because they have no choice, not because they want to.
    C: No. This choice describes people who join a civic organization with the express purpose of contributing to the community. In the passage, the beneficial impact on society was a side effect of people joining an organization for their own enjoyment. Make sure that the answer you select matches the logic and theme of the relevant part of the passage.
    D: Yes. This choice is not perfect, but it is the closest of the four in describing a situation in which people participate in something because they want to, and not for any other reason. Make sure to look for and select the "least wrong" answer.

6. **B**   This is a Type 2 New Information/Strengthen question.
        This question provides the information that as a vehicle for civic engagement (Boy Scout and Girl Scout troops) grows, so does a community's wealth (median income). The author argues that civic engagement and wealth are positively correlated in paragraph 2.
    A: No. This new information is not directly relevant to the history of civic engagement.
    B: Yes. This new information provides an example that strengthens this claim made in the second paragraph.
    C: No. This new information does not suggest that coordination and communication are increased through participation in Boy Scouts/Girl Scouts; therefore, this claim is not directly strengthened by this new information.
    D: No. This new information does not suggest that trust is increased through participation in Boy Scouts/Girl Scouts or that it contributes to future endeavors; therefore, this claim is not directly strengthened by this new information.

7. **C**   This is a Type 2 New Information/Weaken question.
        This new information undermines that author's point made in the fourth paragraph that "dense social ties facilitate gossip and other valuable ways of cultivating reputation—an essential foundation for trust in a complex society."
    A: No. This new information does not have any impact on democracy (a concept that is also never addressed in this passage).
    B: No. While this answer choice is supported by the passage (paragraph 3: "A society that relies on generalized reciprocity is more efficient than a distrustful society"), it does not address the new information about gossip and its impact on trust and reputation. Therefore, this is not the best choice.
    C: Yes. The author states in paragraph 4: "dense social ties facilitate gossip and other valuable ways of cultivating reputation—an essential foundation for trust in a complex society." This new information essentially says the opposite (as gossip increases, trust and reputation decrease). Therefore, this is the best answer choice.
    D: No. Be wary of answer choices such as this one—the new information provided is applicable to the author's assertions about gossip in the fourth paragraph. Therefore, this is not an acceptable choice.

8. **B**   This is a Type 1 New Information question.

This new information suggests that civic engagement has decreased in the past 30 years. The author claims that civic engagement fosters economic development (paragraph 2); therefore a decline in one should result in a decline in the other.

A: No. This choice goes in the opposite direction. If anything, less civic involvement would be consistent with a decrease, not an increase, in organized protests.

B: Yes. Paragraph 2 states: "These communities did not become civic simply because they were rich. The historical record strongly suggests precisely the opposite: They have become rich because they were civic. The social capital embodied in norms and networks of civic engagement seems to be a precondition for economic development, as well as for effective government." Therefore, this is the most likely possible outcome of decreased civic engagement.

C: No. The passage never mentions "sociocultural awareness."

D: No. There is nothing to suggest that a decrease in "the number of Americans who attend public meetings or political rallies" would lead to an increase in participation in other activities. If anything, the new information would suggest that there would be a decrease in participation in other activities.

9. **C**   This is a Type 1 New Information question.

Since the passage mentions nothing about religion, this new information could be translated as saying that religious participation is the most common form of civic engagement today. Therefore, participation in religion can be viewed as "civic engagement," as described in the passage, when evaluating each answer choice.

A: No. There is no indication that civic engagement relies on government.

B: No. While participation in religion can be viewed as a form of civic engagement, which will increase social capital (according to the passage), there is not enough information in the question stem to suggest "active members of a religion have more social capital than those who are not religious." This question stem states that "religion is the most common associational membership among people;" it does not distinguish active from non-active participation, nor does it provide information about other forms of civic engagement (e.g., a non-religious person might engage in three other forms of civic engagement). This is not a logical conclusion from the new information and the passage text, and is not the best choice.

C: Yes. It is reasonable to infer, based on the passage, that membership in associations or organizations qualifies as a form of civic engagement.

D: No. Even though the author ties civic engagement to economic development, this is not a reasonable conclusion from the information provided in the question stem.

Chapter 4 Summary

Know the five steps you should take in answering any question:

1. Read the question carefully and identify the question type.

2. Translate the question into your own words.

3. Identify key words and phrases (when the question stem references a particular issue within the passage) and go back to the passage to find the relevant information.

4. Answer the question in your own words.

5. Use Process of Elimination.

Know the ten basic question types that you will encounter in MCAT CARS:

1. Retrieval

2. Inference

3. Main Idea/Primary Purpose

4. Tone/Attitude

5. Structure

6. Evaluate

7. Strengthen

8. Weaken

9. New Information

10. Analogy

Monitor your progress and improve your accuracy by keeping a Self-Evaluation Log.

CHAPTER 4 PRACTICE PASSAGES

Individual Passage Drills

Do the following two passages untimed. Use these passages to focus on answering the questions in your own words.

Get a stack of Post-it® Notes. Paste one over each set of answer choices, leaving the questions themselves visible. Work the passage as usual, but when it comes time to answer each question in your own words, write your answer on the Note. When finished answering each question in your own words, immediately lift up the Post-it® Note and use your answer as a guide, while actively using POE to eliminate choices that may sound similar but are flawed in some way.

Once you have completed the passages and checked your answers, fill out an Individual Passage Log for each passage.

In your self-evaluation, focus in particular on question types. Did you correctly identify the question type? Did you understand what the question was asking you to do? Did you apply the 5 Steps in a way that was appropriate for the question task? Which question types were easier and harder for you to complete and why? And, what kinds of Attractors did you fall for? Finally, how can you change your approach to answering questions to improve your accuracy and efficiency?

CHAPTER 4 PRACTICE PASSAGE 1

The language of efficiency, or cost-effectiveness, is all around us. We hear it everywhere, in our private lives as well as in public conversation. I recently read an advertisement in a local newspaper for a fully wired kitchen that would allow me to program my microwave and stove from the office simply by flicking a button on my handheld computer. By the time I reach home, dinner will be ready to eat. The alarm system will disengage as I reach the front door. "How efficient!" the ad proclaims in bold lettering.

But the ad misses, not by accident, I suspect, one crucial piece of information. It does not tell me *at what* this newly wired, very expensive kitchen will be efficient. At improving the quality of my food? At saving time? What, I worried, will I be expected to accomplish with the time saved? Is it legitimate to use the twenty minutes I might gain to read a novel I have been longing to read? Or am I expected to engage in "productive" work in the time I save? How will this time-saving kitchen improve my satisfaction? My welfare?

The seduction of efficiency is not restricted to the latest advances in labor-saving devices for the beleaguered working mother. The language of efficiency shapes our public as well as our private lives. Those who provide our public services are expected to do so efficiently. Physicians and nurses in the hospital where my mother was treated are expected to work efficiently. So are teachers, governments, and civil servants. They are constantly enjoined to become efficient, to remain efficient, and to improve their efficiency in the safeguarding of the public trust. Efficiency, or cost-effectiveness, has become an end in itself, a value often more important than others. But elevating efficiency, turning it into an end, misuses language, and this has profound consequences for the way we as citizens conceive of public life. When we define efficiency as an end, divorced from its larger purpose, it becomes nothing less than a cult.

Our public conversation about efficiency is misleading. Efficiency is only one part of a much larger public discussion between citizens and their governments. Efficiency is not an end, but a means to achieve valued ends. It is not a goal, but an instrument to achieve other goals. It is not a value, but a way to achieve other values. It is part of the story but never the whole.

Even when efficiency is used correctly as a means, when it is understood as the most cost-effective way to achieve our goals, much of our public discussion is fuzzy about its purpose. What does effectiveness mean? What, for example, is an effective education? To answer that question, we would first have to discuss the purposes of education, a discussion that is informed by values, and only then could we come to some understanding

of the criteria of effectiveness. At times, however, even the mention of effectiveness is absent, and the conversation slides over to focus only on costs. And when the public discussion of efficiency focuses only on costs, the cult becomes even stronger.

Yet the word "efficiency" is not only misused in public conversation as an end rather than a means. Our public conversation is not merely bedeviled by a simple technical error. The cult of efficiency, like other cults, advances political purposes and agendas. In our post-industrial age, efficiency is often a code word for an attack on the sclerotic, unresponsive, and anachronistic state, the detritus of the industrial age that fits poorly with our times. The state is branded as wasteful, and market mechanisms are heralded as the efficient alternative. This argument, we shall see, is based on a fundamental misunderstanding of the importance of the "smart" state in the global, knowledge-based economy.

Material used in this particular passage has been adapted from the following source:
J. G. Stein, *The Cult of Efficiency*. © 2001 by House of Anansi Press.

1. The author draws an important distinction between:

    A) goals and the ways those goals are accomplished.
    B) efficient and inefficient technology.
    C) representative and misleading advertising.
    D) public and private dialogues about efficiency.

2. The author suggests which of the following to be true of cults?

    A) They can influence society at large.
    B) They promote illogical and unreasonable beliefs.
    C) They are simply groups of like-minded individuals.
    D) They are usually organized around a focus on costs.

3. The author most likely supports a view of government as an institution that:

    A) finds the most cost-effective ways to provide for society's needs.
    B) is wasteful and fits poorly with our times.
    C) has an important role to play in the modern economy.
    D) is not as efficient as market mechanisms.

4. Suppose a public school board were to demand teachers use fewer hours to prepare instruction so that the school board can save money. In response, the author would most likely:

A) praise the board for striving to find more efficient ways to deliver services.

B) support the board's commitment to quality education.

C) withhold judgment and suggest the decision be considered within a larger context.

D) criticize the school board for undermining public education.

Inference

5. Which of the following assertions about language is LEAST supported by the passage?

A) Language has the power to shape how citizens think about their relationships with each other and government.

B) Language can be misused to advance political agendas.

C) Vague language sometimes leaves out important information.

D) Government uses language to mislead us in the public conversation about efficiency. P4

new info!

6. Elsewhere, the author writes in more detail about public hospitals in Canada. Based on the information in the passage, these hospitals are most likely:

A) offering a lower standard of care than private hospitals do.

B) unable to afford efficient, time-saving technology.

C) under pressure to provide better care without increased resources.

D) overly focused on costs rather than patient care.

7. Throughout the passage, the author suggests which of the following to be true of efficiency?

A) It is a deceptively attractive idea.

B) It is the foundation of a well-run state.

C) It is just as important to public life as to private life.

D) It is never a worthy goal.

way

CHAPTER 4 PRACTICE PASSAGE 2

Three basic positions have prevailed on the debate over the Voting Rights Act, distinguished largely by their different views on whether the Act should be rolled back, pushed forward, or simply maintained. Given these differences in orientation, these ideological responses to the act can be called conservative, progressive, and centrist. The conflicting claims of conservatives and progressives set the outer limits of debate, making discussion of minority representation a sharply contested and exceedingly polarized affair. In such a context of mutually exclusive assertions, the centrist attempt to strike a reasonable balance appears immediately appealing.

On the whole, while conservatives and progressives are united in their rejection of the status quo, they diverge sharply in their reasons for seeking change. Where conservatives see a politics that has been held hostage to the demands of civil rights elites, progressives describe a politics increasingly dominated by white racism and retrenchment. It is in this polarized context of claims and counterclaims that the centrists attempt to fashion a reasonable middle position. Dismissing both conservative and progressive claims as exaggerated rhetoric, centrists argue that the debate over the Voting Rights Act is actually quite narrow. While name calling and finger pointing have drawn the lion's share of attention, centrists claim that most of the disputants are actually concerned with achieving a color-blind society. Beneath the barbed polemics, controversies over minority representation amount to a disagreement over means rather than ends. Bernard Grofman and Chandler Davis suggest that the "highly abstract" mode of the current debate only breeds misunderstanding and conflict; a better approach is to be found in a "consideration of the empirical evidence of the actual consequences of the [Voting Rights Act]."

In the centrist view, then, the Voting Rights Act is neither a racially balkanizing nor a broadly empowering document. In essence, the act takes limited steps to ameliorate specific and concrete inequities. The incrementalist, case-by-case nature of voting-rights policy means that remedial measures can be crafted without raising larger issues of democratic theory. Big questions such as "What is fair minority representation?" never need to be asked because judges and other federal officials are simply correcting what is obviously wrong given the specific facts at hand.

What can be made of the centrist attempt to steer a middle course between conservative and progressive claims? Centrists make the claim for a responsive political process largely by insisting that the incrementalism of voting rights policy avoids theoretical questions. The very realism and reasonableness of the Voting Rights Act inheres in its atheoretical design. Thus, the centrist argument amounts to more than a simple

corrective of exaggerated views. If the centrists are right, the entire polarized debate between conservatives and progressives should be set aside as a distraction. We will do just fine if the country and the courts continue to muddle through the issue of minority representation a case at a time.

One could argue that so long as the Supreme Court is effectively constrained by its own canons of statutory construction, voting-rights reform need not plunge into any conceptual morass. The difficulty with such an argument is that the judiciary has historically employed a number of canons, many of which point interpretation in different directions. It is true that some legal commentators have spoken of the judge "worth his salt" or with the right "sense of the situation" who can negotiate among the various canons, consistently producing an accurate rendering of the statute's meaning or purpose. Despite such claims, widespread consensus on what should count as the proper "sense of the situation" has not emerged. Easy agreement has proved elusive because the choice between interpretive strategies itself depends on what Cass Sunstein calls "background principles" —principles that express particular visions of how government ought to operate and, thus, provide the baseline against which statutes should be understood.

In general, one can say that the process of statutory interpretation is critically concerned with normative disputes over how the government ought to operate. By stressing measurable facts and hard evidence, the centrist argument as a whole sidesteps the debate's key issue. The progressive and conservative views are not simply "mistakes" that can be corrected by a more accurate set of facts. Each of these camps anchors its claims in different conceptions of fair representation, which serve as guides for how the Voting Rights Act's promise of equal political opportunity ought to be realized. Thus, conservatives and progressives do not simply disagree on what the "facts" of the debate are. More importantly, they disagree on what the same "facts" mean in light of what fair minority representation is taken to be.

Material used in this particular passage has been adapted from the following source:

K. Bybee, *Mistaken Identity: The Supreme Court and the Politics of Minority Representation.* © 1998 by Princeton University Press.

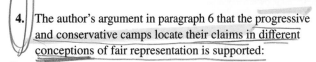

1. Which of the following statements best expresses the main thesis of the passage?

A) Three positions have emerged in the debate over the Voting Rights Act, which may be labeled progressive, centrist, and conservative.

B) While imperfect, the centrist approach is the most reasonable, given that it avoids the ideological extremes embodied in the conservative and progressive positions and that it advocates a case-by-case evaluation of the impact of the Voting Rights Act.

C) The centrist position on the Voting Rights Act, while seemingly a pragmatic middle road between two extremes, fails to address the theoretical issues that underlie questions of minority representation.

D) While the conservative and progressive positions on the Voting Rights Act both seek significant change, the centrist position prefers a more incrementalist approach.

2. The author refers to commentators who speak of judges with the correct "sense of the situation" in order to:

A) illustrate a way in which a common understanding of basic principles of fair representation might be reached.

B) raise and then challenge a consideration that might be used to support the centrist approach.

C) criticize judges for arriving at overly personal solutions to complex theoretical problems.

D) support the claim that the Voting Rights Act turns on the contestable issue of "equal political opportunity."

3. Suppose it were shown that progressives believe fair representation of a minority group can only by achieved through electing representatives who are members of that group, while conservatives believe that minority interests are well protected by any representative who works for the good of society as a whole. If this is true, which claim described in the passage would be most _undermined_?

A) The author's claim that background principles determine how facts are interpreted

B) The conservative claim that the Voting Rights Act should be rolled back

C) The centrist claim that application of the Voting Rights Act need not consider big abstract questions

D) The progressive claim that politics is dominated by white racism

4. The author's argument in paragraph 6 that the progressive and conservative camps locate their claims in different conceptions of fair representation is supported:

A) weakly, because no descriptions or examples of these different concepts are provided.

B) weakly, because this claim conflicts with the centrist argument that the Voting Rights Act is atheoretical.

C) strongly, because it is based on Sunstein's conception of "background principles."

D) strongly, because it implies that the same facts may be interpreted in different ways by different people.

5. In the context of the passage, "incrementalism" (paragraph 4) most likely refers to a policy that:

A) causes fundamental societal change.

B) considers problems on a case-by-case basis.

C) is concerned with achieving a color-blind society.

D) takes a step-by-step approach to reaching agreement on basic theoretical principles.

6. Which of the following would be most analogous to the centrist approach, as it is described in the passage?

correcting what is wrong

A) A physicist who seeks to reconcile two competing theories by finding a middle ground that incorporates aspects of both

B) A physicist who draws on a new field of theoretical mathematics in order to address a longstanding dispute within the field

C) A physicist who delineates three distinct approaches to solving a problem and evaluates their relative strengths and weaknesses

D) A physicist who suggests that a significant experimental discrepancy can be addressed without major reworking of present theories

7. Which of the following, if true, would most support the author's evaluation of the centrist position?

A) Different ideas of what constitutes fair representation are inextricably bound up with differing ideas about the proper role of the state within society.

B) Controversy about how to delineate electoral districts in order to ensure fair representation is often based on disagreements about population statistics.

C) The original writers of the Voting Rights Act did not believe that the implementation of the act would require debate on abstract questions of principle.

D) The conflicting claims set out by progressives and conservatives differ more in terms of vocabulary than on the basic ideas intended to be expressed through the rhetoric employed by each side.

SOLUTIONS TO CHAPTER 4 PRACTICE PASSAGE 1

1. **A**   This is an Inference question.
    - **A:** **Yes. See paragraph 4: "Efficiency is not an end, but a means to achieve valued ends." This answer choice uses different words to refer to "ends" and "means," and this distinction is central to the author's main idea about efficiency.**
    - B: No. While the example of the automated kitchen in paragraph 1 does introduce the idea of efficient technology, the author does not explicitly describe a distinction between different types of technology.
    - C: No. The author does suggest in paragraph 2 that the advertisement referred to in paragraph 1 is intentionally vague—"But the ad misses, not by accident, I suspect, one crucial piece of information"—but no distinction is drawn between different types of advertising.
    - D: No. See paragraph 3: "The language of efficiency shapes our public as well as our private lives." This suggests our public and private views of efficiency are similar, rather than distinct.

2. **A**   This is an Inference question.
    - **A:** **Yes. In paragraph 6, the author says, "The cult of efficiency, like other cults, advances political purposes and agendas." Advancing a political purpose entails making an impact on the political conversation. Cults, as the author defines them, therefore can influence society.**
    - B: No. Be sure to choose answers that are supported by the passage text. This choice is a common-sense view of cults that is not expressed in the passage. The author does not go so far as to call the cult of efficiency "illogical."
    - C: No. The author uses the word "cult" in the context of describing how the "cult of efficiency" "misuses language" in a way that "has profound consequences for the way we as citizens conceive of public life" (paragraph 3). She also writes that the "cult of efficiency, like other cults, advances political purposes and agendas" (paragraph 6). To label cults as *simply* groups of people who agree with each other would be inconsistent with the author's tone.
    - D: No. This choice uses language that is too absolute. The "cult of efficiency" may be based on a discussion of costs, but the passage does not apply this idea to other cults.

3. **C**   This is an Inference question.
    - A: No. The author discusses the value of government in paragraph 6, but does not say that its value lies in cost-effectiveness.
    - B: No. This is the view of "the cult of efficiency" as described in paragraph 6, which the author says "is based on a fundamental misunderstanding of the importance of the 'smart' state in the global, knowledge-based economy."
    - **C:** **Yes. See paragraph 6: "The state is branded as wasteful, and market mechanisms are heralded as the efficient alternative. This argument, we shall see, is based on a fundamental misunderstanding of the importance of the 'smart' state in the global, knowledge-based economy." The author believes the state is still relevant.**
    - D: No. The author defends the value of the state in paragraph 6. While the passage doesn't indicate that the government is as efficient as the market (the author rejects efficiency as a valid stand-alone standard of judgment), neither does the author indicate that it is less efficient.

4. **C**   This is a New Information question.
    - A: No. See paragraph 4: "Efficiency...is not a goal, but an instrument to achieve other goals." The author would not necessarily see cutting costs as an important goal in its own right for the school board.

B: No. In the passage, the author argues that efficiency in and of itself does not equate with quality: "Efficiency is not an end, but a means to achieve valued ends" (paragraph 4). In paragraph 5, the author writes: "What, for example, is an effective education? To answer that question, we would first have to discuss the purposes of education, a discussion that is informed by values, and only then could we come to some understanding of the criteria of effectiveness." Therefore, the author would not automatically equate saving money with quality education (more likely, the opposite).

C: **Yes. Consider paragraph 5: "Even when efficiency is used correctly as a means, when it is understood as the most cost-effective way to achieve our goals, much of our public discussion is fuzzy about its purpose. What does effectiveness mean? What, for example, is an effective education?" So, any discussion of the merits of cutting costs depends on a larger discussion of the *goals* of cutting costs. Thus, this is the author's most likely response.**

D: No. The author's main idea is that efficiency should be used as a means rather than an end, but this answer takes that idea too far by implying the author is opposed to the idea of efficiency (in education) altogether.

5. **D** This is an Inference/EXCEPT question.

A: No. This assertion is supported in paragraph 3: "The language of efficiency shapes our public as well as our private lives." In paragraph 6, the author specifically discusses how the language of efficiency relates to and affects our view of the state.

B: No. This assertion is supported in paragraph 6: "Yet the word 'efficiency' is not only misused in public conversation as an end rather than a means.... The cult of efficiency, like other cults, advances political purposes and agendas." Since the former statement is the author's opinion and the latter the explanation of that opinion, it is reasonable to infer that the cult of efficiency misuses the term.

C: No. In paragraphs 1 and 2, the author states that the phrase "How efficient!" intentionally obscures "one crucial piece of information. It does not tell me *at what* this newly wired, very expensive kitchen will be efficient."

D: **Yes. The passage does not suggest the government itself uses language to mislead. Thus, this is the correct choice.**

6. **C** This is a New Information question.

A: No. The author does not compare public and private hospitals.

B: No. Technology is the subject of paragraphs 1 and 2, not paragraph 3 in which the author discusses the state of hospitals and other publicly funded institutions. There is no evidence in the passage that public hospitals are unable to afford any particular type of technology, only that they are under pressure to be cost-effective.

C: **Yes. See paragraph 3: "Those who provide our public services are expected to do so efficiently. Physicians and nurses in the hospital where my mother was treated are expected to work efficiently.... They are constantly enjoined to become efficient, to remain efficient, and to improve their efficiency in the safeguarding of the public trust." This answer choice paraphrases the idea that hospitals and their employees are under pressure to be more efficient. We are not told what country the author is writing about in the passage; however, this choice represents a reasonable (compared to the other choices) analogy to draw, even if the author is not discussing Canada in the passage text.**

D: No. The author describes the demands placed on public services from the outside. The hospital's own focus is outside the scope of the argument. This choice is also too extreme; the existence of pressure to reduce costs does not necessarily guarantee that costs have taken precedence over patient care within the hospital itself.

7.   **A**   This is an Inference question.
A: **Yes. In paragraph 1, the example of the ad illustrates that efficiency is attractive. In paragraph 2, the author then explains this promise lacks substance. In paragraph 3, she refers to this advertisement process as a "seduction," a process based on attraction.**
B: No. On one hand, the author does say efficiency is important. In paragraph 4, she says it can be "used correctly as a means...to achieve our goals." However, the author also states in the same paragraph that "Efficiency is only one part of a much larger public discussion between citizens and their governments." That is, it would be one means (perhaps among many) to a goal of a well-run state, whatever "well-run" might mean in context.
C: No. The passage makes no comparison between the importance of efficiency itself in public and private life (only that the *language* of efficiency is used in both).
D: No. This is too extreme; it is inconsistent with the author's argument that efficiency can be an important means to an end (paragraph 4).

SOLUTIONS TO CHAPTER 4 PRACTICE PASSAGE 2

1.   **C**   This is a Main Idea/Primary Purpose question.
A: No. This choice is too narrow to be the correct answer to a Main Idea question. While the statement is supported by the passage, it leaves out the heart of the author's argument, which is his evaluation of the validity (or lack thereof) of the centrist position.
B: No. This choice misrepresents the author's opinion. While the author does state that "the centrists attempt to fashion a reasonable middle position" (paragraph 2), and that their position "appears immediately appealing" (paragraph 1), the author argues in paragraphs 5–6 that this position is fundamentally flawed in its assumption that discussion and implementation of the Voting Rights Act can avoid theoretical discussion. Always make sure to take the entire passage into account for a general question and to clearly define the author's opinion.
C: **Yes. After discussing the three positions in paragraphs 1–4, the author argues that the centrists are fundamentally wrong in their assertion that the act can be understood or implemented without confronting abstract issues: for example, what constitutes fair representation. The author's tone is clear in phrases such as "The difficulty with such an argument" and "The centrist position as a whole sidesteps."**
D: No. As in choice A, this answer is supported by the passage (paragraphs 1 and 2), but is too narrow to be the main thesis of the passage. For example, it leaves out the author's negative evaluation of the centrist position.

2.   **B**   This is a Structure question.
A: No. The author suggests the opposite. He states: "Despite such claims, widespread consensus on what should count as the proper 'sense of the situation' has not emerged" (paragraph 5). Furthermore, the commentators themselves are not referring to judges who achieve a common understanding of basic principles, but rather to those who supposedly can come to an accurate understanding of the meaning or purpose of a statute (and how to apply it to a particular case).

B: Yes. A centrist might use the argument that abstract principles need not be considered by voting-rights reform because judges are able "negotiate among the various canons" to interpret and apply statutes without relying on theoretical interpretation. The author goes on to say that this is not in fact the case, because deciding how to interpret a statute requires choosing between basic principles regarding "how the government ought to operate" (paragraph 6). Notice that the author introduces the example of these judges with "it is true that," and that the following sentence begins with "Despite such claims." These phrases indicate that the point of view referenced in the question stem tends to challenge the author's overall position.

C: No. There is no criticism of the judges themselves expressed by the author. The implied criticism is of the commentators who make this argument about judges. Also, the problem identified by the author isn't that their approach is too "personal," but rather that it cannot in fact avoid theoretical issues.

D: No. This is the wrong issue. While the author does reference this argument in paragraph 5, the discussion of judges in that paragraph does not itself give evidence that the act depends or hinges on the particular contestable issue of "equal political opportunity."

3.　**C**　This is a New Information question.

　Note: The new information suggests a disagreement about what constitutes fair representation. This, if valid, would undermine the centrist claim that "Big questions such as 'What is fair minority representation?' never need to be asked because judges and other federal officials are simply correcting what is obviously wrong given the specific facts at hand" (paragraph 3). And, by undermining the centrists, it strengthens the author's critique of the centrist position.

A: No. This new information would strengthen rather than weaken the author's position.

B: No. This new information has no impact on the conservative position. The fact that there are different conceptions of fair representation does not by itself suggest that the act is something that should be maintained or extended rather than rolled back.

C: Yes. The centrist claim that abstract questions do not need to be considered rests in part on their belief that most people agree on basic principles, and that there can be wide agreement on what is "obviously wrong given the specific facts at hand" (paragraph 3). If there is in fact disagreement on what constitutes fair representation, this would weaken or undermine the centrist position. Note that the author states in paragraph 6 that "Each of these camps anchors its claims in different conceptions of fair representation, which serve as guides for how the Voting Rights Act's promise of equal political opportunity ought to be realized." This suggests that the very different ways of conceiving of "fair representation" described in the question stem would qualify as different ends or principles, not just different means.

D: No. The new information gives no evidence one way or the other about the existence or role of white racism in the political process.

4.　**A**　This is an Evaluate question.

A: Yes. This statement is weakly supported. The author makes the claim but gives no supportive evidence to prove the claim. We don't know what those different conceptions are, or how significantly they might differ.

B: No. The first word of the choice is correct, but the rest of it is incorrect. The entire point of the passage is largely to disprove the centrist argument. Simply conflicting with an opposing position is not itself a weakness.

C: No. While the claim cited in the question follows from the discussion of Sunstein's idea (paragraph 5), the concept of the existence of background principles does not itself support the claim that conservatives and progressives have different concepts of fair representation.

D: No. The second part of the choice is accurate (see paragraph 6), but the evaluation ("strongly") is incorrect. This choice essentially reverses the relationship between parts of the argument. The implication of a claim (that is, the conclusion based on it) does not itself provide support for the claim.

5. **B**   This is an Inference question.
   A: No. This is the opposite of what the term expresses in the context of the centrist view. The centrists, who advocate the incrementalist view, believe that application of the act on a case-by-case basis entails simply correcting mistakes on a relatively small scale.
   B: **Yes. "Incrementalism" is essentially defined in the previous paragraph: "The incrementalist, case-by-case nature of voting-rights policy means that remedial measures can be crafted without raising larger issues of democratic theory."**
   C: No. This describes what the centrists believe to be true of most people (paragraph 2), but does not define incrementalism itself.
   D: No. This choice is half-right but half-wrong. Yes, it is a step-by-step approach, but not to reaching agreement on theoretical principles. The centrists (who are identified with incrementalism in the passage) believe that this agreement has already been reached (see paragraph 2).

6. **D**   This is an Analogy question.
   Note: The correct answer will be the one that is most logically similar to the centrist view or approach. In the passage, the author states that according to the centrists, "the act takes limited steps to ameliorate specific and concrete inequities" (paragraph 3), that "Big questions such as 'What is fair minority representation?' never need to be asked because judges and other federal officials are simply correcting what is obviously wrong given the specific facts at hand" (paragraph 3), and that "We will do just fine if the country and the courts continue to muddle through the issue of minority representation a case at a time" (paragraph 4).
   A: No. This choice is immediately attractive because it mentions a middle ground. However, the centrists aren't trying to get the progressives and conservatives to come to some new agreement through compromise. Rather, the centrists argue that there is already basic agreement or mutual understanding on what is fair, and it's just a practical issue of how to achieve that in particular cases.
   B: No. The centrists do make use of any new theory or outside discipline.
   C: No. Although the passage delineates three positions, the question asks for an analogy to the approach of the centrists, not of author of the passage.
   D: **Yes. This choice is analogous to the author's description of the centrists as seeking to focus on a case-by-case approach that does not require engaging deep theoretical questions.**

7.   A   This is a Strengthen question.

A: Yes. In paragraphs 5 and 6, the author critiques the centrist position in part by arguing that agreement on how to apply statutes requires agreement on "background principles" about "how government ought to operate"(that is, the proper role of the state in society). He goes on to say that this means that because each camp has a different idea of what "fair representation" means, they disagree on abstract issues of principle regarding how to interpret "facts." The author, however, never directly states that, or explains how, the operation of government relates to fair representation. If the two are in fact fundamentally interrelated, it would support the author's critique of the centrists' claim that there is no fundamental disagreement on principles within the Voting Rights Act debate.

B: No. This would support the centrists themselves, by suggesting that at least some of the debate is about facts or empirical questions (here, statistics), rather than about matters of principle.

C: No. To the extent that the intent or belief of the writers of the act is relevant, this would go against the author's interpretation.

D: No. This would weaken the author's argument by supporting the centrist claim. This choice suggests that the disagreement between progressives and conservatives is not as stark as it may seem, and there is a fair amount of basic agreement on basic ideas.

Individual Passage Log

Passage # _____

Q#	Q type	Attractors	What did you do wrong?

Revised Strategy _____

Passage # _____

Q#	Q type	Attractors	What did you do wrong?

Revised Strategy _____

Think Like a Test-Writer: Exercise 2

THINK LIKE A TEST-WRITER: EXERCISE 2

There are certain kinds of statements in passage texts that tend to generate questions: transitions, comparisons and contrasts, expressions of the author's opinion or the opinions of others, example indicators, etc. In the passage text on the next page, some of these "question generators" are in red text and some of those are numbered. The purpose of the drill is to sensitize yourself to the kinds of things in passages that the test-writers use to create questions and the right answers to those questions (and attractive wrong answers as well). [Note: the computer-based testing tools do not allow you to change the color of the text, and there will be no red text in your MCAT passages. The red font here is only for the purpose of the drill. The questions attached to a CARS passage on the test will also not usually be presented in the order in which the relevant material appears in the test.]

First, read the entire passage. When you see red text, pay special attention to that part of the passage. Note the logical function and importance of that segment in the context of the paragraph and, as you read further, in the context of the passage as a whole. A series of numbered MCAT CARS-like questions connected to the corresponding number in the text are provided at the end of the passage. Answer the questions in your own words, going back to those parts of the passage as needed, and then check the explanations that follow.

The text on the next page is longer than a CARS passage in order to give you extra practice with these skills.

EXERCISE 2

In 1552, Francisco López de Gómara, who had been chaplain and secretary to Hernando Cortés while he lived out his old age in Spain, published an account of the conquest of Mexico. López de Gómara himself had never been to the New World, but he could envision it nonetheless. "Many [Indians] came to gape at the strange men, now so famous, and at their attire, arms and horses, and they said, "these men are gods!" [Q1] The chaplain was one of the first to claim in print that the Mexicans had believed the conquistadors to be divine. Among the welter of statements made in the Old World about inhabitants of the New, this one found particular resonance. It was repeated with enthusiasm, and soon a specific version gained credence: the Mexicans had apparently believed in a god called Quetzalcoatl, who long ago had disappeared in the east, promising to return from that direction on a certain date. In an extraordinary coincidence, Cortés appeared off the coast in that very year and was mistaken for Quetzalcoatl by the devout. Today, most educated persons in the United States, Europe, and Latin America are fully versed in this account, as readers of this piece can undoubtably affirm. In fact, however, there is little evidence that the indigenous people ever seriously believed the newcomers were gods, and there is no meaningful evidence that any story about Quetzalcoatl's returning from the east ever existed before the conquest. A number of scholars of early Mexico are aware of this, but few others are. The cherished narrative is alive and well, and in urgent need of critical attention.

In order to dismantle a construct with such a long history, it will be necessary first to explain the origins and durability of the myth and then to offer an alternate explanation of what happened in the period of conquest and what the indigenous were actually thinking. In proposing an alternative, I will make three primary assertions: first, that we must put technology in all its forms— beyond mere weaponry—front and center in our story of conquest; [Q2] second, that we can safely do this because new evidence from scientists offers us explanations for divergent technological levels that have nothing to do with differences in intelligence; and third, that the Mexicans themselves immediately became aware of the technology gap and responded to it with intelligence and savvy rather than wide-eyed talk of gods. They knew before we did, it seems, that technology was the crux. ...

Our first task must be to ask ourselves whence came the myths associated with the conquest. The simple truth is that, by the 1550s, some [Indigenous people] were themselves saying that they (or rather, their parents) had presumed the white men to be gods. ... [Q3] Numerous scholars have analyzed these words while ignoring their context. The best known such work is Tzvetan Todorov's *Conquest of America: The Question of the Other.* Although quick to say there is no "natural inferiority" (indeed, he [Q4] aptly pointed out that it is the [Indigenous people] who rapidly learn the language of the Spanish, not the other way around), he insists that it is the Spaniards' greater deftness in manipulating signs that gives them victory. While the Spanish believe in man-man communication ("What are we to do?"), the [Indigenous people] only envision man-world communication ("How are we to know?"). Thus the [Indigenous people] have a "paralyzing belief that the Spaniards are gods" and are "inadequate in a situation requiring improvisation." Popular historians have been equally quick to accept this idea of indigenous reality, often with the best intentions. Hugh Thomas's recent monumental 800-page volume is a case in point. Thomas uses apocryphal accounts as if they had been tape-recorded conversations in his portrayal of the inner workings of Moctezuma's court. ... Thomas does this, I believe, not out of naïveté but out of a genuine desire to incorporate the [Indigenous] perspective. He does not want to describe the intricate politics of the Spanish while leaving the [Indigenous] side vague, rendering it less real to his readers.

With such friends, though, perhaps the indigenous and their cultural heirs do not need enemies. A different approach is definitely needed, or the white gods will continue to inhabit our narratives. And beginning anew, let us first ask what sources we have available. We in fact have only one set of documents that were undoubtedly written at the time of conquest by someone who was certainly there—the letters of Cortés. The *Cartas* are masterful constructions [Q5], loaded with political agendas, but we are at least certain of their origin, and Cortés never wrote that he was taken for a god....

[Another] group of sources were produced by the indigenous themselves, but here is the heart of the problem: we have none that date from the years of conquest or even from the 1520s or 1530s. There are sixteen surviving pre-conquest codices (none from Mexico City itself, where the conquerors' book burning was most intense), and then, dating from the 1540s, statements written in Nahuatl using the Roman alphabet, which was then rapidly becoming accessible to educated indigenous through the school of Tlatelolco. The most famous such document about the conquest is the lengthy Book Twelve of the Florentine Codex. Although it was organized by Sahagún, and the Spanish glosses were written by him, the Nahuatl is the work of his Indian aides. [In addition,] at the end of the century, a few indigenous men wrote histories. …

These, then, are the rather limited documents we have to work with.… It is in this context that we must approach the later understanding that the Aztecs were convinced that their own omens had for years been predicting the coming of the cataclysm, [Q6] and that Cortés was recognized as Quetzalcoatl and the Europeans as gods. The most important source for all these legends is Book Twelve of the Florentine Codex. Lockhart notes that it reads very much as if it were two separate documents: the first part, covering the period from the sighting of the European sails to the Spaniards' violent attack on warrior-dancers participating in a religious festival, reads like an apocryphal fable (complete with comets as portents), while the second part, covering the period from the Aztec warriors' uprising against the Spaniards after the festival to their ultimate defeat over a year later, reads like a military archivist's record of events. Indeed, this phenomenon makes sense: the old men being interviewed in the 1550s would likely have participated as young warriors in the battles against the Spanish, or at least have been well aware of what was transpiring. On the other hand, they would most certainly not have been privy to the debates within Moctezuma's inner circle when the Spaniards arrival first became known: the king's closest advisers were killed in the conquest, and at any rate would have been older men even in 1520.

Still, the fact that the informants for the Florentine were not acquainted with the inner workings of Moctezuma's court only proves that they were unlikely to have the first part of the story straight; it tells us nothing about why they chose to say what they did. It seems likely that they retroactively sought to find particular auguries associated with the conquest. The Florentine's omens do not appear to have been commonly accepted, as

they do not appear in other Nahuatl sources. Interestingly, Fernandez-Armesto notes that the listed omens fall almost exactly in line with certain Greek and Latin texts that are known to have been available to Sahagún's students.

Why would Sahagún's assistants have been so eager to come up with a compelling narrative about omens? [Q6] We must bear in mind that they were the sons and grandsons of Tenochtitlan's most elite citizens—descendants of priests and nobles. It was their own class, even their own family members, who might have been thought to be at fault if it were true that they had had no idea that the Spaniards existed prior to their arrival. … It begins to seem not merely unsurprising, but indeed necessary, that Sahagún's elite youths should insist that their forebears had read the signs and had known what was to happen. In their version, the Truth was paralyzing and left their forebears vulnerable, even more so than they might have been.

The idea that Cortés was understood to be the god Quetzalcoatl returning from the east is also presented as fact in Book Twelve. Moctezuma sends gifts for different gods, to see which are most welcome to the newcomers, and then decides it is Quetzalcoatl who has come. There are numerous obvious problems with the story. First, Quetzalcoatl was not a particularly prominent god in the pantheon worshiped in Mexico's great city. The one city in the empire where Quetzalcoatl was prominent, Cholula, was the only one to mount a concerted attack against Cortés as he made his way to the Aztec capital. Many aspects of the usual post-conquest description of Quetzalcoatl—that he was a peace-loving god who abhorred human sacrifice, for example—are obviously European mythological constructs, thus rendering the whole story somewhat suspect. Furthermore, in the Codex itself, when the earlier explorer Juan de Grijalva lands on the coast in 1518, [Q7] he is taken to be Quetzalcoatl. So much for the explanation that Cortés happened to land in the right year, causing all the pieces to fall into place in the indigenous imagination.

——Adapted from "Burying the White Gods: New Perspectives on the Conquest of Mexico," by Camilla Townsend. *The American Historical Review,* Vol. 108, No. 3. © 2003 by Oxford University Press on behalf of the American Historical Association.

Question #1: Why does the author state that López de Gómara's account "found particular resonance" and "was repeated with enthusiasm"?

_____

_____

_____

Question #2: What can you infer from the author's statement that "we can safely [focus on the role of technology] because new evidence from scientists offers us explanations for divergent technological levels that have nothing to do with differences in intelligence"?

_____

_____

_____

Question #3: What "context" is the author referring to when she writes "Numerous scholars have analyzed these words while ignoring their context" in the third paragraph?

_____

_____

_____

Question #4: What is the author's attitude toward Todorov's work?

_____

_____

_____

Question #5: Why does the author call Cortés's letters "masterful"?

_____

_____

_____

Question #6: Suppose it were shown to be true that both the Spaniards (during their conquest of the New World) and Aztec elites (after conquest) propagated the "white god" myth. Based on the passage, could you infer that they had the same motives in promoting such similar stories?

_____

_____

_____

Question #7: Is the story of Juan de Grijalva consistent or inconsistent with the author's argument regarding the causal factors entailed in the conquest of Mexico presented earlier in the passage?

_____

_____

_____

Bonus question: What is the Primary Purpose of the passage as a whole?

_____

_____

_____

SOLUTIONS TO EXERCISE 2

1. Note that in the beginning of the passage, it at first appears that the author might agree with the story that "the Mexicans had believed the conquistadors to be divine." Remember, however, that just because the author says that other people believe something to be true doesn't by itself mean that the author agrees. Keep an open mind, read on, and you discover that the author makes these statements to indicate that this story is *widely believed, but false*. The author's true position begins to become clear with the phrase "In fact, however…" later in that same paragraph.

2. There are at least two main things that you can infer from this statement. First, and most straightforwardly, the author believes that technology, NOT belief in the divinity of the Spaniards (note the phrase "and then to offer an alternate explanation of what happened" that precedes the cited claim) played a key role in the conquest of Mexico by Spain. Secondly, the author does NOT believe that difference in intelligence played a role in that conquest; she states that we can "safely" focus on technology *because* it has "nothing to do with differences in intelligence."

3. The context being referred to here (paragraph 3) doesn't become fully clear until later in the passage. It is only in paragraph 7 that we learn that the writings of indigenous people regarding the conquest may have been affected by the desire to absolve their predecessors of blame for not understanding the threat presented by the Spaniards. Just as the author emphasizes the importance of context, you must take the full context of the passage, in this case a paragraph much later in the passage, into account when answering this question.

4. The author does say some good things about Todorov: he "*aptly* pointed out that it is the [Indigenous people] who rapidly learn the language of the Spanish…" Meaning, he was correct to do so. As with Thomas, the author does not ascribe bad motives, just the opposite: Thomas did what he did "not out of naïveté but out of a genuine desire to incorporate the [Indigenous] perspective." However, the author of the passage is using Todorov and Thomas as examples of writers who, despite their good intentions, get it wrong by buying into the story that conquest was facilitated by the Aztec's belief in the divinity of Cortés and his men. Therefore, while the author is not condemning Todorov, she is certainly critical of his claims. This negative tone is reinforced by the first sentence of the next paragraph: "With such friends, though, perhaps the indigenous and their cultural heirs do not need enemies."

5. Again, context is key. Taken by itself, the word "masterful" sounds very positive. Here, however, the author's point is that they were written at least in part for political purposes (and that Cortés did a very good job of that). The author isn't making a major point of praising Cortés's political acumen, but neither is she criticizing it. The relevant issue is that while Cortés may not have been writing with the goal of providing a fully honest portrayal of the events, his writings do have some value ("we are at least certain of their origin") as they provide more evidence that Cortés was not seen as a god by the Aztecs. You have to be careful not to over-interpret the word "masterful" or to apply it to the wrong issue in the passage.

6. Paragraphs 6-8 provide an extended discussion of indigenous sources, what they did and did not report, and how they give evidence that the Aztecs themselves asserted the truth of the "white god" explanation for their own conquest. However, while the stories are the same, the

passage indicates that their motives would be very different. The Spaniards may have promoted the story to aid in conquest of the New World, while the Aztecs told it to save or rehabilitate the reputation of their family members. Therefore, this issue represents both a comparison (same story) and a contrast (different timing and motivation).

7.   The story of Juan de Grijalva is consistent with the rest of the author's argument. If read too carelessly, it may seem as if the author is contradicting herself by giving an example of a Spanish explorer who WAS seen as a god, the god Quetzalcoatl. However, when taken in context, you can see that this is yet another piece of evidence AGAINST the "white gods" story. If Juan de Grijalva, who appeared at a completely different time, was hailed as Quetzalcoatl, it is unlikely that Cortés was believed to be Quetzalcoatl returning from the east as well, or that conquest was facilitated by a crazy coincidence of Cortés appearing at just the right time to be hailed as the returning god.

Bonus question: Note the logical structure of the passage. First the author sets up the story of the Spaniards being hailed and welcomed as gods, and then she proceeds to knock that story down piece by piece, and to suggest that the superior technology of the Spaniards was the real cause. The following phrases (among others) indicate that the author's purpose is to reject the "white gods" causal story and to suggest an alternative story:

- "In fact, however, there is little evidence that the indigenous people ever seriously believed the newcomers were gods" (P1)
- "The cherished narrative is alive and well, and in urgent need of critical attention." (P1)
- "In order to dismantle a construct with such a long history, it will be necessary first to explain the origins and durability of the myth and then to offer an alternate explanation of what happened in the period of conquest" (P2)
- "three primary assertions: first, that we must put technology in all its forms—beyond mere weaponry—front and center in our story of conquest" (P2)
- "With such friends, though, perhaps the indigenous and their cultural heirs do not need enemies. A different approach is definitely needed" (P4)
- "There are numerous obvious problems with the story." (P9)

Chapter 5
The Process of
Elimination (POE)
and Attractors

GOALS

1) To learn the principles and steps of working through questions using the Process of Elimination (POE)
2) To recognize patterns in Attractors

5.1 THE PROCESS OF ELIMINATION

As we discussed in the last chapter, there are five basic steps you must take in answering any CARS question.

1) **Read the question word for word and identify the question type.**
2) **Translate the question into your own words: identify what the question task is asking you to do with the information in the passage.**
3) **Identify any key words that refer to specific parts of the passage. If key words are provided, *go back to the passage* to locate that information.**
4) **Answer in your own words: articulate what the correct answer will need to do based on the question type and the information in the passage.**
5) **Use Process of Elimination (POE), and choose the *least wrong* answer choice.**

In this chapter, we'll focus in more detail on Step 5, Process of Elimination or **POE**.

It is more effective to attack the question by eliminating the three wrong answer choices than by searching for the perfect choice. The MCAT writers are highly skilled at hiding the credited response in obscure and convoluted language, and at creating wrong answer choices that at first glance look good, but have a subtle yet fatal flaw. Your mission is to avoid the traps on your way to the correct choice.

Here are the basic steps of POE. In most cases, you will need to take two "cuts" through the choices as you narrow them down.

First Cut

Read Every Word of Every Choice Carefully.

This is not the time to skim! Once you have misinterpreted or skipped over something, it is very difficult to recognize your mistake.

Eliminate Choices Using the Bottom Line of the Passage.

Remind yourself of the Main Point and tone of the passage, and then read through each answer choice, eliminating any that violate, or directly contradict, the author's argument (unless it's a Weaken or EXCEPT/LEAST/NOT question). Understanding the passage's Bottom Line will also allow you to quickly eliminate choices that, although they may not contradict the author's points, are not relevant to the passage and thus are out of scope.

Eliminate Choices Inconsistent with Your Own Answer (When Possible, Given the Question Type).

Use your own answer to the question (which should be based closely on the passage and on the question task) as a guideline for eliminating answer choices. Do not, however, eliminate a choice just because it's not a perfect match. Be flexible.

As you gain experience predicting the answer, trust yourself more and more. Don't let an inconsistent answer make you second guess yourself. Your prediction is your life raft: don't abandon it on a whim! On the other hand, if none of the choices are consistent with your prediction, don't force a round peg into a square hole and talk yourself into one that "kind of sounds like" what you were looking for. Carefully re-read the question and go back into the passage to see what you might have missed the first time.

Second Cut

Reread the Question Stem.

Remind yourself (or improve your understanding) of the question type and issue.

Compare the Remaining Choices to Each Other.

Notice strength of language, scope, content references, and any other relevant differences between them.

Go Back to the Passage Again to Pin It Down (When Necessary).

Keep the differences between the choices in mind to help you find where you need to go.

Choose the Least Wrong Answer Choice.

When making your final choice, it's important to keep two things in mind.

1) **Be highly suspicious of absolute or extreme statements.**
   EXCEPT on Strengthen or Weaken questions, correct MCAT answer choices will rarely make an extreme claim. Do not use this test carelessly, however. Simple declarative statements (such as, *The inquisitorial system is historically superior to the adversarial system.*) are not necessarily extreme. Look for words that may indicate absolute statements such as *any, all, none, never, always, totally, must, only, exactly, impossible*, etc. Look out for statements that make extreme claims even without using any of these words.

Notice the wishy-washy or equivocal wording in the previous statement; these words *may*, not *must*, indicate statements that are too extreme for the passage. Whether or not a particular word or statement is extreme depends on how it is used within the context of the answer choice. The following phrases illustrate the difference between extreme and not so extreme statements, in the context of language that should and should not make you suspicious of answer choices.

Extreme	Not Extreme	Comments
will be	will for a time be	The phrase *will be* predicts the future, which may well be beyond the scope of the passage. The phrase *will for a time be* suggests a temporary condition, which is more moderate and therefore more likely to be supported by the text.
the greatest result	a great result	The use of the definite article *the* in combination with the suffix *-est* makes this a very strong statement. The phrase *a great result* is much less absolute, because it could be one of many great results.
kill all the roaches	kill roaches	The statement *kill roaches* sounds extreme because of the word kill, but in context the statement is not extreme or absolute. *Kill all the roaches* is in fact extreme because the statement is all-inclusive.

2) **If part of an answer choice is wrong, then it's all wrong.**

Pay attention to every word: one incorrect word or phrase will make the entire answer choice wrong. This is one reason why searching for the correct choice—instead of the three wrong choices—may lead you to an incorrect choice. Don't talk yourself into an answer just because you really like one thing about it; something really good about part of an answer can't outweigh a definitively bad part of that same answer. A wrong answer may have something attractive about it, but the credited response won't have anything incorrect in it (or will at least be the best supported of the four).

Any word can make an answer choice wrong. If the answer choice implies that something is true *all* of the time, and the passage suggests that it is true *some* (but *not all*) of the time, then the answer choice cannot be supported by the passage. Pay special attention to words of negation (such as *no, not, none, never,* etc.).

5.2 ATTRACTORS

Usually, if you understand the Bottom Line of the passage, it is easy to eliminate two of the four answer choices. But, students commonly express this lament: "I always get it down to two choices and then I pick the wrong one!" That's because the test is designed to make you do this.

For each question, there is usually at least one **Attractor**: an answer choice designed to tempt you into choosing it. It will have something attractive about it, such as words from the passage or concepts similar to those discussed by the author. If you're in too much of a hurry looking only for the "right" answer, you'll fall for an Attractor much of the time. Remember: the test-writers know how students think and what kind of logical mistakes they tend to make. Take the control away from them by predicting and avoiding the traps.

Typical Attractors

If you look for it, you'll see some patterns appear in the answer choices. The MCAT utilizes a core group of Attractors to tempt those who rush or who do not understand basic ideas presented in the passage. Here are the most common Attractors, grouped into categories. Learn them, look for them, and, thus, defend yourself against them.

Decoys

These choices are written to sound just like the passage. However, they include something that doesn't match up, either with the passage text or the question task.

- **Words out of context**
  This Attractor uses vocabulary right from the passage. It "sounds good," but the meaning of the words is changed. That is, the answer choice uses the right words but carries the wrong meaning. This is a trap in particular for people who are not going back to the passage, or who are not rereading the relevant parts of the passage carefully enough.

- **Half-right/half-wrong**
  These are "bait and switch" answers. Part or most of the choice is exactly what you are looking for, but another part is not supported by the passage (e.g., too extreme or out of scope). This is a trap set for people who make up their minds before they read the entire choice, or who try to "rehabilitate" an answer because part of it sounds so good. Remember that one word is enough to make a choice wrong.

- **Opposite/Negations**
  These choices take a sentence or idea directly from the passage, but add or remove a crucial "not" or "un." The statement therefore sounds just like the passage, but in fact directly contradicts it.

- **Reversals**
  This answer choice extracts a relationship from the passage but then reverses it to go in the opposite direction. It may flip a sequence of cause and effect, or confuse the order of events in a chronology.

- **Garbled language**
  This choice gives you some familiar words, but is difficult or impossible to understand. The test-writers are hoping that you will pick it thinking that because it is confusing it must be correct. However, another version of this trap is to put the correct choice into confusing language, with the hope that you will immediately eliminate it because it doesn't "sound good." So, when you see garbled language, don't automatically pick it, but don't automatically eliminate it either. And, don't spend five minutes trying to decipher it. Use POE aggressively: there may be a better choice, or it may be the only one left after you have eliminated the other three.

- **Right answer/wrong question**
  The statements in these Attractors, unlike in the other members of this category, are in fact directly supported by the passage. However, they aren't relevant to the question being asked. When you are down to two choices, always reread the question stem in order to avoid this trap.

- **Wrong point of view**
  This is a variation on the right answer/wrong question Attractor. If there is more than one point of view described in the passage, a wrong answer might describe a point of view different from the one referred to in the question stem.

Extremes

These choices go too far in one direction or the other.

- **Absolutes**
  This type of wrong answer uses language that is much stronger than the language in the passage. It may include extreme words such as *none, always, never, only,* etc. Keep in mind, however, that a strongly worded passage may support a strongly worded choice. Remember that a choice doesn't have to include one of the standard extreme words to be making a claim that is too extreme or absolute in its meaning.

- **Superlatives**

  These wrong answers include words like *first, last, best, most, worst, least* (or anything else ending in *–est*), or *primary*. For instance, it may describe a theory as the *first* or the *best* theory, but the author simply says that it's an important theory.

- **Judgments and recommendations**

  The choice passes judgment on whether something is good or bad, but that thing is described by the author in a neutral tone. Or, the answer choice states that a proposal should be implemented or rejected when that policy or action is merely described in the passage, or the choice may describe a moderate point of view in overly extreme terms. Finally, a wrong answer may tempt you to intuit the author's state of mind or personal beliefs in a way that is not supported by the passage text.

- **Not strong enough**

  This Attractor is specific to Strengthen and Weaken questions. Rather than being too extreme, it is too wishy-washy to significantly affect the author's argument in the passage. Always compare choices to each other; for this question type, you want the choice that goes farthest in the right direction.

Out of Scope

These answer choices introduce facts, issues, or claims that are never addressed in the passage, or, they do not match the scope of the question task.

- **Not the issue**

  This answer choice brings in ideas or facts that are not discussed in the passage. You will usually eliminate these in your first cut.

- **Outside knowledge**

  The wrong answer makes a statement that is true based on your own knowledge, but isn't directly supported by the text of the passage. Remember that the CARS section tests your ability to read actively and analyze the passage; it does not test your general knowledge.

- **Crystal ball**

  The wrong answer predicts the future (but the passage doesn't) or goes beyond the time frame of the passage.

- **No such comparison**

  This incorrect choice will take something that is mentioned in the passage and compare it to something that is not. Or, it may take two things that are mentioned by the author and compare them in a way that is not supported by the passage (often by stating that one option is better than the other).

- **Too narrow/too broad**

  The "too narrow" Attractor is typical on General questions: it mentions or contains only part of the author's argument. Keep in mind however that correct answers to Specific questions (including Inference questions) can be quite narrow. Wrong answers that are too broad have the opposite problem: they overgeneralize or go beyond the author's argument. They may describe a general category into which the topic of the passage would fit. On General questions, use the "Goldilocks Approach": eliminate any answer choices that are too narrow or too broad, and choose the one that is the best fit.

5.3   POE DOS AND DON'TS

Do

- Read and identify the question carefully—predict the traps.
- Read each answer choice word for word the first time, and consider all parts of every choice.
- Read all four answer choices carefully and with an open mind before deciding.
- Be suspicious—look for traps.
- Notice extreme or absolute wording and compare it to the passage text.
- Eliminate using the Bottom Line.
- Eliminate using your own answer.
- Compare the choices to each other.
- Go back to the passage often.

Don't

- Skim the answer choices.
- Pick the first choice that "sounds good."
- Ignore information in a choice, or add something to it, in order to make it fit. That is, don't force a square peg into a round hole.
- Eliminate choices on Strengthen or Weaken questions because of strong wording.
- Eliminate choices on Inference questions because of moderate wording.
- Pick D without reading it carefully just because you've eliminated answer choices A, B, and C.
- Answer based on memory.

5.4   THE SIX STEPS IN ACTION: MODEL PASSAGE

This exercise is intended to give you a picture of what an "ideal" process of attacking a passage looks like. One of your online CARS passages is reproduced on the next two pages.

- First, work through the passage on your own.
- Next, compare your progress through the passage to the model that follows in the book, which takes you from Previewing the Questions all the way through POE.
- The highlighting and noteboard notes in the sample passage provide a picture of what actual good highlighting and passage notes would look like and why. Keep in mind, however, that it isn't important to have matched them exactly—use the model to see if you caught and highlighted the most important things in the passage text and if you correctly understood the key parts of the author's argument. The questions that follow the highlighted passage are annotated to illustrate the thought process involved in translating the question, using the passage to generate an answer, and doing good POE.

It is strange that a novelist as superbly imaginative as John Fowles should be content to write within the canons of conventional textbook realism. Of the four stories in *The Ebony Tower*, three are simple, linear structures—situation, complication, resolution—the incidents rationally linked through the probable interactions of credible characteristics, the action and theme neatly illustrating each other. The fourth story is somewhat more open-ended and covert: a picnic in the country that ends in a disappearance and, by implication, a suicide. One has to draw the connections for oneself and see the sudden gathering storm at the end as an epiphany. But this is a technique that Joyce was practicing in *Dubliners* at the turn of the century, and it is still being practiced, from week to week, in the pages of *The New Yorker* and elsewhere.

Yet each of these stories [by Fowles] is anything but obvious or thin. However conventionally they begin and proceed, there comes a point when their issues dramatically engage and take on complexity and power—it's as though one had picked up a simple, familiar object, casually examined it, and suddenly found it shaking in one's hands. By the same token, Fowles' seemingly typecast characters—a lascivious old artist meets his decorous young critic, a timid literary scholar is ripped off by an aggressive hippie—have a way of slipping out of their mold, surprising us first as individuals and then as the strange faces that our most intense experiences tend to take on.

The popular writer turns life into clichés, the artist of realism turns clichés back into life. But why start with clichés in the first place and why tie yourself down to the restrictions and reductions of a plot? Why all this outmoded literary law and order? It's as though a brilliant playwright came upon the scene, a master of illusion, who insists upon practicing the three unities.

One may believe Fowles enjoys being so clever and also the rewards it has brought him as a writer of highly intelligent books that manage to be very popular. But judging from *The Aristos*, his "intellectual self-portrait," Fowles has more ambitious goals in view: in his quiet, detached way, just as much as Mailer does in his very different way, Fowles wants to create a revolution in the consciousness of his time. Still, if

this is so, surely he must suspect that his fiction is going about it in the wrong way. Tidy narrative structures, well-rounded characters, consistent point of view, lucid prose, accurate descriptions of times and places—aren't these the techniques at our late state of modernism, that confirm the most retrograde bourgeois tastes, that are valuable only so that they can then be superseded or, better yet, destroyed by the writer's innovations? Learn the rules so that you know what you're doing when you break them—so the young writer is told. Learn the craft so that you can then practice the art: craft being what all writers are supposed to be able to do, art being what only the individual writer can do because true art is the creation of new *forms* of consciousness, which only the individualist can achieve. Right?

Wrong. Partly wrong in theory and increasingly wrong in practice. New consciousness does not necessarily require new forms in literature any more than it does in any other field of writing. When Shakespeare wrote the "Dark Lady" sonnets, he was doing something original in love poetry, and hence for love itself, though he left the sonnet form undisturbed. And while it is true that new literary forms can provoke new consciousness, it tends more often to work the other way around. In any case, modernism, which has tended to identify individuality with formal innovation exclusively, has left the writers who still subscribe to it increasing high and dry: i.e., rarefied and empty. Or as Fowles himself put it in *The Aristos*: "There is a desperate search for the unique style, and only too often the search is conducted at the expense of content. This accounts for the enormous proliferation in styles and techniques…and for that only too characteristic coupling of exoticism, of presentation, and banality of a theme." If you don't think he is right, pick an anthology of current experimental fiction or poetry and see how much genuine new consciousness you find and how much of the same surreal solipsism, forlorn, or abrasive. Talk about conventionality.

Material used in this particular passage has been adapted from the following source:
T. Solotaroff, *A Few Good Voices in My Head: Occasional Pieces on Writing, Editing, and Reading My Contemporaries* © 1987 by Reed Business Information.

1. The author's example of Shakespeare is used to:

A) describe how Shakespeare changed the sonnet form.
B) illustrate how new forms of literature are required to bring new consciousness.
C) support the claim that writers should not necessarily learn the rules with the goal of eventually breaking them.
D) provide an example of a modernist work.

2. The author states that Joyce and other authors use plotlines similar to Fowles' fourth story in *The Ebony Tower* in order to suggest that:

A) Fowles' prose is more conventional than it seems.
B) Fowles' usage of open-ended and covert plotlines contributes to his ambition to create a revolution in consciousness.
C) the impact of Fowles' work comes more from its content than from formal innovation.
D) Fowles' work is just as good as Joyce's *Dubliners*.

3. Which of these characters or plots from novels would exemplify the author's description in paragraph 2 of Fowles' work?

   I. A private investigator falls for his client. He later discovers that she is his long-lost daughter.
   II. A suburban mother watches as her daughter is slowly dying of a mysterious illness. In the final chapter of the novel, it is revealed that the mother has been poisoning her daughter all along.
   III. The son of a small-town pastor leads the church choir to winning a national singing competition.

A) I only
B) II only
C) I and II
D) I, II, and III

4. Some literary theorists claim that the impact of a literary work is defined not by the intent of the author, but rather by the interaction between reader and text, and that different readers may have very different and at times contradictory reactions to and interpretations of the same text. If valid, what impact would this theory have on Fowles' goal of creating a revolution in consciousness?

A) It would suggest that Fowles could not succeed in his goal because for a revolution to occur there must be agreement on what new views should replace the old way of thinking.
B) It would suggest that Fowles succeeded in his goal because the popularity of his work ensured that it had impact on the thinking of a significant number of people.
C) It would suggest that Fowles misunderstood the complexity involved in creating a revolution in consciousness through literature.
D) It would suggest that achieving Fowles' goal of creating a revolution in consciousness depends on factors that go beyond using conventional forms to express original ideas.

5. What is "conventional textbook realism" as it is defined in the passage?

A) A novel with a simple story structure and believable outcome
B) Stories that are based on real-life events
C) A story based on use of stereotypical characters
D) Stories that begin conventionally and then reveal unexpected levels of complexity

6. Which of the following statements, if true, would most *undermine* the author's argument?

A) Rules are not valuable only when they are destroyed by a writer's innovative techniques.
B) Mailer's writing is often described as aggressive.
C) Literature that contributes to a transformation in consciousness is often only recognized as such many decades after it is written.
D) Fowles intended for *The Aristos* to be partially autobiographical.

Ranking the Passage

Abstract passage content + several hard question types = Later/Killer passage

Previewing the Question Stems

Below are the question stems only. The key words to note in the Preview stage are highlighted. Remember: you are only looking for references to passage content at this point in the process.

1. The author's example of Shakespeare is used to:

2. The author states that Joyce and other authors use plotlines similar to Fowles' fourth story in *The Ebony Tower* in order to suggest that:

3. Which of these characters or plots from novels would exemplify the author's description in paragraph 2 of Fowles' work?

4. Some literary theorists claim that the impact of a literary work is defined not by the intent of the author, but rather by the interaction between reader and text, and that different readers may have very different and at times contradictory reactions to and interpretations of the same text. If valid, what impact would this theory have on Fowles' goal of creating a revolution in consciousness?

   Note: When a question is this long, you may want to skip it during the Preview stage.

5. What is "conventional textbook realism" as it is defined in the passage?

6. Which of the following statements, if true, would most *undermine* the author's argument?

   Note: There is no reference to specific passage content here— skip it in the Preview stage.

TONE **LIST INDICATORS—CONTRAST**

QUESTION TOPICS

It is strange that a novelist as superbly imaginative as John Fowles should be content to write within the canons of conventional textbook realism. Of the four stories in *The Ebony Tower*, three are simple, linear structures—situation, complication, resolution—the incidents rationally linked through the probable interactions of credible characteristics, the action and theme neatly illustrating each other. The fourth story is somewhat more open-ended and covert: a picnic in the country that ends in a disappearance and, by implication, a suicide. One has to draw the connections for oneself and see the sudden gathering storm at the end as an epiphany. But this is a technique that Joyce was practicing in *Dubliners* at the turn of the century, and it is still being practiced, from week to week, in the pages of *The New Yorker* and elsewhere.

PIVOTAL WORD

TONE

Yet each of these stories [by Fowles] is anything but obvious or thin. However conventionally they begin and proceed, there comes a point when their issues dramatically engage and take on complexity and power—it's as though one had picked up a simple, familiar object, casually examined it, and suddenly found it shaking in one's hands. By the same token, Fowles' seemingly typecast characters—a lascivious old artist meets his decorous young critic, a timid literary scholar is ripped off by an aggressive hippie—have a way of slipping out of their mold, surprising us first as individuals and then as the strange faces that our most intense experiences tend to take on.

PIVOTAL WORDS— CONTRAST

COMPARISON

PIVOTAL WORD/ LEADING QUESTION

The popular writer turns life into clichés, the artist of realism turns clichés back into life. But why start with clichés in the first place and why tie yourself down to the restrictions and reductions of a plot? Why all this outmoded literary law and order? It's as though a brilliant playwright came upon the scene, a master of illusion, who insists upon practicing the three unities.

SUGGESTED PIVOT

ACTUAL PIVOT

COMPARISON/ CONTRAST

QUESTION TOPIC

SUGGESTED PIVOT/ LEADING QUESTION

One may believe Fowles enjoys being so clever and also the rewards it has brought him as a writer of highly intelligent books that manage to be very popular. But judging from *The Aristos*, his "intellectual self-portrait," Fowles has more ambitious goals in view: in his quiet, detached way, just as much as Mailer does in his very different way, Fowles wants to create a revolution in the consciousness of his time. Still, if this is so, surely he must suspect that his fiction is going about it in the wrong way. Tidy narrative structures, well-rounded characters, consistent point of view, lucid prose, accurate descriptions of times and places—aren't these the techniques at our late state of modernism, that confirm the most retrograde bourgeois tastes, that are valuable only so that they can then be superseded or, better yet, destroyed by the writer's innovations? Learn the rules so that you know what you're doing when you break them—so the young writer is told. Learn the craft so that you can then practice the art: craft being what all writers are supposed to be able to do, art being what only the individual writer can do because true art is the creation of new forms of consciousness, which only the individualist can achieve. Right?

AUTHOR'S/ FOWLES' POSITION

QUESTION TOPIC

PIVOTAL WORDS/ CONTRAST

TONE

Wrong. Partly wrong in theory and increasingly wrong in practice. New consciousness does not necessarily require new forms in literature any more than it does in any other field of writing. When Shakespeare wrote the "Dark Lady" sonnets, he was doing something original in love poetry, and hence for love itself, though he left the sonnet form undisturbed. And while it is true that new literary forms can provoke new consciousness, it tends more often to work the other way around. In any case, modernism, which has tended to identify individuality with formal innovation exclusively, has left the writers who still subscribe to it increasing high and dry: i.e., rarefied and empty. Or as Fowles himself put it in *The Aristos*: "There is a desperate search for the unique style, and only too often the search is conducted at the expense of content. This accounts for the enormous proliferation in styles and techniques… and for that only too characteristic coupling of exoticism, of presentation, and banality of a theme." If you don't think he is right, pick an anthology of current experimental fiction or poetry and see how much genuine new consciousness you find and how much of the same surreal solipsism, forlorn, or abrasive. Talk about conventionality.

Material used in this particular passage has been adapted from the following source:
T. Solotaroff, *A Few Good Voices in My Head: Occasional Pieces on Writing, Editing, and Reading My Contemporaries* © 1987 by Reed Business Information.

Model Noteboard Notes

This is what your noteboard for this passage might look like:

Passage [#], Q 1–6

¶ 1)   Fowles—conventional techniques
¶ 2)   But surprising complexity
¶ 3)   So why use conventions?
¶ 4)   Misguided approach?
¶ 5)   No—new form ≠ new consciousness

BL: Fowles' conventional form for new consciousness (author supports)

Attacking the Questions

The questions below are annotated to represent the thought process you would go through in answering the questions, not to represent the actual appearance of the screen. Remember: on the test, you can only strike out or select entire answer choices; partial strikeouts are not possible. The explanations to the right of each choice model a first cut through the answers: what you may have eliminated and why, and what you might have left in. The "Down to Two" explanations to the left describe the reasoning that you would use to eliminate down to the correct answer in your second cut.

1. The author's example of Shakespeare is used to:

A) describe how Shakespeare changed the sonnet form. **Opposite—he didn't**

B) illustrate how new forms of literature are required to bring new consciousness. **(Left it in)**

C) support the claim that writers should not necessarily learn the rules with the goal of eventually breaking them. **(Left it in)**

D) provide an example of a modernist work. **Words out of context—example makes larger point about literature, not just about modernism**

Question Type: Structure
Translation: Why does the author discuss Shakespeare?
Back to the Passage: Last paragraph—Shakespeare did something original but used existing sonnet form
Answer: To show that position described at end of previous paragraph is wrong

Down to Two—Compare:

B and C are opposites of each other. C fits the Bottom Line, although it is tricky—have to see relationship between paragraphs 4 and 5, and that paragraph 5 is denying validity of the position described at end of paragraph 4 ("Right? Wrong.").

2. The author states that Joyce and other authors use plotlines similar to Fowles' fourth story in *The Ebony Tower* in order to suggest that:

A) Fowles' prose is more conventional than it seems. **(Left it in)**

B) Fowles' usage of open-ended and covert plotlines contributes to his ambition to create a revolution in consciousness. **Contradicts point of the paragraph and Bottom Line—it wasn't his plotlines that did this**

C) the impact of Fowles' work comes more from its content than from formal innovation. **(Left it in)**

D) Fowles' work is just as good as Joyce's *Dubliners*. **Not the issue/No such comparison on quality**

Question Type: Structure
Translation: Why does the author state that other authors use similar plotlines?
Back to the Passage: First paragraph—part of discussion of Fowles' use of conventional textbook realism (later says that issues within them are complex)
Answer: To provide evidence that Fowles did not use innovative techniques to achieve his effect

Down to Two—Compare:

Both have idea of conventional form, but A suggests that it seemed unconventional, while passage argues the opposite. Seeing the validity of C requires connecting paragraph 1 to the Bottom Line.

5.4

3. Which of these characters or plots from novels would
exemplify the author's description in paragraph 2 of
Fowles' work?

I.   A private investigator falls for his client. He later
     discovers that she is his long-lost daughter. **Twist/
     unexpected: yes**

II. A suburban mother watches as her daughter is
     slowly dying of a mysterious illness. In the final
     chapter of the novel, it is revealed that the mother
     has been poisoning her daughter all along. **Twist/
     unexpected: yes**

III. The son of a small-town pastor leads the church
     choir to winning a national singing competition.
     Totally expected: No

A) I only
B) II only
C) I and II
D) I, II, and III

Eliminate anything with III. I and II
are so similar that you can't include
one without the other.

Question Type: Analogy

Translation: Which is most similar to Fowles' work as
it's described in second paragraph?

Back to the Passage: Begins conventionally, but
complex and powerful

Answer: Begins in familiar way, then surprises us with
more complexity (maybe character that does something
unexpected)

4. Some literary theorists claim that the impact of a
literary work is defined not by the intent of the author,
but rather by the interaction between reader and text,
and that different readers may have very different and
at times contradictory reactions to and interpretations
of the same text. If valid, what impact would this
theory have on Fowles' goal of creating a revolution in
consciousness?

A) It would suggest that Fowles could not succeed in his
goal because for a revolution to occur there must be
agreement on what new views should replace the old way
of thinking. **Too extreme/Out of scope**

B) It would suggest that Fowles succeeded in his goal
because the popularity of his work ensured that it had
impact on the thinking of a significant number of
people. **Too extreme/Out of scope**

C) It would suggest that Fowles misunderstood the
complexity involved in creating a revolution in
consciousness through literature. (Left it in)

D) It would suggest that achieving Fowles' goal of creating
a revolution in consciousness depends on factors that
go beyond using conventional forms to express original
ideas. (Left it in)

Question Type: New Information (Strengthen/Weaken)

Translation: If it's true that the effect of work depends
on various reader interpretations, not just author, how
would this affect Fowles' goal?

Back to the Passage: Fowles' goal most directly
discussed in paragraph 4. Passage never discusses role of
readers' interpretations.

Answer: Would have to take this additional factor into
account

Down to Two—Compare:

C indicates that Fowles was unaware of this, but we don't
know that. D only indicates that there are additional
factors. D is more moderate, and within the scope of the
passage and question stem information.

5.4

5. What is "conventional textbook realism" as it is defined in the passage?

A) A novel with a simple story structure and believable outcome **(Left it in)**

B) Stories that are based on ~~real-life events~~ **Out of scope/Outside "knowledge"**

C) A story based on use of ~~stereotypical characters~~ **Fowles' characters only *seem* typecast or stereotypical**

D) Stories that begin conventionally and then ~~reveal unexpected levels of complexity~~ **(Left it in)**

Question Type: Inference

Translation: What is "conventional textbook realism," as described in passage?

Back to the Passage: Paragraph 1—simple, linear structure, credible, not innovative

Answer: What the passage said

Down to Two—Compare:

Both A and D describe Fowles' work, which uses conventional realism. But only A is given as part of the description of realism more generally, while D is specific to Fowles' work. Choice A is a close paraphrase of the passage description.

6. Which of the following statements, if true, would most *undermine* the author's argument?

A) Rules are ~~not~~ valuable only when they are destroyed by a writer's innovative techniques. **(Left it in)**

B) Mailer's writing is often described as aggressive. **No effect on passage (paragraph 4—author already says Mailer different)**

C) Literature that contributes to a transformation in consciousness is often only recognized as such many decades after it is written. **(Left it in)**

D) Fowles intended for *The Aristos* to be partially autobiographical. **Strengthens/Consistent with "intellectual self-portrait" (paragraph 4)**

Question Type: Weaken

Translation: What would be most inconsistent with author's claims in the passage?

Back to the Passage: Bottom Line—Fowles' conventional form for new consciousness (author supports)

Answer: Either that innovative form does/might lead to new consciousness, or that conventional form does not

Down to Two—Compare:

A has tricky wording and connects to tricky relationship between last two paragraphs. But when translated, it's consistent with author's real position in last paragraph: it strengthens, not weakens. Connection of C to passage is less obvious, but it's inconsistent with argument in last paragraph: it suggests that "current experimental fiction or poetry" might eventually lead to a new consciousness.

5.5   DEALING WITH STRESS

In Chapter 2, we discussed some possible ways of dealing with the stress and anxiety that most people experience when preparing for and taking the MCAT. By now, you should have settled on a method that you can use effectively whenever anxiety or loss of concentration becomes a problem. Remember, stress won't go away, but it can be managed so that all that extra adrenaline coursing through your system can work for you, not against you.

In the table below, describe any symptoms of anxiety you may have experienced when taking a practice test or doing homework, and the method or methods you use (or will use in the future) to help manage it.

Symptoms	Management Methods

Many people use music to control and manage anxiety, and just to feel better overall. If you are a music person, create a playlist with a set of songs you can listen to whenever you find yourself feeling negative or non-productive emotions, be it anxiety and fear, or fatigue and lethargy.

When I'm feeling:	I'll listen to:

Along with stress, losing control of your pacing strategy can be a problem, especially toward the end of the test. On your next practice test or timed CARS section, monitor your pacing throughout. If you begin to panic about the time, or rush through questions without feeling reasonably secure in most of your answers, STOP and take three deep breaths. Remind yourself of the strategy and techniques you have spent so much time and effort learning. Don't let yourself lose your form at the finish line. Regain control of yourself and of the test before moving on.

Chapter 5 Summary

- Use POE aggressively.

- Know and eliminate the common Attractors.

- Read carefully—do not skim the questions or the answer choices.

- Continue to manage your stress: make it work for you, not against you!

CHAPTER 5 PRACTICE PASSAGES

Individual Passage Drills

Do this exercise *untimed* at first. Work and Annotate the passages as usual (remember to preview the questions). As you work the questions, for each answer choice you eliminate, write down the reason next to the choice, and/or highlight the word or words within the choice that make it wrong. Keep a list of Attractors nearby, and feel free to refer to it as you work. Take time to remind yourself which Attractors commonly appear on particular question types. If you cannot tell the difference between two choices and must guess between the two, note that next to the question.

When you check your answers, for each question you missed, note down in the Individual Passage Log what was wrong with the incorrect answer you chose, and what you thought was wrong with the correct answer. Look for patterns in your mistakes. Do you consistently choose the same kind of Attractor? Do you tend to eliminate the correct answer too quickly, and then talk yourself into a wrong answer choice further down the list? Do you pick the choice that sounds right, instead of eliminating the wrong answer choices and picking the least wrong choice? Devise a strategy to avoid making those same mistakes in the future.

Continue to do this exercise over the next few weeks, doing at least two passages back to back at a time. Eventually you can do the passages timed, but give yourself an extra minute or two to annotate the answer choices. Continue to monitor your progress and to diagnose any changing patterns in your performance.

CHAPTER 5 PRACTICE PASSAGE 1

The Depression yielded not only misery but also tremendous energy and radicalism. Union-organizing and reform movements of all kinds flourished as the crisis challenged Americans to abandon the constraints of the past and move forward, boldly, into the future. Recovery in the family, as in the economy, would be achieved not simply by returning to ways of the past, but by adapting to new circumstances. The economic crisis opened the way for a new type of family based on shared breadwinning and equality of the sexes.

But by the time the Depression was over and World War II had come and gone, it was clear that millions of middle-class American families would take the path toward polarized gender roles. What caused the overwhelming triumph of "traditional" roles in the "modern" home?

Although most Americans experienced some form of hardship during the Depression, it was the nation's male breadwinners—fathers who were responsible for providing economic support for their families—who were threatened or faced with the severest erosion of their identities. Those who lost income or jobs frequently lost status at home, and self-respect as well. Economic hardship placed severe strains on marriage. Going on relief may well have helped the family budget, but it would do little for the breadwinner's feelings of failure.

With the breadwinner's role undermined, other family roles shifted dramatically. Frequently wives and mothers who had never been employed took jobs to provide supplemental or even primary support for their families. Given the need for women's earnings, the widespread employment of women might have been one of the most important legacies of the Depression era. But discriminatory policies and public hostility weakened that potential. Although many families depended on the earnings of both spouses, federal policies supported unemployed male breadwinners but discouraged married women from seeking jobs. Section 213 of the Economy Act of 1932 mandated that whenever personnel reductions took place in the executive branch, married persons were to be the first discharged if married to a government employee. As a result, 1,600 married women were dismissed from their federal jobs. Many state and local governments followed suit; three out of four cities excluded married women from teaching, and eight states passed laws excluding them from state jobs. These efforts to curtail women's employment opportunities were directly related to the powerful imperative to bolster the employment of men.

If the paid labor force had been more hospitable, and if public policies had fostered equal opportunities for women, young people in the 1930s might have been less inclined to aspire to prevailing gender roles. Viable long-term job prospects for women might have prompted new ways of structuring family roles. In the face of persistent obstacles, however, that potential withered. The realities of family life combined with institutional barriers to inhibit the potential for sustained radical change among white middle-class American families.

The prevailing family ideology was gravely threatened when women and men adapted to hard times by shifting their household responsibilities. In the long run, however, these alternatives were viewed as temporary measures caused by unfortunate circumstances, rather than as positive outcomes of the crisis. Young people learned, on the one hand, to accept women's employment as necessary for the family budget; on the other hand, they saw that deviations from traditional roles often wreaked havoc in marriages. Children who grew up in economically deprived families during these years watched their parents struggle to succeed as breadwinners and homemakers, and they suffered along with their parents if those expectations proved impossible to meet. The sociologist Glen Elder, in his pioneering study of families during the Depression, found that the more a family's traditional gender roles were disrupted, the more likely the children were to disapprove of the altered balance of power in their homes.

Material used in this particular passage has been adapted from the following source:
E. T. May, "Myths and Realities of the American Family," *A History of Private Life*, Volume V. © 1991 by The Belknap Press of Harvard University Press.

1. In paragraph 1, families are compared to the economy. This comparison is based on:

A) a contrast between the workplace and the home.
B) the possibility of new forms of social organization.
C) the actions of radicals hoping to undermine the status quo.
D) the unfortunate results of an economic crisis.

2. The author's argument about the impact of the Depression on male breadwinners would be best supported by research that demonstrated:

A) married men were more likely to lose jobs than unmarried men.
B) government welfare programs helped ease financial hardship for the unemployed.
C) unemployment was a reliable predictor of psychological depression.
D) unfair wages meant many wives were unable to replace the breadwinner's income by entering the workforce.

3. The support for the author's view about government's role in the changing form of marriage is:

A) strong: the author provides several examples suggesting government inhibited change.
B) strong: the author supports his view thoroughly with relevant analogies.
C) weak: the author's examples do not effectively support the author's view.
D) weak: the author does not significantly address the government's role.

4. Which of the following best characterizes the author's attitude towards the effects of the Depression on gender roles?

A) A missed opportunity
B) A tragic development
C) An important legacy
D) A radical change

5. The author most likely feels that marriage based on equality of the sexes:

A) can be successful, given the right circumstances.
B) is untenable because government cannot accept women's equal right to work.
C) is typical in the modern home.
D) inevitably causes conflict within the family.

6. Suppose a study were to find evidence of widespread discrimination in employers' hiring practices during the Depression. Specifically, when less qualified male candidates and more qualified female candidates were in direct competition for jobs, the males were very frequently hired. Furthermore, the government took little to no action to rectify these supposed injustices. How would the author most likely respond?

A) This is consistent with public and government attitudes during the Depression: men's employment was seen as more important than women's.
B) Since prejudices are first shaped by family life, a radical change toward more equitable gender roles in marriage was necessary before society could reject gender discrimination in the workplace.
C) Public and institutional viewpoints such as these, which prevented women from providing supplemental or even primary support for their families, were unfair and regrettable.
D) Government's lack of response is surprising; the Economy Act of 1932 suggested government was interested in employment demographics at the time.

CHAPTER 5 PRACTICE PASSAGE 2

German anthropologists understood nature as a static system of categories that allowed them, in their study of "natural peoples," to grasp an unchanging essence of humanity, rather than the ephemeral changes historians recorded. However, the concept of nature was anything but stable in nineteenth-century Germany. Since the early part of the century there had been a deep tension between Kantian models of natural science and idealist *Naturphilosophie*, conflicts in which many anthropologists themselves were active participants. Furthermore, in nature anthropologists sought a realm free from historical change just as Darwinians began asserting that nature, like humans, did in fact change over time. The boundary between history and nature, which formed an important basis for both humanism and anthropology, came to appear more unstable than ever....

The idea of nature and natural science that informed German anthropology was based on elements from two conflicting approaches, conventionally associated with Immanuel Kant and Friedrich Schelling. The founders of German anthropology belonged to a generation of natural scientists who, in the second half of the nineteenth century, rejected Schelling's romantic *Naturphilosophie* in favor of a return to Kant's more secular and rationalist notion of nature and natural science. As is the case with so many philosophical rejections, however, anthropologists preserved as much *Naturphilosophie* as they cast off, and their understanding of nature was really a synthesis of the two philosophers' approach.

From Kant anthropologists took an idea of nature as a static and objective system that could be conclusively known by scientists. In his *Metaphysical Basis of Natural Science*, Kant had maintained that an "authentic natural science" consisted exclusively of a priori deductions of necessary laws. He thus applauded a version of Newtonian mechanics based solely on mathematics as a perfect natural science and dismissed chemistry as a "systematic art" rather than a science because its laws were derived from sensory experience of "given facts." Unlike Newton, Kant excluded theological considerations from natural science, founding a tradition in Germany of strictly separating natural science and religion, a tradition sharply distinct from British natural theology. While this law-based, objective, totally secular, and perfectly knowable nature would have appealed to anthropologists, they would not have subscribed to the Kantian notion of science as the a priori deduction of mathematical laws. Indeed, anthropology was above all a science of the given facts, which Kant had rejected as a source of natural scientific knowledge.

It was precisely over this issue of the empirical that Schelling had originally broken with Kant, and it was in their empiricist approach to nature that anthropologists retained their allegiance to Schelling. Schelling had justified experience and empirical knowledge of nature against Kant's insistence that true knowledge of nature had to be deductive, a priori, and law-like. Thus, a science of qualities, such as chemistry with its qualitatively different elements, could count as a science for Schelling but not for Kant. For Schelling, the rehabilitation of the empirical in natural knowledge was part of an idealist project to overcome the difference between theological and natural knowledge, mind and nature, and speculation and experience. When anthropologists denounced *Naturphilosophie*, it was not for its empiricism. Worse than the idealism of *Naturphilosophie* was, for anthropologists, its view of nature as becoming rather than being, a view antithetical to the concept of nature that anthropologists wanted to use against historicist humanism. Thus, Virchow asserted that, "while the facts teach that the races of humans and the species of animals are immutable," *Naturphilosophie* (wrongly, in Virchow's view) teaches that they can change. Furthermore, anthropologists separated religious and scientific questions, following Kant's rather than Schelling's understanding of the relation of natural and theological knowledge. Allowing theology and development to enter into discussions of nature would undermine the basic project of anthropology as an antihumanist science of natural peoples outside history. When they spoke of *Naturphilosophie*, anthropologists thought as much about Darwinism as about the philosophical writings of Schelling and his followers.

Anthropologists saw in the science of botany a model for their own antievolutionist synthesis of Kant's systematizing with Schelling's empiricism. There were a number of botanists active in the Berlin Anthropological Society, including the latter-day *Naturphilosoph*, Alexander Braun. Braun argued that the study of plants allowed one to observe the essence of nature relatively directly because plants do not disguise themselves with culture, as humans do. Adolf Bastian extended Braun's understanding of plants to natural peoples, whom he compared to cryptograms, flowerless plants such as algae, mosses, and ferns. As botanists had gained general knowledge about plants by studying the flowerless cryptograms, which had previously been "despised and crushed underfoot," so too would anthropologists solve the "highest questions of culture" by considering natural peoples, who lack the "flowers of culture."

Material used in this particular passage has been adapted from the following source:

A. Zimmerman, *Anthropology and Antihumanism in Imperial Germany.* © 2001 by The University of Chicago.

1. The primary purpose of the passage is most likely to:

A) describe the analogy drawn by German anthropologists between botany and anthropology.

B) criticize 19th century German anthropologists for drawing inspiration from two mutually inconsistent schools of thought regarding natural science.

C) explain the views of 19th century German anthropologists regarding the proper approach to studying human beings in the context of natural science.

D) describe how 19th century German anthropology synthesized Kant's views on theology with Schelling's belief that science consists of a priori deductions of natural laws.

2. Which of the following claims, if true, would most *undermine* the German anthropologists' view that botany is a valid model for anthropology?

A) Human beings inherently exist within a social context, and therefore there is no such thing as a people not influenced by culture.

B) Some botanists believe that the study of flowerless cryptograms can tell us little about the structure and function of flowering plants.

C) Alexander Braun abandoned *Naturphilosophie* early in his academic career, and therefore his ideas about botany have little in common with the views of that school of thought.

D) It is impossible to study theology without taking into account cultural influences.

3. Which of the following statements, based on the passage, most accurately represents a relationship between the German anthropologists' views on natural science and those of Kant and Schelling?

A) The German anthropologists accepted Kant's view that science consists of deductions from necessary laws and rejected Schelling's belief that empiricism requires combining theological and natural knowledge.

B) The German anthropologists accepted Schelling's empiricist approach and rejected Kant's belief that science consists of deductions from mathematical laws.

C) The German anthropologists rejected Kant's inclusion of theological considerations within natural science and accepted Schelling's belief that human beings are mutable.

D) The German anthropologists rejected Kant's systematizing and accepted Schelling's empiricism.

4. Which of the following, based on the passage, would be most analogous to a historicist view of anthropology?

A) A belief that physics consists of a set of unchangeable laws that govern all actions and interactions between objects.

B) A belief that chemistry is a science rather than a systematic art, given that its laws can be discovered through empirical evidence.

C) A belief that political science is the study of how different political systems create and shape, and are themselves shaped by, human beliefs and values over time.

D) A belief that economics is inherently the study of how inherent and consistent human motivations play themselves out in different contexts.

5. Elsewhere, the author of the passage writes that in 19th-century Germany the study of geology, within natural science, was divided into *Geognosie*, the study of the present-day, essential, and inherent characteristics of the earth, and *Geologie*, the study of how geological features evolve and come into being. Based on information in the passage, how would the German anthropologists most likely view these two fields of study?

A) They would accept both as related and equally essential approaches to a scientific understanding of the earth.

B) They would reject both as irrelevant to a scientific understanding of human beings.

C) They would accept *Geologie* as a scientific approach to understanding the nature of the earth, while seeing *Geognosie* as a questionable attempt to impose rigid categories on inherently changeable features.

D) They would see *Geognosie* as a more scientific approach to geology than *Geologie*.

6. With which of the following statements would the German anthropologists discussed in the passage be LEAST likely to agree?

A) Culture can obscure qualities common to all humans.

B) Nature can be described through a set of objective and unchanging categories.

C) Chemistry cannot be legitimately labeled as a science.

D) Newton erred in including theological considerations within natural science.

7. Which of the following statements made in the passage most directly supports the author's assertion that "in nature anthropologists sought a realm free from historical change" (paragraph 1)?

A) The concept of nature was unstable in 19th century Germany.

B) British natural theology combined religion with natural science.

C) According to Virchow, while *Naturphilosophie* teaches that the races of humans and species of animals can change, they are in fact immutable.

D) There was a tension between Kantian models of natural science and idealist *Naturphilosophie*.

SOLUTIONS TO CHAPTER 5 PRACTICE PASSAGE 1

1. **B** This is a Structure question.

   A: No. The author does not contrast (i.e., illustrate differences between) the workplace and the home. Rather, the author states that they are similar in that adaptation to new circumstances was needed (paragraph 1).

   B: Yes. In paragraph 1, the author states that "Recovery in the family, as in the economy, would be achieved not simply by returning to ways of the past, but by adapting to new circumstances."

   C: No. The author does mention "radicalism," but does not describe radicals hoping to make changes to the family.

   D: No. This choice is too negative. This comparison follows shortly after the sentence, "The Depression yielded not only misery but also tremendous energy and radicalism" (paragraph 1). The author also states in that paragraph that "the crisis challenged Americans to abandon the constraints of the past and move forward, boldly, into the future." Therefore, the author recognizes positive as well as negative results of the economic crisis.

2. **C** This is a Strengthen question.

   Note: The author's argument about the impact of the Depression on male breadwinners suggests breadwinners who lost their jobs were personally hurt and that this had a negative impact on families (paragraphs 3 and 6).

   A: No. This evidence would not strengthen the argument. The author's argument is about the effect of unemployment on married men on an individual and family level. Knowing that married men overall were more likely to lose their jobs would not strengthen the author's point about the impact of unemployment on individual men and their families.

   B: No. This answer choice does not strengthen the author's argument about the effects of unemployment on men. The author states in the passage that relief efforts had little impact on unemployed men's feelings (paragraph 3).

   C: Yes. Evidence that unemployment caused depression would strengthen the author's claim in the passage that loss of employment coincided with loss of identity and marriage strain.

   D: No. This choice refers to the discrimination women faced, not directly to men's experience of unemployment. According to the author, men were most affected by their perceived loss of status and identity, not just by a reduction in household income.

3. **A** This is an Evaluate question.

   A: Yes, paragraph 4 provides numerous examples in which the government tries to manipulate the job market in favor of men.

   B: No. The author does not use analogy to support her argument. The only analogy drawn is between the economy and the family (paragraph 1), but there is no direct connection between that comparison and the author's specific discussion of the role of the government.

   C: No. The examples in paragraph 4 do directly support the idea that "federal policies supported unemployed male breadwinners but discouraged married women from seeking jobs," and later, "Many state and local governments followed suit."

   D: No. The author does address government's role in paragraph 4, on a federal, state, and local level.

4. **A**   This is a Tone/Attitude question.

    Note: This question is essentially asking about the author's overall attitude toward the events of the passage. Thus, use your sense of the author's overall purpose in writing the passage.

    A: **Yes. See paragraph 4: "Given the need for women's earnings, the widespread employment of women might have been one of the most important legacies of the Depression era. But discriminatory policies and public hostility weakened that potential." The word choice in paragraph 5 also suggests the author might have supported changes to traditional roles in marriage: "Viable long-term job prospects for women might have prompted new ways of structuring family roles. In the face of persistent obstacles, however, that potential withered."**

    B: No. While there was reason to believe the author might like to have seen more lasting change take place (see the explanation for choice A), the word "tragic" is too strong to describe the tone of the passage.

    C: No. This contradicts the author's attitude as expressed in the passage. In paragraph 4, the author states that the employment of women might have been an important legacy, but it was not allowed to take root.

    D: No. This choice represents a misreading of the main idea of the passage. The potential for radical change to gender roles in marriage did not turn into lasting change during the Depression.

5. **A**   This is an Inference question.

    A: **Yes. The author believes external obstacles (i.e., government and social resistance) prevented family roles from changing. In paragraph 5, the author says if those obstacles were removed, we might have seen real change.**

    B: No. The use of the word "cannot" implies government still holds this view; the attitudes of government today are beyond the scope of this passage. Also, government did not discourage women from working because it "could not accept" women working, but because men's employment was seen as more important.

    C: No. This choice contradicts paragraph 2, which refers to the "overwhelming triumph of 'traditional' roles in the 'modern' home."

    D: No. This choice is too extreme. The word "inevitably" is absolute, whereas paragraph 6 says "deviations from traditional roles *often* [emphasis added] wreaked havoc in marriages."

6. **A**   This is a New Information question.

    Note: Questions that give new information are often most relevant to a specific part of the passage. This one corresponds most closely to paragraph 4; the credited answer will reflect that.

    A: **Yes. See paragraph 4: "But *discriminatory policies and public hostility* [emphasis added] weakened that potential. Although many families depended on the earnings of both spouses, federal policies supported unemployed male breadwinners but discouraged married women from seeking jobs."**

    B: No. This answer choice puts forward a general theory—changes to the family are required for changes to the workplace—while the author suggests the opposite. That is, that government action in the workplace limited the possibility of change within the family (see paragraph 5).

    C: No. This choice suggests the author's general approach is to criticize or lament obstacles to women's progress. It would be more accurate to say the author is explaining why more equitable gender roles did not take hold at the time. Secondly, the passage suggests that women were able to provide financial support for their families at the time, at least to some extent (paragraph 4); "prevented" is too strong to be supported by the passage.

    D: No. This choice uses familiar language but is inconsistent with the passage. Government would not be expected to stop such discrimination; its inaction would not be a surprise. In fact, government institutionalized discrimination in the Economy Act of 1932 (paragraph 4).

SOLUTIONS TO CHAPTER 5 PRACTICE PASSAGE 2

1. **C** This is a Main Idea/Primary Purpose question.

   A: No. This choice is too narrow. While the analogy described in the last paragraph is part of the author's discussion of the views of German anthropologists, it is one piece of evidence supporting the larger argument, not the main point or primary purpose of the passage as a whole.

   B: No. This choice has the wrong tone. The author is not criticizing the anthropologists, but rather is giving a neutral description of their views and of some of the sources of those views.

   C: **Yes. This choice is broad enough to cover the content of the passage without going beyond its scope, and it has an appropriately neutral tone. Paragraph 1 introduces the idea that the anthropologists studied "humanity" and "natural peoples," as well as the idea that this study occurred within the larger context of natural science. The rest of the passage relates to the views of these German anthropologists, and/or sources of inspiration for those views.**

   D: No. While German anthropology was based on a synthesis of views of these two men (paragraph 2), this choice partially misrepresents the pieces from each that were synthesized. The anthropologists did follow Kant's "exclu[sion] of theological considerations from natural science" (paragraph 3). However, it was Kant, not Schelling, who believed that science consists of a priori deductions of natural laws, and the passage states that the anthropologists "would not have subscribed to the Kantian notion of science as the a priori deduction of mathematical laws" (paragraph 3).

2. **A** This is a Weaken question.

   Note: According to the last paragraph, anthropologists saw botany as a model because as botany "allowed one to observe the essence of nature relatively directly because plants do not disguise themselves with culture, as humans do," the study of so-called "natural peoples" (analogized to flowerless cryptograms) allowed anthropologists to understand culture and humanity through studying people who supposedly had no culture.

   A: **Yes. The anthropologists saw botany as a model, according to the passage, largely because they believed that one could learn about an "unchanging essence of humanity" (paragraph 1) by studying people with no culture, just as botanists can learn about an "essence of nature" by studying plants with no flowers. If there is no such thing as a people without culture, however, this would significantly undermine the validity of botany as a model for anthropology.**

   B: No. This choice does not go far enough to undermine the anthropologists' view. "Some botanists" could be two or three, and we don't know from the answer choice that their claim is valid. Beware of choices that are too weak to have a significant impact when answering Strengthen and Weaken questions.

   C: No. While Braun is identified as a "latter-day *Naturphilosoph*," the relevance of his views to those of the anthropologists does not depend on Braun representing that school of thought (keep in mind that the anthropologists rejected much of *Naturphilosophie* (paragraph 2)).

   D: No. This choice is not relevant to the question. The anthropologists believed that theology was not a legitimate part of natural science (paragraph 4). Therefore, even if the study of theology requires the study of culture, this has no impact on the anthropologists' views on the study of humanity within natural science.

3. **B** This is an Inference question.

A: No. The first part of this choice is incorrect. The anthropologists rejected Kant's view that science consists of deductions from necessary laws (see end of paragraph 3).

B: **Yes. Both parts of this choice are supported by the passage. The passage states in paragraph 4 that "it was in their empiricist approach to nature that anthropologists retained their allegiance to Schelling." In paragraph 3, the author writes that the anthropologists "would not have subscribed to the Kantian notion of science as the a priori deduction of mathematical laws. Indeed, anthropology was above all a science of the given facts, which Kant had rejected as a source of natural scientific knowledge."**

C: No. This choice is accurate up until the very last word. However, it was the idea that "the facts teach that the races of humans and the species of animals are immutable" or unchangeable that the anthropologists accepted, rather than an idea that humans are mutable or changeable (an idea that Schelling did not, according to the passage, propose).

D: No. The first part of this choice is incorrect: "Anthropologists saw in the science of botany a model for their own antievolutionist synthesis of Kant's systematizing with Schelling's empiricism" (paragraph 5). Thus, they accepted rather than rejected Kant's systematizing.

4. **C** This is an Analogy question.

Note: The non-historicist view of the German anthropologists was that nature is "a static system of categories that allowed them, in their study of 'natural peoples,' to grasp an unchanging essence of humanity, rather than the ephemeral changes historians recorded" (paragraph 1). The author also states that "in nature anthropologists sought a realm free from historical change" (paragraph 1). Later in the passage the author states: "Worse than the idealism of *Naturphilosophie* was, for anthropologists, its view of nature as becoming rather than being, a view antithetical to the concept of nature that anthropologists wanted to use against historicist humanism" (paragraph 4). Therefore, a historicist view of anthropology would be based on studying changes over time rather than some unchanging "essence of humanity." To answer the question, you need to eliminate choices that would be similar to the German anthropologists' approach, and to find the answer that represents studying changes or development over time.

A: No. This, in its study of unchanging laws, would be a non-historicist approach.

B: No. There is no suggestion that this approach to chemistry involves studying changes over time. The reference to the discovery of empirical laws, in fact, suggests the opposite.

C: **Yes. This approach to political science would involve studying how political systems and human beliefs and values interact and change over time, or, through history.**

D: No. A belief in the existence of inherent and consistent human motivations (similar to an "unchanging essence of humanity") suggests consistency rather than change over time.

5. **D** This is a New Information question.

Note: The German anthropologists saw nature as a "static and objective system that could be conclusively known by scientists" (paragraph 3), and believed that "Worse than the idealism of *Naturphilosophie* was…its view of nature as becoming rather than being, a view antithetical to the concept of nature that anthropologists wanted to use against historicist humanism." While the anthropologists studied human beings, they saw this study as existing within the realm of natural science. Therefore, we can infer that they would accept "*Geognosie*, the study of the present-day, essential, and inherent characteristics of the earth" as a more legitimate scientific approach than "*Geologie*, the study of how geological features evolve and come into being."

A: No. The passage suggests that they would prefer *Geognosie* over *Geologie*, as more scientific.

B: No. There is no evidence in the question stem or in the passage that the anthropologists would see either, especially *Geognosie*, as totally irrelevant.

C: No. The passage suggests that the anthropologists themselves were looking for strict categories to apply to humanity (paragraph 1). Therefore, there is no reason to infer that they would see categorization as a problem. Furthermore, the anthropologists believed natural science should look for unchanging, rather than changeable, elements.

D: Yes. *Geognosie* fits better with the anthropologists' view of legitimate natural science.

6.   **C**   This is an Inference/LEAST question (that is, it asks which statement is least supported by the passage).

A: No. This statement is supported by paragraph 5, where the author writes: "Braun argued that the study of plants allowed one to observe the essence of nature relatively directly because plants do not disguise themselves with culture, as humans do." Braun's ideas were part of the reason why the anthropologists saw botany as a model for their own approach.

B: No. In paragraph 1, the author states that "German anthropologists understood nature as a static [or unchanging] system of categories." In paragraph 3, the author claims: "From Kant anthropologists took an idea of nature as a static and objective system that could be conclusively known by scientists." Therefore, the anthropologists would agree with this statement.

C: Yes. While Kant believed chemistry was not a science, the anthropologists disagreed on this point. For Schelling and for the anthropologists (who followed Schelling's empirical approach), "a science of qualities, such as chemistry with its qualitatively different elements, could count as a science" (paragraph 4). Therefore the anthropologists would least agree with this statement.

D: No. In paragraph 3, the author states that "Unlike Newton, Kant excluded theological considerations from natural science" and that "this law-based, objective, totally secular, and perfectly knowable nature would have appealed to anthropologists." In paragraph 4, the passage states that "anthropologists separated religious and scientific questions, following Kant's rather than Schelling's understanding of the relation of natural and theological knowledge. Allowing theology and development to enter into discussions of nature would undermine the basic project of anthropology as an antihumanist science of natural peoples outside history." Therefore, the anthropologists would agree, not disagree, with this choice.

7.   **C**   This is a Structure question.

Note: All of the claims cited in the choices are in the passage. The question is, which claim is used by the author to most directly support the assertion cited in the question stem.

A: No. The existence of a debate over the concept of nature doesn't itself directly support or explain the author's claim about the anthropologists' own views. The fact that this statement appears in the same paragraph is not enough to show that it acts to logically support the assertion cited in the question.

B: No. The fact that British natural theology, unlike the anthropologists' approach to natural science, combined religion with science doesn't by itself support the author's claim about the actual content or nature of the anthropologists' views on historical change.

C: **Yes. Virchow is quoted in paragraph 4, in the context of the author's explanation of the anthropologists' view that "Worse than the idealism of *Naturphilosophie* was, for anthropologists, its view of nature as becoming rather than being, a view antithetical to the concept of nature that anthropologists wanted to use against historicist humanism." (Note the word "thus" at the beginning of the next sentence, which indicates that the Virchow quote is part of the discussion of the anthropologists' view.) This is a continuation of the discussion that begins in paragraph 1 of the anthropologists' antihistorical approach. Therefore, even though Virchow's statement appears in a different paragraph, it still acts to support and explain the assertion made in paragraph 1.**

D: No. While discussion of this tension is part of the author's overall argument, it doesn't itself directly support the author's claim about the specific assertion cited in the question stem. The fact that it appears in the same paragraph as the assertion doesn't guarantee that it acts to support that assertion.

Individual Passage Log

Passage # _____

Q#	Q type	Attractors	What did you do wrong?

Revised Strategy _____

Passage # _____

Q#	Q type	Attractors	What did you do wrong?

Revised Strategy _____

Think Like a Test-Writer: Exercise 3

THINK LIKE A TEST-WRITER: EXERCISE 3

Just as there are certain kinds of statements in passage texts that tend to generate questions, there are particular aspects of the logical structure of a passage text that the test-writers use to create attractive wrong answers (that is, "Attractors"). For example, if two things are compared or contrasted and a question asks what is true of one, the test-writers will likely create a wrong answer that is true of the other. If the author describes a point of view and then *disagrees* with it, a wrong answer may describe the author as *agreeing* with that point of view. If the author stakes out a moderate position, a wrong answer may describe it as much more extreme than it actually is. And, if a question asks for the main idea or primary purpose of the passage as a whole, a wrong answer may state something that is true based on the passage, but is only one theme among many in the text.

The purpose of this drill is to sensitize you to the aspects of a passage that may generate predictable wrong answers, so that you are able to predict, recognize, and eliminate them more effectively when doing a CARS passage.

In the text on the next page, you will see parts of the passage in red font. These are some of the kinds of things that test-writers may use to create attractive wrong answers. A short description of a type of Attractor this text might inspire follows, *italicized and in [brackets].*

First, read the entire passage, paying close attention to the parts in red but also tracking the author's argument in each paragraph and through the passage as a whole. Then address the questions that follow; for each question, a guide to the right answer is provided. Your task is to think about what kind of wrong answer the test-writers might create for that question, perhaps tied to a part of the passage with the text in red. You might come up with anything from a general idea about the type or category of Attractor (e.g., "the opposite of what the right answer would be") to a specific statement that could be the actual Attractor choice. Once you have completed the drill, take a look at the explanations that follow.

[Note: the computer-based testing tools do not allow you to change the color of the text, and there will be no red text in your MCAT passages. The red font here is only for the purpose of the drill. The questions attached to a CARS passage on the test will also not usually be presented in the order in which the relevant material appears in the test.]

The text on the next page is longer than a CARS passage in order to give you extra practice with these skills.

EXERCISE 3

Is it *possible* to write literary history, that is, to write that which will be both literary and a history? [*An Attractor might give the wrong answer to this rhetorical question*] Most histories of literature, it must be admitted, are either social histories, or histories of thought as illustrated in literature, or impressions and judgements on specific works arranged in more or less chronological order. [*An Attractor might mix up these views, or the views of the authors referenced next*] A glance at the history of English literary historiography will corroborate this view. Thomas Wharton, the first "formal" historian of English poetry, gave as his reason for studying ancient literature that it "faithfully records the features of the time and preserves the most picturesque and expressive representations of manners" and "transmits to posterity genuine delineations of life." Henry Morley conceived of literature as "the national biography" or the "story of the English mind." Leslie Stephen regarded literature as "a particular function of the whole social organism," "a kind of byproduct" of social change. W.J. Courthope, author of the only history of English poetry based on a unified conception of its development, defined the "study of English poetry as in effect the study of the continuous growth of our national institutions as reflected in our literature," and looked for the unity of the subject "precisely where the political historian looks for it, namely, in the life of a nation as a whole."

While these and many other historians treat literature as major document for the illustration of national or social history, those constituting another group recognize that literature is first and foremost an art, but appear unable to write history. [*An Attractor might take this overly literally or misrepresent these views on literature*] They present us with a discontinuous series of essays on individual authors, [*An Attractor might misrepresent the passage authors' criticism*] attempting to link them by "influences" but lacking any conception of real historical evolution. In his introduction to *A Short History of Modern English Literature* (1897), Edmund Gosse professed, to be sure, to show the "movement of English literature," to give a "feeling of the evolution of English literature," but he was merely paying lip service to an ideal then spreading from France. In practice, his books are a series of critical remarks on authors and some of their works, chronologically arranged…. [*An Attractor might misrepresent the nature of the passage authors' criticism*] Most leading histories of literature are either histories of civilization or collections of critical essays. One type is not a history of *art*; the other, not a *history* of art.

Why has there been no attempt, on a large scale, to trace the evolution of literature as art? One deterrent is the fact that the preparatory analysis of works of art has not been carried out in a consistent and systematic manner. Either we remain content with the old rhetorical criteria, unsatisfactory in their preoccupation with apparently superficial devices, or we have recourse to an emotive language describing the effects of a work of art upon the reader in terms incapable of real correlation with the work itself.

Another difficulty is the prejudice that no history of literature is possible save in terms of causal explanation by some other human activity. [*An Attractor might represent the passage authors' opinion as the opposite of what it really is*] A third difficulty lies in the whole conception of the development of the art of literature. Few would doubt the possibility of an internal history of painting or music. It suffices to walk through any set of art galleries arranged according to chronological order or in accordance with "schools" to see that there is a history of the art of painting quite distinct from either the history of painters or the appreciation or judgement of individual pictures. It suffices to listen to a concert in which compositions are chronologically arranged to see that there is a history of music which has scarcely anything to do with [*An Attractor might indicate that the opposite is true*] the biographies of the composers, the social conditions under which the works were produced, or the appreciation of individual pieces. Such histories have been attempted in painting and sculpture ever since Winckelmann wrote his *Geschichte der Kunst im Altertum* (1764) and most histories of music since Burney have paid attention to the history of musical forms.

Literary history has before it the analogous problem [*An Attractor might misrepresent the nature or purpose of this analogy*] of tracing the history of literature as an art, in comparative isolation from its social history, the biographies of authors, or the appreciation of individual works. Of course, the task of literary history (in this limited sense) presents its special obstacles. Compared to a painting [*An Attractor might misrepresent this comparison, or the comparison with music*], which can be seen at a glance, a literary work of art is accessible only through a time-sequence and thus is more difficult to realize as a coherent whole. But the analogy of musical form shows that a pattern as possible, even when it can be grasped only in a temporal sequence. There are, further, special problems. In literature, there is a gradual transition from simple statements to highly organized works of art, since the medium of literature, language, is also the medium of everyday communication and especially the medium of sciences. It is thus more difficult to isolate the aesthetic structure of a literary work. Yet [*An Attractor might ignore the shift indicated with this word "yet"*] an illustrative plate in a medical textbook and a military march are two examples to show that the other arts also have their borderline cases and that the difficulties in distinguishing between art and non-art in linguistic utterance are only greater quantitatively.

Theorists there are, however, who simply deny that literature has a history. W. P. Ker argued, for instance, that we do not need literary history, as its objects are always present, are "eternal," and thus have no proper history at all. T.S. Eliot also will deny the "pastness" of a work of art. "The whole of the literature of Europe from Homer," he says, "has a simultaneous existence and composes a simultaneous order." Art, one could argue with Schopenhauer, has always reached its goal. It never improves, and cannot be superseded or repeated *[An Attractor might misrepresent this claim, perhaps by taking it too literally]*…. So literary history is no proper history because it is the knowledge of the present, the omnipresent, the eternally present. One cannot deny, of course, that there is some real difference between political history and history of art. *[An Attractor might misrepresent the nature of this contrast]* There is a distinction between that which is historical and past and that which is historical and still somehow present.

As we have shown before, an individual work of art does not remain unchanged *[An Attractor might take this too literally]* through the course of history. There is to be sure a substantial identity of structure which has remained the same throughout the ages. But this structure is dynamic; it changes throughout the process of history while passing through the minds of readers, critics, and fellow artists. The process of interpretation, criticism, and appreciation has never been completely interrupted

and is likely to continue indefinitely, or at least as long as there is no complete interruption of the cultural tradition. One of the tasks of the literary historian is the description of this process. Another is the tracing of the development of works of art arranged in smaller and larger groups, according to common authorship, or genres, or stylistic types, or linguistic tradition, and finally inside a scheme of universal literature.

But the concept of the development of a series of works of art seems an extraordinarily difficult one. In a sense each work of art is, at first sight, a structure discontinuous with neighboring works of art. One can argue that there is no development from one individuality to another. One meets even with the objection that there is no history of literature, only one of men writing. Yet according to the same argument we should have to give up writing a history of language *[An Attractor might indicate that the author believes this, or the claim about "personalism" below, to be true]* because there are only men uttering words or a history of philosophy because there are only men thinking. Extreme "personalism" of this sort must lead to the view that every individual work of art is completely isolated, which in practice would mean that it would be both incommunicable and incomprehensible. We must conceive rather of literature as a whole system of works which is, with the accretion of new ones, constantly changing its relationships, growing as a changing whole.

—Adapted from Rene Wellek and Austin Warren, *Theory of Literature.* Copyright © 1956, 1949, 1942 by Houghton Mifflin Harcourt Publishing Company, renewed 1984, 1977, 1975 by Rene Wellek and Austin Warren.

Question #1: What answer to the question posed in the first sentence is suggested by the rest of the passage?

Right answer: Yes, it is possible to write a true "literary history."

Predicted Attractor: _____

_____

_____

Question #2: The authors state that Leslie Stephen believes literature to be which of the following?

Right answer: "A particular function of the whole social organism" (most likely a paraphrase of this statement).

Predicted Attractor: _____

_____

_____

Question #3: When the authors state in paragraph 2 that some writers on literature "appear unable to write history," they most likely mean that these writers:

Right answer: The authors of the passage mean that these writers may claim to be writing a literary history, but what they are really producing are assessments of individual writings with no real discussion of the evolution of literature over time, or of what links those pieces together.

Predicted Attractor: _____

_____

_____

Question #4: What can be inferred from the authors' statement in paragraph 4 that "Another difficulty is the prejudice that no history of literature is possible save in terms of causal explanation by some other human activity"?

Right answer: The authors indicate here that a history of literature CAN be written on its own terms, without reference to other aspects of human existence (for example politics or social institutions).

Predicted Attractor: _____

_____

_____

Question #5: With which of the following statements regarding the history of music would the authors be most likely to agree?

Right answer: The authors draw an analogy between literary history and musical history in paragraph 4. The authors' point is that you CAN write a history of music without reference to "the biographies of the composers, the social conditions under which the works were produced, or the appreciation of individual pieces."

Predicted Attractor: _____

_____

_____

Question #6: Which of the following would most *weaken* the passage's claim regarding the difference between literature and painting presented in paragraph 5?

Right answer: Anything that indicates that the way we perceive a work of literature and a painting is similar in a relevant way would *weaken* the contrast drawn in the passage; for example, that one DOES in some way view aspects of a painting sequentially rather than all at once "at a glance" or that we do NOT perceive a work of literature "through a time-sequence."

Predicted Attractor: _____

_____

_____

Question #7: The authors of the passage most likely refer to an illustrative plate in a medical textbook in order to:

Right answer: The authors refer to a medical illustration to suggest that (1) it may not be purely aesthetic in nature and therefore (2) literature is not unique in this way. Thus, the purpose is to (3) refute a possible objection to the authors' argument.

Predicted Attractor: _____

_____

_____

Question #8: Which of the following would be most analogous to T.S. Eliot's claim that a work of art has no true "past"?

Right answer: To understand this statement it helps to take it in the context of W. P. Ker's similar argument that the objects of literary history are "always present, are 'eternal,' and thus have no proper history at all." That is, that literature takes as its subject eternal aspects of human existence. One valid analogy, for example, might describe the field of ethics as presenting questions that are always at issue in human life and that do not fundamentally change over time.

Predicted Attractor: _____

_____

_____

Question #9: By "an individual work of art does not remain unchanged" (paragraph 7) the authors most likely mean:

Right answer: Taking this statement in the context of what follows it in the passage, the authors mean that art "changes" as others interpret it. As in, it is perceived and understood in different ways by different people in different times, and this in a sense transforms that work of art.

Predicted Attractor: _____

_____

_____

Question #10: What is the primary purpose of the passage?

Right answer: The primary purpose of this passage is to argue that it is possible to write a true evolutionary history of literature without explaining it through extraneous factors (like politics, or the author's biography or the social context in which it was written).

Predicted Attractor: _____

_____

_____

SOLUTIONS TO EXERCISE 3

1. Predicted Attractor—A wrong answer might state that no, one cannot write a true literary history, perhaps because it has not yet been accomplished, or because the two genres are supposedly mutually exclusive.

2. Predicted Attractor—A likely wrong answer would reference other views described in paragraph 1 that are not focused on change: that it "faithfully records the features of the time and preserves the most picturesque and expressive representations of manners" and "transmits to posterity genuine delineations of life" (Thomas Wharton), or that it is "the national biography" and the "story of the English mind" (Henry Morley).

3. Predicted Attractor—An answer choice that takes this statement too literally would be tempting. For example, that they are intellectually incapable of writing literary history, or that it is literally impossible to write about literature and to write history at the same time.

4. Predicted Attractor—When an author states an opposing position in order to debunk it, a wrong answer that describes the opposing position rather than the author's position often sounds great. Here, that wrong answer would suggest that literature *cannot* be explained on its own terms, and that any causal explanation would have to refer to some other human activity as well.

5. Predicted Attractor—If you got turned around in the beginning of the paragraph and thought the opposing position was the authors' position and vice versa, that mistake might carry through to this part of the paragraph as well. The test-writers know this, so they may well present the claim that you CANNOT write about music without reference to "the biographies of the composers, the social conditions under which the works were produced, or the appreciation of individual pieces" as a wrong answer.

6. Predicted Attractor—One of the most predictable Attractors on a Weaken question is something that strengthens. Add to this that one of the most predictable Attractors for a question about a contrast in the passage is something that indicates a similarity. Add those together, and the most predictable Attractor for this question would be something that *strengthens* that part of the passage by indicating that painting and literature are in fact *different* in this way.

7. Predicted Attractor—Especially given the abstract nature of this part of the passage, the test-writers know that it is hard to follow the twists and turns in the authors' argument. Therefore, they may present you with a choice that (1) indicates that the medical illustration (and the military march) are *counterexamples* to the authors' argument or that they (2) are given to support a different claim in the passage (for example the earlier argument about time sequence).

8. Predicted Attractor—One possible way in which an answer may go wrong is to present a scenario in which something "has no past" for an opposite reason. For example, it might describe a technological innovation that has fundamentally changed the nature of human existence and that has no antecedent and therefore "no pastness."

9. Predicted Attractor—A wrong answer may take this statement too literally, for example as if the authors are saying that an individual literary work may be rewritten or edited later in time. Or, a wrong answer may interpret the statement in the context of some other part of the passage; for example, as if the authors were still discussing the issue of time sequencing, or the possibility of tracing the evolutionary history (change over time) of literature.

10. Predicted Attractor—One of the most predictable Attractors tied to a particular question type is the "too narrow" answer to a general question. Here, the wrong answer could be any sub-point in the passage, such as "Literature, unlike a painting, cannot be perceived through a single glance," or "Art is always changing" or "Most histories of literature are histories of society or else assessment of individual works of art." These are all true according to the passage, but none of them capture the passage as whole.

Chapter 6
Ranking and Ordering
the Passages

GOALS

1) To understand the organization of the MCAT CARS section
2) To learn to assess the difficulty levels of passages
3) To learn a strategy for attacking the section as a whole

6.1 WHY RANK THE PASSAGES?

As we have discussed, to maximize your efficiency and accuracy within each passage you must take control of the material and not let the material control you. In the same way, you'll maximize your score by taking control of the section *as a whole*, working through the passages in a way that helps you get the easy questions right instead of wasting time on the most difficult questions.

This chapter outlines what you need to know about how the MCAT CARS section is organized in terms of level of difficulty and how you can assess the nine passages to design your best plan of attack.

How Are the MCAT CARS Passages Organized?

The MCAT does not follow a strict pattern in how they organize the nine passages; they are presented more or less randomly. Needless to say, the AAMC will not disclose specific information concerning how the passages are chosen, how many are at an easy, medium, or difficult level, etc. Moreover, each administration is different, and every time the test is administered there are multiple forms of the test. So, where does that leave us?

Let's begin with what we know. During the many years that we have been developing these materials, we have discovered some patterns. A lot of experience has led us to the following conclusions about the structure of the CARS section.

Passage Organization

Although one might think that the nine passages would be arranged in order of level of difficulty (that is, easy passages first, medium next, and difficult last), this is generally *not* the case. What would be the point of putting all the difficult passages at the end in a section that students sometimes don't finish? In fact, the passages are in a seemingly random order; often, the last passage in the section is an easy or medium passage that you want to be sure to complete, and the hardest passage is in the middle of the section.

Many CARS sections will have at least one passage that merits the rank of Killer, meaning it's so difficult that spending even 30 or 40 minutes wouldn't allow you to answer all—or even most of—the questions correctly. Killer passages are not worth your valuable time—guess on the questions or, at least, do them last.

Therefore, it's up to you to strategically reorganize your nine passages in order to address them most effectively.

Passage Division

Division of the nine passages generally breaks down into

- 2–3 easy passages
- 3–5 medium passages
- 1–2 difficult passages

Unless your reasonable goal is to score at the very top of the scale, you probably should be randomly guessing on at least one passage; that is, the one or two most difficult passages in the section. And if your reasonable goal is to score in the 98th or 99th percentile, you may still do best by guessing on a few of the most difficult questions you encounter.

6.2   ASSESSING DIFFICULTY LEVEL: NOW, LATER, AND KILLER

Your first objective when beginning the section is to assess the relative difficulty of the passages. A passage should be ranked Now if it seems relatively straightforward. The passages that appear to be more challenging should be ranked as Later. The most difficult passage or passages (the ones on which you may be randomly guessing) get a rank of Killer.

Although it's tempting to associate topic or subject matter with difficulty level, remember that—unlike the science sections—the CARS section of the MCAT does not test outside knowledge. Everything you need to correctly answer the questions is in the passage. In fact, bringing in outside knowledge can actually hurt your score.

Students will often want to skip easier passages simply because they're about, say, poetry or opera (or any other topic that tends to be unfamiliar). However, what really makes a passage difficult is the way it's written (and in some cases the types of questions that are asked about it). Just because a topic is boring or foreign to you doesn't mean the passage is written in an inaccessible way, and even though a topic may be interesting or familiar, the passage can be written in a dense, convoluted way.

The Passage Text

What Should You Look For?

The following criteria should be used to evaluate the difficulty of the passage text itself.

1) **Level of concreteness or abstraction:** Passages that are highly theoretical and that discuss abstract concepts will be much harder to follow than passages that are concrete and descriptive. Would you rather read a passage about the "philosophic contemplation of the Not-Self" or one on the "doubling of the cost of living in the last ten years"? And again, subject matter is not the key to difficulty. For example, an art passage that is essentially a painter's biography may be very concrete and factual, and therefore quite easy to comprehend.

2) **Language level:** While the CARS section cannot expect you to know technical language specific to a particular discipline (without defining the terms in context), difficult passages will often include esoteric language that no one really uses in everyday conversation. If the author uses many such words as *lugubrious*, *phlegmatic*, *synesthesia*, or *flagitious* in the first few sentences, she's probably not going to start using "plain English" in the next few. Lots of unfamiliar vocabulary will make the passage more difficult to understand, regardless of the topic.

3) **Sentence structure:** Extremely long, convoluted sentences are harder to read, especially under a time constraint. Short, direct sentences will be easier to follow.

How to Evaluate the Passage Text

Skim the first few sentences of the first or second paragraph. Try to paraphrase what you have just read. If your reaction is essentially "huh???," and all you can do is repeat the exact wording of the passage because the meaning of those words is so unclear, this indicates a more difficult passage. If, on the other hand, you can easily put the meaning of those lines into your own words, the passage is likely to be fairly straightforward.

Think of it this way: if, in 15 seconds, you could explain to your six-year-old sister what those two sentences are saying, then the passage will probably make sense to you, too.

Do NOT rank a passage solely on the basis of its length. The few moments it may take you to read five or six extra lines will not significantly affect your performance, but choosing a short yet difficult passage over a longer but easier passage certainly will.

The Questions

Adapting to Difficulty Level

Given that the questions are displayed one at a time, on separate screens, for most test-takers it is too cumbersome and time-consuming to click through and look at each question, evaluate the difficulty level of the set, and then incorporate that into a ranking decision. Therefore, most of your ranking decisions should be based on the apparent difficulty of the passage text.

However, once you have decided to do a passage and are Previewing the Questions, if you notice a high percentage of very difficult question types (in particular, Application and Structure-Evaluate questions) or unusually lengthy question stems and/or answer choices, you may decide at that point to skip over that passage (Flagging the questions for review, guessing on the questions and making a clear noteboard note) and move on to the next. Do not, however, employ this strategy more than once or twice during a CARS section. Otherwise, you will spend too much time previewing questions without answering them, and your efficiency and pacing will suffer.

6.3   ORDERING THE SECTION

Now that you have the criteria with which to rank your passages, let's discuss the overall ordering of
the section.

The Two-Pass System

1) For the first passage, write down the passage number and question range on your noteboard
   (e.g., "Passage 1 Q 1-7").

2) Read the first two or three sentences of the passage and try to paraphrase. If it's a Now passage, do it now. If it's a Later or Killer passage, write "SKIPPED" under the passage heading
   on your noteboard, Flag for Review and randomly guess on each question, and move on to
   ranking the next passage. Go through the entire section in the same way: writing the passage
   heading on your noteboard, completing the Now passages, and noting, Flagging, and guessing on the Later or Killer passages. This is your first pass.

3) Once you've completed all the Now passages, take a second pass through the section and do
   all the Later passages. You can use the Review function, if necessary, to find the passages you
   have Flagged and guessed on.

At or before the 5-minute mark (ideally before you begin your last passage), inspect the section to make
sure that you haven't left any questions blank.

If you have a few extra minutes left over for a Killer passage, quickly read the first and last sentence of
each paragraph. Identify the easiest questions (especially Retrieval questions and Inference questions with
paragraph references and/or lead words), and do as many as you can by going to the relevant sections of the
passage text. Again, be careful to leave time to fill in random guesses for the questions you cannot complete.

6.4 CARS EXERCISES: RANKING

Exercise 1: Evaluating the Passage Text

Each of the following paragraphs represents the first two sentences of a CARS passage. Using the criteria described earlier, decide if these are likely to be Now, Later, or Killer passages. You can find answers at the end of the exercise.

Passage I

It is often argued that the attempt to regulate the behavior of corporations through legislation is at best futile and at worst deleterious; in making their argument, advocates of nonregulation assume a distinction between the morality of duty and the morality of aspiration. They argue that duties, which specify the minimum standards of human conduct, lend themselves to legal enforcement better than do aspirations, which exhort one to realize one's full potential.

Passage II

A fundamental element of the American criminal justice system is trial by impartial jury. This constitutionally protected guarantee allows the defendant to challenge prospective jurors who are clearly prejudiced in the case.

Passage III

Imagining a primal state of existence, one in which there is no notion of space or time as we know it, pushes most people's powers of comprehension to the limit.... We run up against a clash of paradigms when we try to envision a universe that is, but somehow does not invoke the concepts of space or time.

Passage IV

The KT boundary, as it is called, marks one of the most violent events ever to befall life on Earth. Sixty-five million years ago, according to the current theory, the Cretaceous period was brought to a sudden conclusion by the impact of an asteroid or comet ten kilometers in diameter.

Passage V

A satisfactory explanation of the deepest significance of the fluoridation controversy remains elusive. Despite decades of research on the topic, the persistence and the passion of the fluoridation debates are yet incompletely understood by social scientists and social philosophers.

Passage VI

Trust and its violation have intrigued sociologists for decades. Trust is no more than an attribute of individuals; trust also describes a form of social organization, and interorganizational dynamics of trust violations offer a challenge to regulatory models that are largely intercorporate and involve individual or organizational self dealing.

Passage VII

The events of the author's life as they appear in poetry cannot be taken as literally true. As we move through life, our memory of what happened in the past changes and becomes more positive; events that were full of anxiety when they occurred now seem much more enjoyable in retrospect.

Passage VIII

Mention the word "surrealism" today, and certain visual images spring immediately to mind, and these images inevitably lead to certain assumptions about Surrealism: that it was primarily concerned with the visual arts, that it was about jokes, and that it was designed with a beady eye to the market. Nothing could be further from the truth, however.

Passage IX

Punishment appears to have unintended consequences. According to social theory, for example, punishment may increase the incidence of aggression because the target may imitate the behavior of the punishing agent, and offenders who are labeled are likely to behave consistently with expectations associated with that label.

Passage X

Nietzsche sees morality in much the same way that he sees epistemology. There is a gradual emptying out of that which is living in morality.

Explanations for Exercise 1: Evaluating the Passage Text

1. **Difficult:** This paragraph includes abstract concepts such as "the morality of duty and the morality of aspiration" that are difficult to paraphrase. Also, the vocabulary level is high—"deleterious," "nonregulation," "aspiration"—and will likely remain so throughout the passage.
2. **Easy:** This passage seems straightforward and factual.
3. **Medium:** This passage is fairly abstract. "Primal state of existence" and "paradigms" are red flag phrases.
4. **Easy:** This passage seems straightforward, and it seems to have a clear viewpoint.
5. **Medium:** A passage about the "deepest significance" of a controversy is likely to be fairly abstract. This is also indicated by the fact that social scientists and philosophers are trying to understand it, meaning the passage may be a challenge for test-takers to understand as well.
6. **Difficult:** The second sentence in particular is very abstract with a complex structure that makes it difficult to follow—the passage is likely to continue in the same vein.
7. **Easy:** Even though this passage is about a perhaps unfamiliar topic (poetry), the description is straightforward and easy to follow.
8. **Easy:** Although it is about art, which is usually considered an abstract topic, the paragraph is fairly descriptive and concrete rather than being highly theoretical.
9. **Medium:** There are some fairly abstract references here (e.g., "aggression," "the target," and "the punishing agent") which may muddy up the clarity of the passage.
10. **Difficult:** Try doing the six-year-old sister test on this paragraph. The vocabulary level, the sentence structure, and the abstractness of the subject matter indicate that this will be an extremely difficult passage.

Exercise 2: Evaluating the Questions

In most cases, your passage ranking will be based only on the passage text. However, to be able to adapt your ranking, if needed, to an usually difficult set of questions during the preview stage, you need to be able to recognize what tends to make questions easier or harder. Classify each of the following CARS questions as Easy or Hard. You can find answers at the end of the exercise.

1. It can be inferred from the passage that the availability of temperature-depth records for any specific area of the United States depends primarily on the:

2. In order to support his view with respect to Wilson's *Declining Significance of Race*, Hill would be most likely to discuss which one of the following?

3. Which of the following statements would most *weaken* the author's claim that voir dire fails to ensure a jury's impartiality?

4. Suppose it was demonstrated that social media has a less significant effect on political opinion than previously thought. What impact would this have on the author's claims in the second paragraph?

5. According to the passage, which of the following was most important in creating the modern trend toward redistribution?

6. The phrase "potent political opposition" (paragraph 1) refers to:

7. The author's attitude toward insider trading can best be described as:

8. In their evaluation of the fossil record, the author states that Cutler and Behrenmeyer did all of the following EXCEPT:

9. Of the following, which would be most logically similar to the way in which a majority of fatalities from malaria occur, as the process is described in the passage?

10. The author claims that the art market rises and falls in concert with the stock market. How well is this claim supported by the author?

Explanations for Exercise 2: Evaluating the Questions

1. **Easy:** Inference questions with specific references to the passage often have straightforward answers. In this case, you would probably just need to find where these records are discussed in the passage.

2. **Hard:** This is a Strengthen question that involves two speakers—you need to keep both of their perspectives in mind and conclude what approach Hill would take to support his or her own position in comparison (or contrast) to Wilson's.

3. **Hard:** A Weaken question requires taking new information provided in the answer choices and using reasoning to apply it to the passage.

4. **Hard:** The word "suppose" indicates that this question is going to require evaluating new information in the question stem and then taking multiple steps to answer the question. Also, the question stem is quite lengthy.

5. **Easy:** This is a Retrieval question, so the answer can be found in the passage text.

6. **Easy:** This question tells you where to go to find the information you need. As long as you remember to read above and below, it should not be difficult to answer.

7. **Easy:** The author's attitude can usually be determined with little difficulty.

8. **Easy:** The wording "The author states" tells you that this is a Retrieval question. The fact that it is an "EXCEPT" question shouldn't make it significantly more difficult, as long as you keep track of the question format, and of why you are eliminating each choice.

9. **Hard:** The phrase "logically similar" indicates that this is an Analogy question, which involves a higher level of reasoning and abstraction than do most question types.

10. **Hard:** This is an Evaluate question: you will have to decide if the support given is strong or weak and why.

Exercise 3: Evaluate Your Ranking

Ranking is a skill, like any other, that needs to be learned, practiced, and refined over time. If you ever rank an easy passage as Later (or Killer), or a difficult passage as Now, review the passage to see what made it easy or difficult and how you could have evaluated it better the first time through.

Compare the ranking you gave each passage to your eventual performance (taking into account both your accuracy and your efficiency/pacing) on that passage. Determine the order of attack that would have worked best for you.

- Were there any Killer passages that you should have skipped and guessed on? How could you have known it was a Killer before you wasted any time on it?
- Did you fail to get to any easy passages lurking at the end of the section?
- How will you change your approach on the next MCAT Practice Test you take?

Chapter 6 Summary

- The nine passages in the MCAT CARS section are "organized" in a seemingly random way. The level of difficulty of each passage depends on both the reading level of the passage text and on the difficulty level of the question types.

- To maximize your score, you must attack the passages strategically. Don't waste your time on Killer passages!

CHAPTER 6 PRACTICE PASSAGES

Individual Practice Drills

Rank the two passages that follow. Do the passage that you rank as easier first. Keep track of the time you spend on each passage, but don't give yourself a set time limit.

Once you have completed the passages and checked your answers, fill out an Individual Passage Log for each passage. In particular, decide if you ranked and ordered them correctly. If not, define what you could have recognized about the passage text and/or the questions in order to rank and order the passages more accurately and effectively.

By now, you should be taking full timed CARS sections and full practice tests from online or other resources. Always evaluate your ranking after completing a CARS test section.

Don't agonize over your decisions or panic if every choice you make isn't perfect. Ranking is simply another way to gain more control over the test (and to take that control away from the test-writers).

CHAPTER 6 PRACTICE PASSAGE 1

While I would certainly not want to disparage the efforts of vegetarians to limit violence toward animals in their personal lives and in public institutions and practices involving the slaughter and consumption of animals, I think it is important also to underscore that vegetarianism is itself fundamentally deconstructible. Vegetarianism is not just a passion for other animals but a series of practices involving animals and a series of discourses about animals. And if we follow the logic of Derrida's thought on the question of the animal, then it is necessary both to support vegetarianism's progressive potential but also interrogate its limitations. I have already shown how animal ethics in general (and animal rights theory, in particular) tends to reinforce the very metaphysics of subjectivity it seeks to undercut inasmuch as animal ethicists rely on a shared subjectivity among human beings and animals to ground their theories. But there are other limitations in vegetarian and pro-animal practices that should be noted. First, no matter how rigorous one's vegetarianism might be, there is simply no way to nourish oneself in advanced, industrial countries that does not involve harm to animal life (and human life, as well) in direct and indirect forms.... Simply tracking the processes by which one's food gets to the table is enough to disabuse any consumer of the notion that a vegetarian diet is "cruelty free." As such, a vegetarian diet within the context of advanced, industrial societies is, at best, a significant challenge to dominant attitudes and practices toward animals, but it remains far from the kind of ethical idea it is sometimes purported to be. Second, there are other ethical stakes involved in eating that go beyond the effects consumption of meat and animal byproducts has on animals. All diets, even organic and vegetarian diets, have considerable negative effects on the natural environment and the human beings who produce and harvest food. Consequently, if we consider ethical vegetarianism to constitute an ethical stopping point, these other concerns will be overlooked. And it is precisely these other concerns, concerns about the other, often-overlooked forms of violence, that should *also* impassion a deconstructive approach to the question of the animal.

Although these critical points are certainly in line with the logic of a deconstructive approach to animal ethics, they do not form the focus of Derrida's analysis. Derrida draws attention, instead, to a different limitation to pro-animal ethics and politics, one that he associates with "interventionist violence" against animals. The violence at issue here takes a *symbolic* rather than literal form, and this symbolic violence against animals, Derrida seems to think, is one of the most pressing philosophical and metaphysical issues facing thought today. In view of this notion of symbolic violence, he makes the following statement: "Vegetarians, too, partake of animals, even of men. They practice a different mode of denigration." What does he mean by this? Clearly, ethical vegetarianism aims at avoiding consumption of animal flesh—and presumably human flesh, as well. So, in what manner do vegetarians partake of animals and other beings toward which they aim to be nonviolent? Derrida's remark here is part of a complicated argument about the ethical questions concerning eating, incorporation, and violence toward the Other. While Derrida, like Levinas, posits a nonviolent opening to the Other...he does not believe that a wholly nonviolent relation with the Other is possible. On his line of thought, violence is irreducible in our relations with the Other, if by nonviolence we mean a thought and practice relating to the Other that respects fully the alterity of the Other. In order to speak and think about or related to the Other, the Other must—to some extent—be appropriated and violated, even if only symbolically. How does one respect the singularity of the Other without betraying that alterity? *Any* act of identification, naming, or relation is a betrayal of and a violence toward the Other. Of course, this should not be taken to mean that such violence is immoral or that all forms of violence are equivalent.... [Within vegetarianism] the ethical question should not be "How do I achieve an ethically pure, cruelty-free diet?" but rather, "What is the best, most respectful, most grateful, and also most giving way of relating" to animals and other Others?

Material used in this particular passage has been adapted from the following source:

M. Calarco, *Zoographies: The Question of the Animal from Heidegger to Derrida.* © 2008 by Columbia University Press.

1. Which of the following assertions is/are made in the passage?

   I. Derrida believes that symbolic violence against animals is currently one of the most important issues in metaphysical thought.
   II. Symbolic violence against the Other is as bad as literal violence.
   III. Eating in an advanced industrialized society inherently entails harming others.

   A) II only
   B) I and II only
   C) I and III only
   D) I, II, and III

2. The author most likely believes that:

   A) vegetarianism is pointless since it cannot be freed from a relation of cruelty with the Other.
   B) Levinas is short-sighted in believing a non-violent relationship with the Other is possible.
   C) vegetarianism is noble in its efforts to limit violence against human and nonhuman animals, but it is not above questioning and criticism.
   D) Derrida is overly extreme in asserting that "vegetarians partake of animals, even men."

3. Suppose that a young girl rescues a formerly abused greyhound dog from an animal shelter. She names him Odysseus after the Greek explorer to honor the dog's past and celebrate his arrival in a safe and loving home. Based on information provided in the passage, how would Derrida respond to this situation?

   A) Derrida would allow that, even though the act of naming entails treating the animal as Other, the respect signified by the name balances against the violence done to the dog in the past.
   B) He would point out that even naming the Other is an act of violence, albeit a symbolic one, no matter what the intention behind the name.
   C) He would praise the girl for choosing such a historically significant and noble name, saying that this reflects her love of animals.
   D) Derrida would criticize the girl for committing an act of violence as severe as those committed by the dog's former owners.

4. What definition of the word "disabuse" (paragraph 1) best fits in the context of the passage?

   A) Treating something kindly and/or healing it after a period of abuse
   B) Chastising someone for misguided views
   C) Affirming someone's views
   D) Convincing a person that his or her views are fallacious

5. What is the primary purpose of the passage?

   A) To question the Derridian view of animals as Others to whom we owe an ethical responsibility, whether we are vegetarians or not
   B) To critique, with the help of Derrida's philosophy, the central motivations of vegetarianism and to suggest a new basis for a discussion concerning how best to treat animals
   C) To suggest that vegetarianism is fundamentally misguided since nobody can practice a completely "cruelty free" diet
   D) To interrogate the notion of "ethical purity" and argue that such a state of being is impossible

6. All of the following are claims made by the author EXCEPT:

   A) ethical vegetarianism aims to avoid the consumption of animal and human flesh.
   B) vegetarianism remains far from the ethical ideal it is purported to be.
   C) animal ethicists rely on a shared subjectivity between humans and animals to ground their theories.
   D) vegetarianism is fundamentally deconstructive.

7. The author provides the most support for which of the following claims?

   A) Derrida draws attention to a limitation of pro-animal ethics which is associated with "interventionist violence."
   B) There is simply no way to feed oneself in advanced, industrialized countries without causing some harm to animal life.
   C) All diets have considerably negative effects on the environment and on the humans who produce and harvest food.
   D) Vegetarians are not as ethically pure as vegans, who avoid all animal byproducts in their diets, thereby reducing their environmental harm.

CHAPTER 6 PRACTICE PASSAGE 2

Hispanics are the fastest growing minority in the United States. "Hispanics," "Latinos," "Chicanos," "Mexican Americans," "Puerto Ricans," "Cuban Americans," and so on, are all designations used to describe this large, heterogeneous population with different cultural, ethnic, geographic, and social backgrounds. There is still no clear definition of the term "Hispanic." The data available regarding the incidence, morbidity, and mortality from cancer in "Hispanics" are scarce, scattered, outdated, and often incomplete.

From the studies looking at the accessibility and availability of medical care to this population, few have examined in detail the variability within the entire Hispanic population. The aggregation of culturally distinct subgroups, which have resided in the United States for different periods of time, into a more inclusive "Hispanic" category assumes that all persons of Mexican, Central and South American, Cuban, and Puerto Rican extraction have similar perceptions, true or not, of cancer risks and share needs and experience similar barriers in using health services. There is, however, no clear evidence for this assumption.

On the contrary, there is evidence that each group has specific characteristics that make them different and independent from one another, despite the fact that they also share some commonalities. Recruitment of minorities, specifically Hispanics, to clinical trials has been a significant problem that can potentially be overcome by adequate protocol development and investigator education regarding specific knowledge, attitudes, and needs of minority populations. It is timely and refreshing to see a recent anthropological evaluation of the problem of cancer in (female) Hispanics. It reviews the knowledge, attitudes, and barriers (KAB) for breast and cervical cancer in four different groups of women of Hispanic/Latino origin and compare them among themselves and against a group of physicians' KAB.

Unfortunately, there are no complete data regarding cancer in all Hispanic groups. We currently do not know the true number of cancer cases in Hispanics, nor do we have accurate morbidity, mortality, and survival data from these groups. As a result, we are not really able to fully understand or appreciate the physical, emotional, and financial impact of cancer in Hispanic patients and their families. Mortality from cancer in Hispanics is difficult to assess because of the limited data that are available. Utilizing existing community groups and organizations and helping to create strong community bonds could improve the potential for success of minority cancer control efforts and patient recruitment to clinical trials. These programs can become networks of information with inherent trust from their respective communities. In developing these interventions, we should increase our awareness of the needs of all different Hispanic groups and assure that programs are developed together with these communities, in order to assure that they are culture- and community-sensitive, respecting and complementing the Hispanic heritage.

[The recent anthropological study reminds] us that perhaps there are no true knowledge deficits, but rather misconceptions regarding the true cancer risks. Thus, it emphasizes two facts: (1) we must get to know and understand the population(s) with whom we plan to work; and (2) there is a strong need for education, not only of the communities with whom we work but, perhaps more important, of the scientific teams (physicians, nurses, anthropologists, social workers, etc.) that will work in and with those communities. Preliminary data from our group have shown that community-based lay health educators ("Promotoras de Salud"), working together with local health departments can be successful in reaching, educating, and increasing recruitment of Hispanic (Mexican-American) women to cervical cancer screening programs and to cancer clinical trials. This program is now being piloted through the Southwest Oncology Group in San Antonio's (Texas) Hispanic community. The time has come to revise and update our sources of information and data gathering. Careful study of each Hispanic subgroup is essential in order to have a realistic picture of the overall cancer problem in the United States today. These studies must include a clearer definition of the differences among the many Hispanic subgroups with their respective problems and barriers to cancer care.

Material used in this particular passage has been adapted from the following source:

M. R. Modiano, "Breast and Cervical Cancer in Hispanic Women," *Medical Anthropology Quarterly*, © 1995, the American Anthropological Association.

1. The primary purpose of the passage is to:

A) prompt others to create a better, more accurate definition of "Hispanics."
B) promote a better understanding of Hispanic populations in order to recognize and serve their cancer health needs.
C) advocate for the term "Hispanic" to be discarded for its ineffectively inclusive description of diverse peoples.
D) educate Latino cancer patients about available resources.

2. The author characterizes Hispanics as which of the following?

A) A large, diverse minority of Spanish-speaking people in the United States with unusually strong community bonds
B) A population whose various members face similar obstacles in the health care system
C) A group whose known epidemiological cancer data may be lacking
D) A heterogeneous people who are represented well in clinical trials

3. Which of the following are limitations that exist currently, as stated by the passage?

   I. The view of Hispanics as a culturally monolithic people
   II. Language barriers between health care professionals and patients
   III. Interference by medically untrained community groups

A) I only
B) I and II only
C) I and III only
D) II and III only

4. It can be inferred that the author would be in favor of a program with all of the following aspects EXCEPT:

A) a careful study of each Hispanic subgroup focusing on commonalities between them.
B) a community-based initiative that is congruent with Hispanic cultures.
C) an emphasis on cancer screening in women.
D) education of medical professionals about the populations they serve.

5. The author deems all of the following as positive aspects of the recent study discussed EXCEPT:

A) pointing out potentially helpful ways in which clinical trial recruitment can be improved.
B) separating "Hispanic" women in the study into specific groups.
C) utilizing an anthropological approach in analyzing cancer data in Hispanics.
D) gathering data on all of the different Hispanic subgroups.

6. The tone of the passage can best be described as:

A) derisive and accusatory.
B) distressed but indifferent.
C) optimistic and analytical.
D) clinical and regretful.

7. The intended audience of this passage is most likely:

A) cancer hospitals or research center administrators.
B) the American public at large.
C) Hispanic women with breast or cervical cancer.
D) the Southwest Oncology Group.

SOLUTIONS TO CHAPTER 6 PRACTICE PASSAGE 1

1. **C**   This is a Retrieval/Roman numeral question.

   I: **True. In paragraph 2, the author states: "The violence at issue here takes a *symbolic* rather than literal form, and this symbolic violence against animals, Derrida seems to think, is one of the most pressing philosophical and metaphysical issues facing thought today."**

   II: False. Near the end paragraph 2, the author states: "Of course, this should not be taken to mean that such violence is immoral or that all forms of violence are equivalent." There is no statement made that equates symbolic violence with literal violence.

   III: **True. While this answer choice may sound extreme, its language is backed up in paragraph 1, when the author says, "there is simply no way to nourish oneself in advanced, industrial countries that does not involve harm to animal life."**

2. **C**   This is an Inference question.

   A: No. This answer choice is too extreme. While the author critiques vegetarianism, he never goes so far as to dismiss it as "pointless." Note that in paragraph 1, the author states: "It is necessary both to support vegetarianism's progressive potential but also interrogate its limitations."

   B: No. The author does not evoke such critical language with regards to Levinas. Also, we don't know from the text that Levinas does in fact believe that a nonviolent relationship with the Other is possible, only that Levinas, like Derrida, "posits a nonviolent opening to the Other."

   C: **Yes. The author expresses admiration for vegetarians' efforts to limit their role in violence against animals, but spends the passage highlighting some flaws in the reasoning behind vegetarianism. See paragraph 1: "It is necessary both to support vegetarianism's progressive potential but also interrogate its limitations."**

   D: No. The author does not criticize Derrida in any way. Note that when the author asks in the middle of paragraph 2, "What does he mean by this," and goes on to say that clearly vegetarians eat neither animals nor people, he is not suggesting that this (literal consumption) is in fact what Derrida is referring to. Rather, the author goes on to explain that Derrida uses "partake" in the sense of symbolic violence towards "the Other."

3. **B**   This is a New Information question.

   A: No. Derrida believes that the act of naming "the Other" is itself an act of violence (see middle of paragraph 2). Although Derrida would most likely allow or admit that this act of violence is less severe than physical abuse, it is still (symbolic) violence. Therefore the naming adds to, rather than balances against, the violence done to the dog.

   B: **Yes. In paragraph 2, the author discusses Derridian thought and states: "*Any* act of identification, naming, or relation is a betrayal of and a violence toward the Other." This answer choice is therefore the most appropriate one based on information from the passage.**

   C: No. There is no evidence in the passage to support this interpretation of Derrida's reaction. There is no suggestion that Derrida would care what the name is or what the intentions of the namer are.

   D: No. The author, in the context of explaining Derrida's argument, makes an effort to acknowledge that not all forms of violence are equivalent: "Of course, this should not be taken to mean that such violence is immoral or that all forms of violence are equivalent" (paragraph 2).

4. **D**   This is an Inference question.

   A: No. This answer is inappropriate given the context in which the word appears. The word is used in relation to changing one's mind about an opinion: in this case, the author is talking about exposing the reality that vegetarian diets are not in fact "cruelty free."

   B: No. This answer is too strong in tone: there is no personal chastising or reprimanding of the people who held views that vegetarian diets are "cruelty free."

   C: No. This answer choice is antithetical to the context of the word "disabuse" in the passage: disabusing is not about affirming someone's views but rather changing or eliminating them.

   D: Yes. This answer is the best fit according to the passage. The author suggests that thinking about how food gets to us is enough to convince anyone that a vegetarian diet is not in fact "cruelty free."

5. **B**   This is a Main Idea/Primary Purpose question.

   A: No. The author does not question Derrida's views about animals but rather employs them to make his analysis.

   B: Yes. This answer choice best captures the ideas presented in the passage and the purpose of the author's use of Derrida's philosophy. In paragraph 1, the author begins the discussion of vegetarianism's limitations by saying: "And if we follow the logic of Derrida's thought on the question of the animal, then it is necessary both to support vegetarianism's progressive potential but also interrogate its limitations." Paragraph 2 follows in kind, focusing on Derrida's views on the Other and how they relate to vegetarianism. The last sentence suggests a new way of approaching the issue: "[Within vegetarianism] the ethical question should not be 'How do I achieve an ethically pure, cruelty-free diet?' but rather, 'What is the best, most respectful, most grateful, and also most giving way of relating' to animals and other Others?"

   C: No. The words "fundamentally misguided" are too extreme given the tone of the passage. For example, the author states: "it is necessary...to support vegetarianism's progressive potential" as well as to look into its limitations (paragraph 1).

   D: No. This answer is too broad, since it does not address the idea of vegetarianism which is central to the passage. Furthermore, the author does not argue that ethical purity is never possible, but only that vegetarianism cannot itself be an ethically pure position (which relates back to the issue of the choice being too broad).

6. **D**   This is a Retrieval/EXCEPT question.

   A: No. This claim is made in paragraph 2: "Clearly, ethical vegetarianism aims at avoiding consumption of animal flesh—and presumably human flesh, as well."

   B: No. This statement is made in paragraph 1: "A vegetarian diet within the context of advanced, industrial societies is, at best, a significant challenge to dominant attitudes and practices toward animals, but it remains far from the kind of ethical idea it is sometimes purported to be."

   C: No. This statement is made word for word in paragraph 1 of the passage.

   D: Yes. In paragraph 1 the author states that "Vegetarianism is fundamentally deconstructible." This is different from saying it is "deconstructive," since the former term indicates that vegetarianism can be deconstructed, while the latter suggests it can deconstruct other things.

7. **A** This is an Evaluate question.

A: **Yes. After the author mentions Derrida's concept of "interventionist violence" in paragraph 2, he elaborates upon this term and defines it by means of discussion and example (i.e., naming the Other). Therefore, this, out of the four claims, is the one for which the author provides the most support within the passage.**

B: No. This claim is made in the passage (paragraph 1) but the author does not elaborate upon it by providing an explanation of how a vegetarian diet entails harm to animals. First, the following reference to the process by which food arrives at the table still does not explain what the direct or indirect harm might be. Second, the later reference to harm done to the environment hints at an explanation, but only a vague one (there is still no discussion of what that harm might be). Therefore, when comparing this choice to choice A, the statement in choice A is much more strongly supported within the passage.

C: No. This claim is made in the passage (paragraph 1) but the author does not offer specific examples or further explanation of the negative effects mentioned.

D: No. This statement is not made in the passage. The author mentions animal byproducts (second half of paragraph 1), but does not connect this to veganism (which itself is never mentioned—making this connection would require using too much outside knowledge) or suggest that people who avoid animal byproducts are more ethically pure than vegetarians.

SOLUTIONS TO CHAPTER 6 PRACTICE PASSAGE 2

1. **B** This is a Main Idea/Primary Purpose question.

A: No. The focus on simply the definition of "Hispanics" is too narrow. This answer choice ignores many of the central ideas of the text, including using community organizing and education to gain understanding about cancer information in Hispanic populations and to provide proper care.

B: **Yes. The correct answer will be the one of the four choices that best captures and covers all the major themes of the passage. The last four lines of the passage describe what the author believes is important (understanding the Hispanic populations) and the changes he believes should be made to help the affected people by creating "a realistic picture" of the situation. The rest of the passage explains why this better understanding is needed, and suggests ways in which it might be achieved.**

C: No. This choice is both too extreme and too narrow. While the author agrees that the use of the overly inclusive term "Hispanic" results in barriers to discovering important information about cancer in those populations, he never advocates discarding the term. He simply believes that each subgroup of the population should be examined separately. Furthermore, while the term "Hispanic" may be problematic in some ways, this is not the focus of the entire passage.

D: No. The passage states that education is an important facet that needs to be addressed, but the text itself does not offer much educational information regarding using cancer resources. The examples of the "Promotoras de Salud" and "Southwest Oncology Group" are only to illustrate the author's argument about the need for such organizations and programs.

2. **C**   This is an Inference question.

A: No. "Hispanics" are described as a large, diverse group of people (paragraph 1). However, the author never states or suggests that Hispanics speak Spanish. Be careful not to use outside knowledge or assumptions when picking an answer choice. Furthermore, while the author does discuss measures that would help to "create strong community bonds" (paragraph 4), the passage does not suggest that Hispanics have unusually strong community bonds compared to other groups.

B: No. The passage states the opposite of this statement: the use of the "'Hispanic' category" assumes all the people "experience similar barriers" in health services (paragraph 2). However, "each group has specific characteristics that make them different and independent from one another" (paragraph 3).

C: Yes. The last line of paragraph 1 states that "The data available regarding the incidence, morbidity, and mortality from cancer in Hispanics are scarce, scattered, outdated, and often incomplete."

D: No. The author states that the Hispanic population is indeed heterogeneous, but notes in paragraph 3 that they are actually underrepresented in clinical trials. This is another example of an "opposite" Attractor.

3. **A**   This is a Retrieval/Roman numeral question.

I: True. The passage states that clumping together the culturally diverse groups that make up the Hispanic population results in a limited and inaccurate picture of "the physical, emotional, and financial impact of cancer in Hispanic patients and their families" (paragraph 4).

II: False. While barriers, in general, are mentioned within the passage, specific language barriers are not addressed and are outside of the scope of the passage.

III: False. The author states that "community-based lay health educators" working with "health departments…can be successful" (paragraph 5).

4. **A**   This is an Inference/EXCEPT question.

A: Yes. The correct answer choice will have the *least* support from the passage text. While the first part of this choice is supported, the second part is not. The author calls for study and understanding of "variability" or differences between the subgroups. The author argues throughout the passage that a focus on, or assumption of, commonalities is misguided.

B: No. Paragraph 4 emphasizes the importance of both a community-based approach and a program "complementing the Hispanic heritage."

C: No. Paragraph 5 mentions, positively, the successful "cervical cancer screening programs" carried out by community based coalitions.

D: No. Paragraph 5 highlights the importance of the education of "physicians, nurses, anthropologists, social workers, etc."

5. **D**   This is an Inference/EXCEPT question.

A: No. Paragraph 3 states, "Recruitment of minorities, specifically Hispanics, to clinical trials has been a significant problem that can potentially be overcome by adequate protocol development and investigator education regarding specific knowledge, attitudes, and needs of minority populations."

B: No. In paragraph 3, the author mentions that the subjects were divided into "four different groups of women of Hispanic/Latino origin."

C: No. The author states in paragraph 3 that "it is timely and refreshing to see a recent anthropological evaluation of the problem of cancer in (female) Hispanics."

D: Yes. The correct answer choice will have the *least* support from the passage. The study in question divided the women into four categories. However, the author does not suggest that there are only four subgroups, or that the study covered all existing subgroups.

6. **C** This is a Tone/Attitude question.

A: No. While the author points out the inefficiencies of the health care system stemming in part from the inclusive term "Hispanics," he does not point fingers or accuse anybody specifically. He simply notes that the term is one with flaws: "There is still no clear definition of the term 'Hispanic'" (paragraph 1). In addition, there are no words that indicate contempt or ridicule as the word "derisiveness" would.

B: No. The author feels that there is a problem, but the word "distressed" is too extreme to describe his attitude. In addition, the author is not indifferent. He promotes ideas that he hopes will cause change. This can be noted through statements like: "The time has come to revise and update our sources of information and data gathering" (paragraph 5).

C: Yes. The author describes, in paragraph 5, progress that is occurring already, and what more improvements can be made. This indicates optimism. His explanation of the problem and situation is analytical—he discusses different aspects of the problem and provides supportive evidence.

D: No. "Clinical" does describe the relatively objective tone of the author. The text lacks passionate claims, but is, instead, professional, as the term "clinical" may indicate. However, the word "regretful" is too extreme to describe the author's attitude. While he would like the health care system to be reformed, the author does not use words that would indicate regret or disappointment. If one part of the choice is incorrect, the whole choice is wrong.

7. **A** This is an Inference question.

A: Yes. The author's intent is to encourage enactment of changes that will positively benefit Hispanics. Note wording such as "In developing these interventions, we should increase our awareness of the needs of all different Hispanic groups" (paragraph 4) or "we must get to know and understand the population(s) with whom we plan to work" (paragraph 5), which suggests that the passage is intended for people working within the field of health care. Administrators at cancer institutes or researchers have the ability to utilize his suggestions and advice, such as by carrying out useful research, or coordinating community based initiatives to reach more Hispanics.

B: No. The tone and content of the passage indicate that it is not intended for the general reader, but rather for people with a specific interest, and role to play, in this particular issue.

C: No. The primary purpose of this passage (as noted in the solution for question 1) is not to educate Hispanic women, but to create changes in our understanding of how cancer affects Hispanics and in how Hispanic people are educated, tested, and treated. While one could imagine that Hispanic women with breast or cervical cancer might be interested in this information, this group is too narrowly defined to be the "intended audience." The passage is geared towards people who would be able to carry out research, education, and treatment, rather than towards potential subjects of research, education, or treatment.

D: No. The Southwest Oncology Group already participates in the practices advocated by the author (paragraph 5). There would be little or no benefit seen by presenting the group with the information of the passage.

Individual Passage Log

Passage # _____   **Time spent on passage** _____

Q#	Q type	Attractors	What did you do wrong?

Revised Strategy _____

Passage # _____   **Time spent on passage** _____

Q#	Q type	Attractors	What did you do wrong?

Revised Strategy _____

Chapter 7
Strategy and Tactics

GOALS

1) To make the most of your time
2) To find ways to improve through self-evaluation
3) To refine your pacing strategy

7.1 MAXIMIZING YOUR PERFORMANCE

Now is the time to ask yourself a serious question: are you diligently and consistently implementing and refining a strategic approach to the test? Or, are you just doing passage after passage and taking test after test in the belief that simple repetition will continue to improve your score? If it's the latter, you must ask yourself WHY you are making the mistakes that you are and HOW you can change to improve your performance.

The Big Picture

Imagine two students. The first (say, the one who isn't using these materials) approaches the CARS section as she would any test in college. The second, a student using this book, uses the strategies she has learned. How will these students use their time on the test?

First Student, with No Specialized Test Strategy

- **On Easier Passages:** Overconfident and complacent, this student rushes through the easier passages, relying on her memory and failing to check her answer choices back to the passage text. She chooses the first answer that sounds good, and is perfectly happy with her choices, not realizing that she has fallen into all of the test-writers' traps.
- **On Harder Passages:** This student, doing the passages in the order given by the test-writers, hits a difficult passage in the middle of the section. Frustrated and confused, she slows down, reading everything three times, trying to understand exactly what the author is saying. She spends five minutes on a question, believing that she can't move on until she is sure of the correct answer. She becomes more and more anxious about the time, which makes it even harder to focus on the passage. This student tries to use sheer effort where strategy would be more effective.

Second Student, with MCAT-Appropriate Strategies

- **On Easier Passages:** Knowing that the majority of her correct answers will come from the easier passages, this student works through them with steadiness and focus. She clearly articulates the Bottom Line of the passage before answering the questions. She answers the questions in her own words before attacking the answer choices, and checks each choice against the passage.
- **On Harder Passages:** This student knows that not all passages will be completely comprehensible, and has an appropriate strategy for the harder passages. She uses POE to the fullest, remembering that she is looking for the "least wrong" choice, not an ideal answer. She asks questions of the answer choices (such as, *Is the language too extreme to be an inference? Is this choice too narrow for a Main Idea question?*) based on her knowledge of question types and common Attractors. This student gains points based on her intelligent, test-appropriate strategy.

Narrowing It Down

Let's revisit our first student. When asked why she misses questions, she responds, "I don't know. I always get it down to two choices, and then I pick the wrong one."

The second student, having done an extensive evaluation of her own performance to date, might respond, "On Inference questions, I tend to forget to look for absolute language, and I pick choices that are too extreme. Sometimes I get too impatient to define the Bottom Line, and then I pick Main Point answer choices that are too narrow. I also sometimes have too much confidence in my own memory, don't go back to the passage, and then miss easy Retrieval questions by choosing answer choices from the wrong part of the passage." The second, self-aware student knows exactly what she needs to work on over the next few weeks, and has a clear path to continued improvement. The first student will most likely continue to make the same mistakes over and over again. Remember, those who don't know and understand their own history are doomed to repeat it.

If you are identifying a bit too much with our first student, now is the time to ask yourself the following questions:

1) **Are you having trouble articulating the Bottom Line?**
   Is it difficult to locate the relevant parts of the passage when you are working the questions?
   The Diagnosis
   Both of these issues go back to articulating the main point of each paragraph or chunk, and synthesizing those themes as you read. If you don't identify the author's main points as you read, separating out the claims from the evidence, it is almost impossible to distill it down at the end to a core argument. And, if you aren't identifying the location of these different themes, the passage runs together in your mind as an undifferentiated block of information, and you will have trouble remembering and locating where different topics appeared.

   The Cure
   Review Chapter 3 on Active Reading.
   Break the argument into chunks and define the Main Points as you read; don't wait to think about it until after you have finished reading the passage. If you haven't been using your noteboard much (or at all), make yourself write down the Main Points as you go. Articulate how each new chunk logically relates to what you have already read. Preview the questions for content, so that you have some context within which to translate what you are reading, and you are alerted to some of the important issues in the passage.

2) **Do you tend to miss certain question types?**
   The Diagnosis
   Use your passage and practice test logs to identify which types give you the most trouble. Is it an overall category (e.g., Specific questions)? Is it a few particular question types or formats?

   The Cure
   Review Chapter 4 on Question Types.
   Identifying these patterns is the first step towards figuring out the exact causes of your mistakes. Here are some common problem areas and solutions.
   - Main Point/Primary Purpose: Pay attention to tone, and break down the passage by defining its logical structure. Avoid choices that are too narrow.
   - Specific questions: Keep track of the specific reference in the question stem, and go back to the passage *before* you take the first cut through the answer choices.

- Structure: Pay attention to words in the passage that distinguish claims (*therefore, thus, in conclusion*) from evidence (*for example, in illustration, in these three cases*).
- New Information: Treat the new information in the question stem like a paragraph of the passage: what is the main point of this chunk, and how does it relate to the logic of the author's argument? Use your noteboard to translate complicated questions.
- Strengthen and Weaken: Clearly define what the correct answer needs to do: what is the relevant issue, and must the correct answer be consistent or inconsistent with the passage? With what part of the passage? Keep close track of direction.
- EXCEPT/LEAST/NOT: Define not only what the right answer needs to do but what kind of choices you will be eliminating. Use your noteboard to keep track of POE.

3) **Do you tend to fall for certain types of Attractors?**

The Diagnosis
Use your logs and look for patterns!

The Cure
Review Chapter 5 on POE.
Each time you do a new passage or test section, pick out ahead of time two types of Attractors you will be on the lookout for. Define a specific tactic for recognizing and avoiding these traps, such as the following:

- Extreme wording: Look out for words like *only, most, all, must, never*, etc. Also, evaluate the strength of the statements in each choice; an answer choice can be too extreme even if it doesn't use these particular words.
- Partially correct: Force yourself to read the entire choice word for word. Actively look for that one word that can make it incorrect. Suspend all judgment on the validity of the choice until you have read every word.
- Right answer/wrong question: Always go back to the passage, with the specific reference in the question clearly in mind. Reread the question before you take your second cut through the choices.

4) **Are you going too slow or too fast?** Problems with pacing can underlie all of the above issues. So, let's move on to discuss it in more detail.

7.2 FOCUS ON PACING

By this point, you should begin timing yourself on your practice passages. If your reasonable goal is to complete eight passages with high accuracy and randomly guess on one passage, as a rule of thumb it should take you about 11 minutes per passage. If your reasonable goal is to complete all 9 (which is only reasonable if you are already scoring well), that entails taking around 10 minutes per passage. Keep in mind that this is only an approximation. A passage with seven questions will take you a bit longer than a passage of equal difficulty with only five questions, and a more difficult passage will legitimately take you a little longer to complete than an easier passage.

Here are some specific guidelines to help you to decide on an appropriate pacing plan for your target score.

Pacing Guidelines

The sections on the following pages describe the appropriate pacing for various CARS target score levels. Use your CARS score on your most recent practice test to determine which targets are most appropriate. If you are not hitting the accuracy goals for your current target level, you should not be trying to speed up or answer more questions. Once you are consistently hitting those targets, you may be ready to attempt the next level.

Current Score Level: Below Average

Target Score: Average

Pacing and Accuracy Goals: 7–8 Passage Pace

In this score range, it is critical that you identify easier (Now) passages and perform with high accuracy. Do not waste time on Killer passages, or spend too much time on Later passages. Plan to skip over at least three or four passages on your first pass through the section.

Now Passages (4):

You should spend 11–12 minutes on each of these passages. The reading should take 4–5 minutes and each question should take on average 1–1.5 minutes. Work carefully and use POE in order to avoid errors.

Accuracy Goal:

0–1 mistakes per passage.

Later Passages (3):

You should spend 13–14 minutes on each of these passages. The reading should take 3–4.5 minutes and each question should take on average 1–2 minutes. If you are taking a very long time on a question or just don't understand it, guess on that question and move on.

Accuracy Goal:

0–2 mistakes per passage.

Killer Passages (2):

You should mostly be guessing on these passages. If, after finishing the other passages, you have a few minutes left, pick another passage and read just the first and last sentences of the text. Then look for Specific questions with paragraph references or lead words. Use aggressive POE. Don't spend too much time on any one question. Make sure you have guessed on every question before time runs out.

Accuracy Goal:

At least 1 correct answer.

Current Score Level: Average

Target Score: Average-High

Pacing and Accuracy Goals: 8–9 Passage Pace

In this score range, it is critical that you not become distracted by the Later or Killer passages early in the test. Plan to skip at least two or three passages on your first pass through the test. Make sure you start with a Now passage and at your target pace.

Now Passages (5):

You should spend 10–11 minutes on each of these passages. The reading should take 3–4 minutes and each question should on average take 1–1.5 minutes. Work carefully and use POE in order to avoid errors.

Accuracy Goal:

0–1 mistakes per passage with ideally at least two perfect passages.

Later Passages (3):

You should spend 11–12 minutes on each of these passages. The reading should take 4–5 minutes and each question should on average take 1–1.5 minutes. If a question is taking a very long time, or you don't understand it at all, use aggressive POE, pick an answer, and move on. You may also choose to randomly guess on several of the hardest questions in some of the passages that you complete (see "Cherry Picking" in Section 7.5 of this chapter).

Accuracy Goal:

0–2 mistakes per passage.

Killer Passages (1):

You should be mostly guessing on one passage. If you start working on a passage early in the test and realize it is a Killer, immediately move on to easier passages. If you have time after completing the Now and Later passages, you should go to the remaining passage and read just the first and last sentence of each paragraph. Then look for Specific questions (or, if there are no Specific questions, Structure questions) with paragraph references and/or lead words from the passage. Use aggressive POE. Don't spend too much time on any single question. Make sure you have guessed on every question before time runs out.

Accuracy Goal:

At least 1 correct answer.

Current Score Level: Average-High

Target Score: High

Pacing and Accuracy Goals: 9 Passage Pace

You should only be attempting a 9–passage pace if you have consistently achieved the accuracy goals of previous levels. At this pace, plan to skip at least one or two passages on your first pass through the test. Make sure that you start with a passage that is not too difficult and to hit a good pace at the beginning.

Now Passages (6–7):

You should spend 8–9 minutes on each of these passages. The reading should take 2.5–3.5 minutes and each question should on average take 1 minute or less. Work carefully and use POE in order to avoid errors.

Accuracy Goal:

0–1 mistakes per passage with at least three perfect passages.

Later Passages (1–2):

You should spend 10–11 minutes on each of these passages. The reading should take 3.5–4.5 minutes and each question should on average take 1 minute or less. If a question is likely to take longer than 1.5 minutes or is confusing, skip it and look at it again before moving on to the next passage. You may also choose to "cherry-pick," that is, randomly guess on 2–3 of the hardest questions in these passages (see "Cherry Picking" in Section 7.5 of this chapter). If you employ this strategy, you will need to get almost every other question correct in order to achieve the target score.

Accuracy Goal:
0–1 mistakes per passage, with at least two perfect passages.

Killer Passages (1):
Your approach to your last passage will depend on how much time you have left. To get a score at the top of the scale, you have to attack every passage and get almost all of the questions correct. However, you don't necessarily have to attempt every single question. You should not spend more time than usual reading the passage; instead keep your focus on main points and tone. Use aggressive POE and don't spend too much time on any single question. However, don't rush through all the questions if you are running out of time. Make a good attempt at most of them, and if needed, guess on one or two particularly difficult questions within the set. Make sure you have answered every question before time runs out.

Accuracy Goal:
At least 3 correct answers.

Diagnosing Pacing Problems
If you are not hitting the right pace to achieve your target score, you must

1) diagnose what is wrong with your current pace, and
2) adjust accordingly

First, let's look at four basic pacing issues.

1) **Going too fast**
   There are three signs that your score will improve if you slow down and do fewer questions.
   - If you are finishing nine passages but consistently missing two or more questions on every passage, or if you often miss more than half of the questions for a passage (that is, you do well on some passages but crash and burn on others).
   - If you realize that you often miss easy questions. This means that when you go over a test, many or most of the questions that you got wrong look obvious in retrospect. You can't imagine why you didn't pick the credited response, and you can't really remember why you liked that wrong answer so much.
   - If you are completing all nine passages and not getting a significantly above-average score.

2) **Going too slow**
   If one or more of the following describes you, increasing your speed and efficiency will improve your score:
   - You consistently answer all or almost all of the questions that you do correctly, but you are doing eight or fewer passages.
   - You spend a disproportionately high amount of time on a few passages or a few questions.
   - You spend 6 or more minutes reading the passage text the first time through.
   - You find yourself over-thinking the passage and/or the questions and spending a lot of time talking yourself into wrong answers.

3) **Getting bogged down on a Killer passage**
Let's return to our two students and compare their different approaches to the Killer passage:
- **What the first student, untrained in strategy, does with the Killer passage:**
    She slows down, gets lost and distracted while reading, and spends too much time going back and rereading long sections of the passage. She gets caught up in deciphering fancy vocabulary words.

    When she moves onto the questions, she goes even slower; she has spent so much time reading the passage that she feels that she has to get all of the questions right to justify it. At some point, the student realizes anxiously that too much time has passed and she guesses on the last two or three questions of the passage before moving on, stressed out and perspiring. She then speeds through the other easier passages, trying to make up for lost time, making foolish errors, and throwing away easy points.
- **What the second, trained student does with the Killer passage:**
    Skips it (or does it last of all).
    By randomly filling in all of the answer choices on the Killer Passage, the second student frees up at least 10–15 minutes that would have been wasted on getting questions wrong. And if she does complete it, she does it last so that it doesn't negatively affect how she does on the easier passages.

4) **Getting bogged down on a Killer question**
Even Now and Later passages can have a question that is extremely hard for you. You can't allow yourself to get sucked into that one question if doing so means you are losing the opportunity to answer two or more easier questions down the road.

7.3 REFINING YOUR PACING
Once you have decided if you need to slow down or speed up, the next question is HOW?

Slowing Down
This is not as obvious as it seems. Don't spend the time that you save by doing fewer questions or passages on excessive rereading. Also, don't sit and ponder difficult parts of the passage at great length, or come up with elaborate justifications for why a variety of answer choices might be correct. It is still important to be tightly focused and efficient, even when slowing down your pace.

Instead, invest the extra time in the following:

- translating the question and clearly identifying the question type and task,
- reading the answer choices more carefully: that is, word for word,
- comparing choices to each other and specifically looking out for common traps,
- and—most importantly—in going back to the passage to find the relevant information and defining what the correct answer needs to do.

Speeding Up

There are four common ways in which students get bogged down and lose time. To pick up your pace, focus on avoiding these traps.

1) **Reading the passage too carefully the first time through**

    If you are reading every word and highlighting the passage heavily, then you're reading the passage like a college course book rather than a CARS passage. You may feel safer going into the questions having consistently spent 6 or more minutes with the passage, but the test doesn't allow you the time to do so. Cut to the chase the first time through, and save the more careful rereading for answering the questions. (Review Chapters 3 and 7.)

2) **Not reading and translating the question carefully**

    If you go back into the passage without a clear idea of what you're looking for, you are likely to get lost and waste precious time backtracking to reread the question, or getting stuck in the answer choices because nothing fits what you first thought the question was asking. Spend a few more seconds translating the question, and the correct answers will come a lot more quickly. (Review Chapter 4.)

3) **Not aggressively using POE**

    You can waste a huge amount of time looking for a perfect answer instead of the "least wrong" answer. Trying to make a watertight case for the credited response when it is one of those "not great, but the best of what I've got" answers will not only suck up a lot of time and energy, it will also often cause you to talk yourself out of the correct choice. Maintain a critical focus through the entire POE process. (Review Chapter 5.)

4) **Overcommitting to one question or one passage**

    - Learn to recognize quickly whether you understand a test question or not. Are you rereading it over and over? Are you bouncing repeatedly (three or more times) from passage to question and back again? If so, these are clear signs that this question is not working for you (that is, it's very difficult). Many people become stubborn about seeing a question through; they think that because they have devoted some time already to the question, they can't abandon that question because doing so means they have wasted time. But spending even more time on a question that is particularly difficult means nothing more than wasting more time. You can't change the past, but you don't have to continue in an effort that is unlikely to yield a point.

        If you doubt this logic, consider the following analogy. If you have dated someone for six months and realize that the person is a jerk, do you say, "Well, I don't want to have wasted the past six months, so I better get married to the jerk?" No! You move on, chalk up the episode to experience, and look for someone easier to get along with. Bringing it back to the world of the MCAT, in this situation use POE, take your best shot, and move on.

    - However, don't go to the opposite extreme. If you are getting it down to two and then guessing on a majority of questions, your accuracy will significantly suffer and your score will go down, not up.

    - Don't spend a high percentage of your resources on a single passage. More difficult passages should take a bit more time, but you need to keep moving. Remember that in many cases hard passages have been edited in such a way that some things are never fully explained or clarified; you could read it ten times over and still not really "get it." Luckily, in most cases you don't need to understand every aspect of the passage to get most of the questions right.

Try Pacing Exercise 1 at the end of this chapter if your accuracy is good but you need to increase your speed. Also see Section 7.5 "Variations on a Theme: Refining Your Strategy" for more specific pacing suggestions.

Avoiding KILLER Passages

Use your previous experience to refine your ranking technique. Each time you rank a passage as Now, and it turns out to be a Later or Killer, go back and re-evaluate the passage and the questions to see what made it harder than you expected, and how you could have recognized it earlier.

Conversely, every time you misidentify an easy passage as a difficult passage, do the same. Look in particular for passages with unfamiliar subject matter that you ranked as Later or Killer that were relatively easy once you got into them.

It is dangerous to rank passages on the basis of familiarity; it is really the difficulty of the language and of the question types that makes for a hard passage.

Review Chapter 6 if you are having trouble ranking passages accurately. See section 7.5 "Variations on a Theme: Refining Your Strategy," as well, for more ranking suggestions.

7.4   CARS EXERCISES: PACING AND SELF-EVALUATION

Exercise 1: Speeding Up

Do this exercise if you have excellent accuracy on the passages that you actually complete, but can only complete a limited number of passages under timed conditions. You may wish to spread this exercise out over a few days or weeks.

Do a full CARS section (or look at your most recent practice test), and note the average time spent per passage here._____

Now do four more passages back-to-back (or, an entire CARS test section), but give yourself one less minute for each passage you attempt. Use the suggestions in this chapter to diagnose areas where you may be wasting time, and to work through those areas more efficiently. If you complete those passages with good accuracy, reduce your time per passage by another 30–60 seconds and do another set of passages.

Continue this process until your accuracy begins to suffer. Note the average time spent per passage here._____

Carefully diagnose the reasons for your mistakes, and continue to work at that pace until your accuracy improves to your previous level.

Continue this exercise until you hit the appropriate pace for you.

Exercise 2: 5-Minute Drill

If you have about 5 minutes left when you've finished a passage, do not begin to carefully read the next Later or Killer passage in your ranking. If you do, you will run out of time with few or no questions answered. Instead, quickly read the first and last sentence of each paragraph. If it's a two-sentence paragraph, just read the first sentence. Next, click through the questions and pick out the easier Specific questions (such as Retrieval, and Inference questions with lead words and/or paragraph references) and do those first, going back to the passage to hunt down and read the relevant sections. You have a good chance of getting those easier questions right, even with little time remaining.

If you have time left after doing these Specific questions, take a shot at any Main Idea or Primary Purpose questions, using what you have now learned about the major themes of the passage. Be sure to rely heavily on POE, thinking actively about identifying and avoiding common Attractors. Even if you only have a minute left, you can probably at least eliminate one or two answer choices on one General question, or even a Reasoning or Application question.

So, imagine that the 5-minute warning has come up on the screen, just as you have completed a passage. Your goal now is to get what you can out of the seven questions for the passage on the next pages in the few minutes you have left.

Formal and informal reactions to crime are distinguished by whether they are administered by representatives of the state. Government officials administer formal reactions, such as penal sanctions. Informal reactions are sanctions imposed by non-state functionaries, usually ordinary citizens. These sanctions include all the detrimental consequences that convicted offenders experience that are not formally specified by law or pronounced by a judge in the disposition. To lose one's job or be ridiculed by others are examples of informal sanctions. Since equality before the law is such a symbolically important part of the criminal justice system, many investigators have examined the legal and extralegal determinants of formal sanctions. For example, the effects of offense and offender characteristics on variations in criminal sentences have been investigated extensively. By contrast, informal reactions to crime have received minimal analytic attention. This failure to explore the determinants of informal sanctions distorts understanding of the links between social structure and social control.

Position in the stratification hierarchy is one of the factors that determine susceptibility to law. Those in low positions are more susceptible to law in that, among other things, their crimes are more harshly sanctioned. The same is true for non-governmental forms of social control. Just as inequality in wealth and power influences decision-making in courtrooms, it also affects how offenders are treated in workplaces and in the community. Criminal conviction has been shown to reduce the employment opportunities of working-class defendants. Case studies of powerful corporate executives who have committed egregious offenses find that they often continue to hold respected positions in both the economic and social worlds. These studies suggest that the "stigmatizing effects" of criminal conviction are not damaging for some white-collar offenders.

Less powerful white-collar offenders may be more stigmatized by criminal conviction than business executives. For example, professionals and public-sector workers convicted of white-collar crimes lose occupational status more often than business executives convicted of similar offenses. The consequences of legal stigma may be influenced more by the offender's class position than by his or her criminal conduct.

The extent of social condemnation presumably varies directly with the seriousness of offense and severity of the criminal sentences received. In theory, those who commit minor offenses provoke little censure from the community-at-large and receive lenient treatment in the legal system. Those who commit more serious offenses do not fare as well: they may receive both stronger social condemnation and harsher punishment. Since judges supposedly deem informal sanctions, such as loss of status, sufficient punishment for white-collar offenders, they may impose less severe sentences on those who experience those sanctions. Consequently, formal and informal reactions to white-collar crime may not be consistent.

Material used in this particular passage has been adapted from the following source:

M. L. Benson, "The Influence of Class Position on the Formal and Informal Sanctioning of White-Collar Offenders," *Sociological Quarterly.* © 1989, Midwest Sociological Society.

1. It can be inferred from the passage that the courts would treat social isolation of an accused business executive as:

A) an expected consequence of public accusations but not relevant to the judicial process.
B) a more potent form of punishment than even a prison sentence.
C) a situation that, since not truly measurable, cannot be considered punitive.
D) a legitimate form of punishment that is often considered before a sentence is determined.

2. According to the passage, which of the following is a ramification of the failure to examine the determining factors of informal sanctions?

A) A misunderstanding of the relationship between the structure of society and sanctions that are used to control criminal behavior
B) A reduction of employment opportunities for working-class defendants
C) An inability to establish effective punitive measures using formal sanctions on criminal behavior
D) The ability of numerous business executives convicted of criminal offenses to maintain respectable positions

3. Which one of the following best describes the author's reaction to the two forms of sanctions discussed in the passage?

A) Frustration that class position is a factor in the severity of both formal and informal sanctions
B) Concern about the injustices frequently occurring because governmental and non-governmental sanctions against offenders are both solely determined by the hierarchy of class position
C) Advocating further study of non-governmental sanctions to address inconsistent treatment of criminal offenders
D) Favoring formal sanctions as the fairest method of punishing criminal offenders

4. The phrase "'stigmatizing effects' of criminal conviction" (paragraph 2) refers to which one of the following?

A) The severity of formal sanctions imposed upon working-class defendants after criminal convictions
B) The less severe formal sanctions received by white-collar criminals after criminal convictions
C) The informal sanctions a defendant receives as a result of being convicted of a crime
D) The inequality of treatment before the law of working-class and white collar offenders

5. Which of the following questions about the two forms of sanctions could not be answered by using the information provided in the passage?

A) What is the difference between formal and informal sanctions?
B) Why have formal sanctions received extensive analytic treatment?
C) Why have informal sanctions not received thorough investigation?
D) Why are formal and informal sanctions of white-collar crimes sometimes inconsistent?

6. Which of the following sentences would best serve as a completion to the passage?

A) As the justice system progresses, the determinants of informal sanctions should receive more investigation.
B) Accordingly, judges should not consider informal sanctions when imposing sentences on criminal offenders, regardless of their position on the social hierarchy.
C) If this trend continues, it will remain impossible for criminal defendants to receive fair sentences until more attention is paid to the study of informal sanctions.
D) It is clear that the seriousness of the offense alone should determine the formal sanctions imposed upon criminal conviction.

7. Which of the following best expresses the main idea of the passage?

A) The extent to which a person is stigmatized by criminal conviction depends in large part on their social status or class.
B) To understand how individual behavior is influenced by society, we must learn more about the effect of social stigma on criminal offenders.
C) Informal sanctions have an even greater effect than formal sanctions on those accused or convicted of crimes and so must be studied in more depth.
D) The workings of law and society cannot be studied in isolation from each other; the two are inherently intertwined in our institutions and cultural beliefs.

Answers to 5-Minute Drill

1. **D**
2. **A**
3. **C**
4. **C**
5. **C**
6. **A**
7. **B**

7.4

Exercise 3: Test Assessment Log

This Log should look familiar; there is a copy of it in Chapter 2. If you haven't been using it to evaluate your practice tests, now is the time to start.

In particular, use it to evaluate your pacing. Are you spending the time you need on the easier passages in order to get most of those questions right? Keep track of how much time you spent (roughly) on the Now passages and on the Later passages. If you find that you are spending the bulk of your 90 minutes on the harder passages with a low level of accuracy, you need to reapportion your time. At the same time, evaluate your ranking: are you choosing the right passages?

Now Passages

Now Passage #	Q # and Type (for questions you got wrong)	Attractors (for wrong answers you picked or seriously considered)	What did you do wrong?

Approximate time spent on Now passages _____

Total Now passages attempted _____

Total # of Qs on Now passages attempted _____

Total # of Now Qs correct _____

% correct of Now Qs attempted _____

7.4

Later Passages

7.4

Later Passage #	Q # and Type (for questions you got wrong)	Attractors (for wrong answers you picked or seriously considered)	What did you do wrong?

Approximate time spent on Later passages _____

Total Later passages attempted _____

Total # of Qs on Later passages attempted _____

Total # of Later Qs correct _____

% correct of Later Qs attempted _____

Final Analysis

Total # of passages attempted (including partially completed) _____

Total # of questions attempted _____

Total # of correct answers _____

Total % correct of attempted questions _____

Revised Strategy

Pacing	
Passage choice/ranking	
Working the Passage	
Attacking the Questions	

7.5 VARIATIONS ON A THEME: REFINING YOUR STRATEGY

Through your preparation you are learning a standard approach to the CARS section that has been tested and refined over decades, based in part on the experience and input of hundreds of thousands of students. However, different people process information somewhat differently. Once you have mastered the approach, you may benefit from experimenting with variations on those techniques in order to make them work optimally for you.

Unfortunately, there are no secret "tricks" to the CARS section. Making score improvements in this section requires a lot of practice, hard work, and vigilant review. It is easy to get into a rut, doing the same thing over and over without thinking about how to further improve your line of attack. This section is intended to spark, or add fuel to, that thought process.

Pacing and Accuracy

As we discussed in the previous sections, the way for many students to maximize their score is to attempt eight of the nine passages, randomly guessing on the hardest passage in the section. However, if your reasonable goal (based on your performance to date) is to score significantly above average, you will most likely need to attempt some or all of a ninth passage. And, if you are currently completing six or seven passages, unless you have close to perfect accuracy, you will need to pick up the pace in order to achieve an average or bit above-average score. The question is then, how can you speed up without a significant loss of accuracy?

Ironically, you might find that going a bit faster not only gets you through more questions, but also improves your accuracy. This may be the case if you tend to overthink the passage or the questions, by making the passage more confusing than it needs to be, or talking yourself out of correct answers.

On the other hand, if you are missing a large number of questions because you did not read carefully enough, or did not think enough about the meaning of what you read, then slowing down (especially if you are doing all nine passages) may pay off. No one really wants to randomly guess on questions (everyone would prefer to do all of the questions and get them all right); however, many students have found that once they do slow down, focusing more on accuracy and less on speed, they not only have the time to do what needs to be done, but they also think more clearly and efficiently.

Below are suggestions and variations on the standard approach that may improve your speed, your accuracy, or both. Always try new approaches on multiple passages and tests to gather enough data to see if they are really working for you. But be sure to test one new approach at a time, rather than trying to do a massive overhaul.

A. Ranking and Ordering: The Three-Pass System

Most test-takers do best with the Two-Pass system of ordering the passages; that is, doing the Now passages the first time through as you find them, then coming back for a second pass to do the Later passages. However, if you find that you struggle with separating out the Nows from the Laters from the Killers, AND that you are often making bad choices in the passages you attempt to the extent that it hurts your score, it is worth trying the Three-Pass system.

1) First Pass: Rank all nine passages Now, Later, or Killer
2) Second Pass: Do the Now passages
3) Third Pass: Do the Later passages and check the Review screen for incompletes.

The Three-Pass system may take a bit more total time than the Two-Pass system. However, if you are consistently making bad ranking decisions and wasting time struggling with difficult passages, comparing all nine passages before beginning your Nows may pay off.

B.   Working the Passage

1) **Push the Pace**

   a) It is comforting to read the whole passage word for word, translating and understanding every point and nuance within the author's argument. However, most questions don't require a deep understanding of the passage. And, many parts of the passage never become relevant to the questions. Try pushing yourself through the passage faster on your first reading, accepting the fact that there will be some sections that you do not fully understand. If you know what was discussed, even if you don't really get the author's meaning, you can always find it again if you need it.

   b) If your reading speed is very slow and you have problems with reading comprehension, one technique to try is to read just the first and last sentence of each paragraph the first time through the passage. You may also want to try this approach if you commonly get bogged down in the passage text, losing too much time and/or comprehension.

   CAUTION: This generally only works well on easier passages. This is also quite risky, as there may well be important information in the middle of the paragraph (and neither the first nor the last sentence of the paragraph is guaranteed to be a topic sentence). However, some people find that it gets them through the passage fast enough (with at least a basic comprehension of the Bottom Line and understanding of the location of different parts of the author's argument) that they can spend their time more productively on the questions. They may also get to more questions this way, and their overall percentage correct increases. This is definitely a strategy that you want to test on a wide range of passages and on multiple practice tests before you settle on it, but for a few people, it does pay off. Make sure that you evaluate your accuracy, not just the number of questions you are able to attempt. If you come out behind score-wise and in terms of overall percentage correct (taking guessing into account), this is not the strategy for you.

2) **Separate Claims From Evidence**

   One way to push the pace is to vary your reading speed, paying attention to the major claims (often the main point of the paragraph or chunk) and skimming through (that is, reading faster, not word for word) the evidence supporting those claims. Look for topic sentences (if they exist) to help you make these decisions. Use "MAPS" (see Chapter 3) to help out as well. If you see data, studies, examples, descriptions, explanations, anecdotes, etc., they are highly likely to be evidence in support of a larger claim. As long as you know where they are and what they are supporting, the details are of little importance the first time through the passage.

For example, here is a sample paragraph (with highlighting).

"Sedentarization is also having a perverse effect on the roles and position of women. For example, in their traditional nomadic state, with men away on caravans or other business, the domestic domain, including the tending of goat herds, education of children, etc., was the preserve of women. The transition from tent to village is being associated with a marked diminution of the domestic responsibilities and authority of women."

The first sentence of the paragraph sets out the main claim being made by the author. The rest of the paragraph supports that claim. If you understand that the paragraph is about the negative effects of sedentarization on women, you don't really need the rest of the details unless they appear in the questions.

3) **Write Less**

You should be writing down the main point of each paragraph (or chunk) and the Bottom Line of the passage on your noteboard for the first several weeks of your preparation. You are training yourself to read differently, and writing it all down at that stage is crucial. However, once defining those aspects of the passage comes more easily to you, and you are more and more accurate in your understanding, you can cut down the amount that you are writing to a couple of words per paragraph and for the Bottom Line. You may even find that it becomes a tool you can use on the harder passages or more confusing paragraphs only, while the rest of the time you do it as a mental step (while still highlighting within the text). This can be especially useful if you find that you usually have a good understanding of the chunks and how they relate to each other (i.e., the logical structure of the passage), but you struggle and get bogged down when putting it into your own words.

This is one area in which there is significant variation between students. Some people who consistently get high scores are writing brief notes for every paragraph and passage because it contributes both to their speed and to their accuracy, while others in the same scoring range use writing more selectively. Find what level of writing works best for you.

4) **Visualize**

a) Visualizing as you read engages a different part of your brain. When you hit an important part of the passage (especially when you go back to the passage as you answer the questions) and it isn't really making sense, create a visual image in your head. Imagine people waving signs and blocking the streets while the city stagnates around them, or elitist historians thumbing their noses at the common people, or humanists admiring Greek statues while turning a group of robed scholars away from a church, or an adult artist frowning in concentration as she paints while a carefree child spontaneously creates artwork next to her. By the way, the difficulty in visualizing an abstract argument, compared to a concrete and descriptive one, is one thing that tends to make abstract passages Laters or Killers.

b) Another way of using visualization is to create a picture in your mind of the structure of the passage. When you hit a pivotal word, imagine a detour sign. At a continuation, think of a bridge. When the author expresses an opinion, picture a smiley or frowny face. Of course, these are all things that you should also be highlighting. You may even choose to write down some quick symbols on your noteboard, such as a "+" or "−" for positive and negative tone, or a Δ (delta) for a significant shift or change. One reason students often find it harder to process a passage on the computer screen than on paper is that it is easier to have a visual map of a whole page than of a scrolled passage. If you put some effort into creating visual map markers as you read, it takes little time and can really pay off when you use them to efficiently find information in the passage as you answer the questions.

5) **To Preview or Not to Preview**
Previewing the Questions is one way of moving faster through the passage; knowing the question topics ahead of time helps you to prioritize. However, if you are spending an appropriate amount of time previewing (20–30 seconds) and still not retaining enough information to make it useful, there are a few things you can try.

a)   First, make sure you are focusing on and highlighting the lead words that indicate passage content, not the question type (question types, while crucial to define as you are answering the questions, are irrelevant at this stage). Picture the lead words as little bursts of information. Focus on each burst as a distinct chunk, rather than skimming through every word of the question with equal attention. Engage your visual memory and your pattern recognition skills. You don't need to fully understand the words at this stage; you just need to fix them in your memory so that you can recognize them in the passage. And, if the question is long and complicated, or if it looks like a New Information question (which usually start with the words "Suppose" or "If"), skip over it during the preview.

b)   Second, if you still can't retain the information, try jotting down a word or two for each content-containing question on your noteboard. While this will take a bit of time, if you are getting bogged down in the passage, or if you are spending an inordinate amount of time hunting for information as you work the questions, it can pay off in the long run.

c)   Third, if no matter what you do, you can't make the preview work for you, then don't do it. That is, if you have practiced it for at least a month, and used it on at least three practice tests and at least 25 practice passages, and it is still not paying off, then those 20-30 seconds are better spent on answering the questions.

C.   Attacking the Questions
1) **Simplify**
Even difficult questions can be amazingly straightforward when you look at them with clear eyes and a calm brain. If you are struggling with a question, stop and remind yourself that you may be overcomplicating it. Imagine a triangle connecting the question stem, the relevant part of the passage, and the correct answer. When you are stuck, ask yourself: "What was the question asking, what did the author say about it, and what answer is most closely connected to both of those things?" Staying with the geometrical theme, also ask yourself if you have left the world of the "MCAT CARS box." Are you bringing in outside knowledge? Are you speculating about what the author might think, rather than basing your answer on what the author explicitly said? Are you debating an imperfect answer, rather than asking, "Is it the least wrong of the four?" Sometimes when you just relax, use your brain, and relocate yourself within the passage and the question task, things look a lot clearer.

7.5

2) **Use Aggressive POE**

If you are going back to the passage multiple times to prove the right answer right, or cycling through the choices multiple times, remember that eliminating the other three choices is a perfectly legitimate way to get the right answer. Use the Bottom Line, tone, the main point of the relevant chunk or chunks, the strength of the language in the passage and in the answer choices, and when possible your own answer (based on the passage) to weed out what you can. If you are left with one choice still standing, a choice you can't find anything wrong with, pick it and move on, even if you aren't thrilled with it.

3) **Triage**

Some questions are not worth saving. Unless your reasonable goal is to get a perfect score, you are going to miss some questions. It can be useful to think of this as a strategy, not a failure. That is, your strategy is to allow yourself to miss some questions in order to maximize your score, rather than to try to get every single question right. If you are the kind of person who can't move on until you are 100% sure you have a question right, push yourself to take your best shot and move on (once you have been through the appropriate procedure). If you have carefully reread the question, compared the remaining choices, gone back to the passage again, looked for Attractors, and you are still stuck between two choices, pick one and move on. Even if three more minutes on that one question would produce a correct answer, it isn't worth sacrificing the two or three other questions you could have answered correctly in those three minutes.

4) **Cherry Pick**

Cherry picking is a somewhat extreme form of triage. Generally, you want to work through every question attached to a passage. Otherwise, you are wasting some of your investment of time in reading and working the passage. However, if you ALWAYS (or almost always) get the hardest question on a passage wrong no matter what you do, then take an educated guess on that question once you recognize it. If you ALWAYS (or almost always) get a particular type of Reasoning or Application question, or the longest questions, wrong, then try guessing on that type when you find it. Compare your performance on several tests, some doing eight passages working all of the questions, and others doing nine passages using cherry picking, and follow the strategy that has the best outcome.

5) **Tone Questions**

If you tend to get Tone/Attitude questions wrong, or if you miss other question types because you missed or mistook the tone of the passage, this often goes back to how you are working the passage, and to whether or not you are looking for and highlighting tone indicators as you read. However, this can also be due to how you are doing POE on questions where tone is particularly relevant. Make sure to identify the "attitude words" in each choice. For example, imagine that you have four answer choices that begin as follows:

A) To defend…
B) To recommend…
C) To show…
D) To contradict…

Make sure that you are focusing particular attention on those tone words. While you should always read all four choices carefully and fully, if you are stuck on the question and you know that the passage was entirely neutral, choice C is your best shot.

Use Exercise 1 in Section 8.2 the next chapter to work on your Attitude skills.

6) **Order the Questions Within a Passage**
If you are always doing every question in order, regardless of question difficulty, consider taking a consistent "two-pass" approach within the set of questions for a passage. As described in the Ranking and Ordering section, first preview the questions for a passage from first to last. Then, while on the last question, work the passage. Next, work backwards through the set for that passage, skipping over the harder questions and completing the easier ones. Finally, click forward through the set, completing the harder questions (and making sure that you are not leaving any blank).

D. Dealing With (or Not Dealing With) Killer Passages
Identify a set of difficult passages from your practice materials. Do at least five of them giving yourself five minutes per passage, and at least five other passages at ten minutes per passage. Compare the results.

1) If you do about the same with five or ten minutes, and your accuracy is low (that is, if you miss a majority of the questions), and if you are completing nine passages during a test without approaching your target score, that is a clear sign that you should slow down to seven and a half or eight passages. That is, your payoff on that last hard passage is very low, and you would be better off spending much or all of that time on improving your accuracy on the other passages.

2) If you do about the same on both sets and your accuracy is high (you miss on average one or zero questions per passage) and you are normally completing eight or fewer passages in a test, these are signs that you may well be able to speed up without losing accuracy.

3) If you do significantly better on a Killer passage when you have ten minutes as opposed to five minutes (getting all or almost all of the questions right in ten minutes) and you have a high level of accuracy overall, you may well want to try Cherry Picking or aggressive triage in order to get to all nine passages.

4) If you do better on hard passages when you spend five minutes than when you spend ten minutes, and you are doing eight or fewer passages, that is a very clear sign that you should try speeding up. You may well be overthinking the passages and the questions, especially the more difficult ones, and the faster pace may be forcing you to simplify and stick to the information in front of you.

7.5

Chapter 7 Summary

- Manage your 90 minutes well by maintaining a steady pace throughout the entire section. Take your time to get most of the easier questions right. Don't spend too much time on difficult passages; use POE and your knowledge of Attractors to help you through.

- Evaluate your own performance so that you can refine your pacing strategy appropriately.

- If you have an awkward amount of time left over after completing a passage (e.g., 5 minutes), shift your strategy to make sure that you can get to at least one or two easier questions on another passage. Make sure that you select random guesses for any questions that you don't have time to complete.

CHAPTER 7 PRACTICE PASSAGES

Individual Passage Drills

Complete the two passages back-to-back, timed, giving yourself a total of 22 minutes.

Once you have completed the passages and checked your answers, fill out the Individual Passage Logs. Focus in particular on the following:

1) Evaluating your pacing. Were you going too fast or too slow?
2) Identifying types of mistakes that you have also made in the past and strategizing on how to avoid making those same mistakes in the future.

CHAPTER 7 PRACTICE PASSAGE 1

No empirical studies show what proportion of the United States population would have to participate in disruptive and violent demonstrations to seriously threaten the political system. Surely the level of anti-regime violence of recent years has not been sufficient to undermine the viability of the American system. Although the actual participants in peaceful demonstrations or violent protests are far fewer in number than the individuals who approve of these activities, most Americans do not approve of either peaceful or violent protests. In both 1968 and 1972, less than one in five Americans approved of peaceful demonstrations and less than one in ten approved of violent, disruptive protests. Although the level of support for these activities did not increase between 1968 and 1972, the level of opposition declined. Increasing numbers of people seem to be willing to tolerate demonstrations and protests under some circumstances.

If the present relationships persist into the future, increasingly greater tolerance but not necessarily more widespread participation can be anticipated. Among college graduates under age thirty, more than 50 percent approve of peaceful demonstrations, and only 10 percent disapprove. These relationships suggest that as education levels increase, approval of demonstrations will increase. These attitudes suggest a growing unwillingness to be repressive against political interests expressed through peaceful demonstrations, perhaps because the claims of participants are granted some legitimacy.

In these terms, there is some uneasiness about the public support for American democracy—and perhaps for any democratic regime. It is possible to view the United States as a democratic system that has survived without a strong democratic political culture because governmental policies have gained a continual, widespread acceptance. If that satisfaction erodes, however, as it has begun to do, the public has no deep commitment to democratic values and processes that will inhibit support of anti-democratic leaders or disruptive activities.

It is argued that in the absence of insistence on particular values and procedures, democratic regimes will fail. Clearly, a mass public demanding democratic values and procedures is stronger support for a democratic system than a mass public merely willing to tolerate a democratic regime. This does not mean, however, that the stronger form of support is necessary for a democratic system, although superficially it appears desirable. Quite possibly, strong support is nearly impossible to attain, and weaker support is adequate, given other conditions.

In our view, the analysis of support for democratic regimes has been misguided by an emphasis on factors contributing to the establishment of democracy, not its maintenance. Stronger public support probably is required for the successful launching of a democracy than it is for maintaining an already established democracy. Possibly, preserving a regime simply requires that no substantial proportion of the society be actively hostile to the regime and engage in disruptive activities. In other words, absence of disruptive acts, not the presence of supportive attitudes, is crucial.

On the other hand, the positive support by leaders for a political system is essential to its existence. If some leaders are willing to oppose the system, it is crucial that there be no substantial number of followers to which the leaders can appeal. The followers' attitudes, as opposed to their willingness to act themselves, may provide a base of support for antisystem behavior by leaders. In this sense unanimous public support for democratic principles would be a more firm basis for a democratic system. The increasing levels of dissatisfaction, accompanied by a lack of strong commitment to democratic values in the American public, appear to create some potential for public support of undemocratic leaders. In this light, the public's loyalty to political parties and commitment to traditional processes that inhibit aspiring undemocratic leaders become all the more important.

Material used in this particular passage has been adapted from the following source:
W.H. Flanigan and N.H. Zingale, *Political Behavior of the American Electorate.* ©1979 by Allyn Bacon.

1. Elsewhere, the authors describe factors that led to the founding of American democracy. If their account is consistent with the information in the passage, such a discussion would most likely include which of the following?

A) Heroic descriptions of violent uprisings against the British such as the Boston Tea Party
B) Anecdotes concerning George Washington's idealistic motivations
C) Data suggesting vigorous support for democracy was widespread in America at the time
D) A suggestion that more peaceful forms of protest would have given way to a more effective democracy

2. Which of the following, if true, would most strengthen the authors' assertion that public support for peaceful protest is likely to increase over time?

A) A hunger strike by a charismatic dissident leader gains some public support
B) Clashes between protestors and police lead to increased participation in violent protests
C) Five years prior to the survey of college graduates cited by the author, 70 percent of college graduates were shown to approve of nonviolent demonstrations
D) Increased government funding will allow colleges to admit larger classes in the future

3. The authors suggest all of the following are generally necessary for a democracy to thrive EXCEPT:

A) public distaste for violent antigovernment activity.
B) leaders committed to the pursuit of democratic ideals.
C) an electorate that insists upon democratic values in government.
D) an insufficient dissident population to support an undemocratic leader.

4. The primary purpose of the passage is to:

A) contrast the relative merits of violent and nonviolent protest.
B) describe conditions in which a government would fail.
C) argue that free speech has deleterious effects.
D) consider factors that determine the stability of a certain type of political system.

5. Suppose a set of American national politicians were to renounce their loyalty to existing political parties and create a new party founded on communist ideals. Given the information in the passage, their success at creating political change would most likely depend on:

A) acceptance of their ideas among a critical mass of the populace.
B) support among more educated Americans.
C) a loyal following willing to actively campaign on their behalf.
D) a clearly delineated party platform.

6. The authors imply that between 1968 and 1972:

A) acceptance of protest increased and opposition to protest did not decline.
B) social unrest led to greater acceptance of protest as a necessary part of political life.
C) Americans' objection to certain types of protest decreased.
D) there was no change in Americans' attitudes toward protest.

7. The American populace is portrayed as generally:

A) distrustful of government and prone to take political action against its violations of democratic ideals.
B) accepting of America's long history of violence and unrest.
C) willing to passively accept a government that meets its basic requirements.
D) patriotic and unwilling to tolerate dissent.

CHAPTER 7 PRACTICE PASSAGE 2

The most famous sentence in Igor Stravinsky's autobiography reads: "Music is by its very nature powerless to express anything at all." When it appeared, this sentence surprised his audience. After all, Stravinsky had composed some of the most expressive music of the twentieth century, from the lyrical *Petrouchka* to the dramatic *Le sacre du printemps* (The Rite of Spring) to the elegiac *Symphony of Psalms*. But ever the polemicist, Stravinsky was in actuality blasting those whom he regarded as his aesthetic opponents, such as the followers of Richard Wagner; such "impurists" were always marshaling music in the service of extramusical ends, from national solidarity to religious freedom. Seeking to repair a perceived imbalance, Stravinsky portrayed the musician as a craftsman whose materials of pitch and rhythm in themselves harbor no more expression than the carpenter's beams or the jeweler's stone.

Stravinsky may have been right that in the absence of an externally imposed "program," music is simply music. He spoke of the "poetics" of music, which in its literal sense refers to the making (*poiesis*) of music. Unintentionally, however, Stravinsky vividly illustrated a different point through his own life: the extent to which the making of music is *not* possible without the externally triggered factor of politics. All creative individuals—and especially all musicians—must deal with a set of associates who not only help the creators realize their vision but also, eventually, with a wider public, determine the fate of the creators' works. Stravinsky's embroilment in personal and professional politics was extreme for an artist of any sort, yet by throwing the political aspects of creation into sharp relief, Stravinsky reveals the extent to which an artist must work with the field that regulates his chosen domain. Whether they do so well or poorly, eagerly or reluctantly, nearly all creative individuals must devote significant energies to the management of their careers.

Stravinsky's early training came in the form of an apprenticeship with Nikolay Rimsky-Korsakov, the dean of Russian composers. Rimsky-Korsakov guided Stravinsky in orchestration, teaching him how to compose for each instrument; they would each orchestrate the same passages and then compare their versions. Stravinsky was an apt pupil, whose rapid advances pleased his mentor; and, perhaps for the first time in his life, Stravinsky found himself in a milieu that fully engaged him.

A dramatic turning point in Stravinsky's career occurred shortly after his mentor's death when Stravinsky was approached by Serge Diaghilev to compose a nocturne for his theatrical project, *The Firebird*. Suddenly, instead of working alone, Stravinsky had almost daily intercourse with the ensemble—a new and heady experience for someone who had craved the companionship of individuals with whom he felt comfortable. Stravinsky turned out to be a willing pupil, one who learned quickly and reacted vividly to everything. He was sufficiently flexible, curious, and versatile to be able to work with the set designers, dancers, choreographers, and even those responsible for the business end of the enterprise. From Diaghilev young Igor learned two equally crucial lessons for ensemble work: how to meet a deadline and how to compromise on, or mediate amongst, deeply held but differing artistic visions. Yet, he may have learned Diaghilev's lessons too well. As Stravinsky gained in knowledge and confidence, he found himself engaged in strenuous disputes about characterization, choreography, and instrumentation.

The most notable creators almost always are perfectionists who have worked out every detail of their conception painstakingly and are unwilling to make further changes unless they can be convinced that such alterations are justified. Few intrepid creators are likely to cede any rights to others; and even if they are consciously tempted to do so, their unconscious sense of fidelity to an original conceptualization may prevent them from following through. Stravinsky was no exception in this, and his goals were well-defined and impassioned. Suppressing whatever revolutionary impulses may have existed in his own person and animated his earlier music, ignoring the rich emotional associations of his early masterpieces, Stravinsky stressed the importance of conventions and traditions, and the utility of self-imposed constraints. He loathed disorder, randomness, arbitrariness, the Circean lure of chaos. Music was akin to mathematical thinking and relationships, and one could discern powerful, inexorable laws at work. In the paradox-packed closing lines of *The Poetics of Music*, Stravinsky declared: "My freedom will be so much greater and more meaningful, the more narrowly I limit my field of action and the more I surround myself with obstacles. Whatever diminishes constraints, diminishes strength. The more constraints one imposes, the more one frees one's self of the chains that shackle the spirit."

Material used in this particular passage has been adapted from the following source:

H. Gardner, *Creating Minds: An Anatomy of Creativity Seen Through the Lives of Freud, Einstein, Picasso, Stravinsky, Eliot, Graham, and Gandhi.* © 1993 by Basic Books.

1. Which of Stravinsky's learning experiences or observations is most *inconsistent* with the author's statement in the last paragraph that "the most notable creators are almost always perfectionists"?

A) Orchestration techniques learned while working with Rimsky-Korsakov
B) Lessons learned from Diaghilev and involvement in the ensemble
C) The need to engage in protracted political battles
D) The observation that "the more constraints one imposes, the more one frees one's self of the chains that shackle the spirit"

2. The word "political" is used in paragraph 2 in order to refer to:

A) collaboration and artifice.
B) greed and expediency.
C) interpersonal relations.
D) cleverness and guile.

3. We can reasonably infer that the perceived imbalance that Stravinsky was seeking to repair was one of:

A) an over-dependence on inspiration rather than craftsmanship in making music.
B) some composers' tendency to inject extraneous elements into their music.
C) too great an involvement in the political side of theatrical staging and production.
D) an over-emphasis on choreography as compared to instrumentation in theatrical productions.

4. The author's discussion of Stravinsky's actions and statements suggests that which two aspects of Stravinsky's character or career may have been at odds with each other?

A) His desire to create music and his involvement with choreography and set design
B) The artistic independence expressed in *The Poetics of Music* and his dependence on others in managing his career
C) His desire to create and his inability to escape interpersonal politics
D) His desire for a strict approach to making music and his willingness to work in a highly collaborative setting

5. In the author's view, Stravinsky's collaboration with others in musical composition and theater can best be summarized as:

A) productive yet contentious.
B) accepted with reluctance.
C) onerous and ultimately destructive.
D) fruitful and harmonious.

6. According to the passage, Stravinsky believed which of the following to be a condition necessary for creativity in music?

A) A willingness to collaborate and compromise
B) Situations of total freedom
C) Openness to new and revolutionary ideas
D) Limitations to lend it structure

7. A study shows that painters who hire agents and business managers early in their careers tend to be more prolific. What effect would this information have on the author's argument regarding an artist's involvement in his own career?

A) It would be contrary to the author's claim that artists need to manage their own careers.
B) It would be relevant to evaluating the notion that the essence of Stravinsky's artistic vision was shaped by collaboration.
C) It would support the author's implication that artistic fields of endeavor are also businesses.
D) It would justify Stravinsky's engagement in strenuous disputes regarding theatrical elements.

SOLUTIONS TO CHAPTER 7 PRACTICE PASSAGE 1

1. **C** This is a New Information question.

   A: No. Nowhere do the authors suggest the conditions for starting a democracy require violence. Nor does the authors' tone suggest violence is "heroic."

   B: No. First, although the authors discuss in paragraph 6 the importance of leaders being committed to a democratic system for the existence or maintenance of democracy, this is not described as "idealism," and the motivation of those leaders is not the issue but rather their behavior. Second, this idea is not explicitly tied to the requirements for *founding* a democracy. Third, this choice, in its reference to George Washington, relies on too much outside knowledge for its relevance to the information in the question stem.

   C: **Yes. In paragraph 5, the authors say, "Stronger public support probably is required for the successful launching of a democracy than it is for maintaining an already established democracy."**

   D: No. The authors do not equate peaceful protest with a stronger democracy.

2. **D** This is a Strengthen question.

   A: No. An isolated incident such as this one is not enough evidence to suggest a trend will continue. Also notice the mild wording; the fact that it gained "some public support" is not enough to "most strengthen" the authors' claim.

   B: No. There is no connection made by the authors between some level (we don't know if it's a significant level) of increased participation in violent protest and increased support for peaceful protest.

   C: No. Because it suggests the number of educated people who support peaceful protest is in some level of *decline*, this answer choice would weaken the argument. Note that even if you were thinking that "more than 50 percent" could be 70 percent, this answer still gives no evidence of an increase over time, or of a likely increase in the future.

   D: **Yes. The authors explain in paragraph 2 that "as education levels increase, approval of demonstrations will increase," but do not explicitly support the premise that education levels will increase. If colleges were to accept more applicants, it is fair to assume education levels would increase, thus strengthening the premise.**

3. **C** This is an Inference/EXCEPT question.

   A: No. One part of the main idea of the passage is that widespread acceptance of disruptive antigovernment activity can threaten democracy (see paragraph 5). Since the question stem asks you to find an answer choice that is not a requirement for democracy, this cannot be the answer.

   B: No. See paragraph 6: "the positive support by leaders for a political system is essential to its existence."

   C: **Yes. Paragraphs 4 and 5 explain that the population does not need to actively campaign for democratic ideals for democracy to work. In fact, such strong support for democratic values may be "impossible" (paragraph 4). At the end of paragraph 5, the author states that "absence of disruptive acts, not the presence of supportive attitudes, is crucial." Although paragraph 6 suggests public support for democracy is necessary when antigovernment leaders come to prominence, this is a specific situation, as opposed to the "general" view that the question stem asks for. Because this idea is not supported by the passage, it is the *correct* answer to this "EXCEPT" question.**

   D: No. See paragraph 6: "If some leaders are willing to oppose the system, it is crucial that there be no substantial number of followers to which the leaders can appeal."

4. **D**   This is a Main Idea/Primary Purpose question.
    A: No. The authors make no such evaluation of different forms of protest. Be sure not to be overly influenced by paragraph 1 of the passage when determining the authors' primary purpose.
    B: No. This answer uses language that is too extreme; the authors do not go so far as to assure us democracy will fail under certain circumstances.
    C: No. This answer choice is too broad. The correct answer must focus on the key issues of the passage: protest, public support, and the stability of democracies. Furthermore, this answer is too negative. While the passage does suggest that free speech is related to peaceful protest (paragraph 2), the authors don't go so far as to suggest that it has harmful effects.
    D: Yes. Although it uses vague language to do so, this answer does address the main focus of the passage. The factors that would influence stability of a democratic political system (a "certain type of political system"), according to the passage, would be the level and type of support and/or dissent.

5. **A**   This is a New Information question.
    A: Yes. Paragraph 6 states, "If some leaders are willing to oppose the system, it is crucial that there be no substantial number of followers to which the leaders can appeal. The followers' attitudes, as opposed to their willingness to act themselves, may provide a base of support for antisystem behavior by leaders."
    B: No. It would be too large of an inference to take the authors' claim that educated Americans are more likely to be tolerant of protest (paragraph 2) to mean their support would be the key to such an insurgent political group's success.
    C: No. The correct answer must be supported by the passage text, rather than by common sense or real world experience. The passage says in paragraph 6 that "it is crucial that there be no substantial number of followers to which the leaders can appeal" and that the "followers' attitudes, as opposed to their willingness to act themselves, may provide a base of support for antisystem behavior by leaders." While you might think that campaigning by a loyal following would help create widespread public support for the dissidents, there is no evidence for this in the passage. Compare this answer to choice A, which does have direct support in the passage text.
    D: No. The passage gives no evidence, in paragraph 6 or elsewhere, that having a clear party platform would influence the public one way or the other.

6. **C**   This is an Inference question.
    A: No. This is a reversal of the information in paragraph 1. Acceptance or support of protest stayed the same, while opposition to protest declined.
    B: No. Although this may be historically accurate, the answer must be supported by the text of the passage. There is no suggestion in the passage that social unrest lead to this kind of change in attitude.
    C: Yes. In paragraph 1, the authors state: "Although the level of support for these activities did not increase between 1968 and 1972, the level of opposition declined."
    D: No. Paragraph 1 clearly states there was such a change; opposition to protest declined.

7.   **C**   This is an Inference question.
  A: No. Paragraph 1 establishes that "most Americans do not approve of either peaceful or violent protests."
  B: No. The passage does not address America's history of violence or public attitudes towards it.
  C: Yes. In paragraph 1, Americans are portrayed as quietly accepting the status quo. Most oppose antigovernment protest and the majority of those who tolerate dissent don't participate. Also, in paragraph 3, the authors describe the American populace as merely "satisfied": "It is possible to view the United States as a democratic system that has survived without a strong democratic political culture because governmental policies have gained a continual, widespread acceptance."
  D: No. The passage does not describe Americans as patriotic. Furthermore, the authors state in paragraph 1 that "Increasing numbers of people seem to be willing to tolerate demonstrations and protests under some circumstances." Even if this is still a minority of the population, it would be too extreme to describe Americans as a whole as "unwilling to tolerate dissent."

SOLUTIONS TO CHAPTER 7 PRACTICE PASSAGE 2

1.   **B**   This is an Inference question.
  Note: The author makes this statement in the context of discussing Stravinsky's faithfulness to his own artistic vision. The passage states that perfectionists "have worked out every detail of their conception painstakingly and are [often] unwilling to make further changes" or "cede any rights to others," and that "Stravinsky was no exception in this."
  A: No. This choice may be tempting, but we have no basis for supposing compromise or acceptance of "imperfection" was required, as we're only told that they composed separately for later comparison.
  B: Yes. It was from Diaghilev that Stravinsky is said to have learned "to compromise on, or mediate amongst, deeply held but differing artistic visions" (paragraph 4). The quote cited in the question stem, in the context of paragraph 5, relates to an unwillingness to "cede any rights to others" or to diverge from the artist's own "original conceptualization."
  C: No. Paragraph 2 indicates that Stravinsky had to engage in political battles in order to "realize [his] vision" and to manage his career. However, there is no indication that these battles involved compromising or going against his perfectionism about the work itself.
  D: No. This answer is consistent with the statement in the question stem. This observation appears in paragraph 5, in the context of the author's description of Stravinsky's dedication to realizing his own goals.

2.   **C**   This is an Inference question.
  A: No. While "collaboration" fits, "artifice," or falsehood, does not. Be careful not to import your own associations with politics into the passage.
  B: No. While "expediency" is not clearly wrong, there is no suggestion of greed. The fact that political battles were necessary in the management of an artist's career doesn't by itself show that the artists are greedy or money-hungry.
  C: Yes. Paragraph 2 says, in the context of discussing the necessary role of politics, that artists "must deal with a set of associates who...help the creators realize their vision."
  D: No. While "cleverness" is not clearly wrong, there is no suggestion of "guile" or deception.

3. **B** This is an Inference question.

A: No. There is no suggestion in paragraph 1, or elsewhere in the passage, that Stravinsky discounted the importance of inspiration ("expression" is not equated with "inspiration"), or that he believed that he himself or other composers displayed insufficient craftsmanship.

B: Yes. This choice is supported by information in the lines above the reference to the "imbalance" in paragraph 1, in which the author refers to Stravinsky's intention of "blasting...his aesthetic opponents" whose goals were extra-musical, attempting to further such things as national solidarity or religious freedom.

C: No. The author does not suggest that Stravinsky tried to reduce his, or others', involvement in the political aspects specifically of presenting music or theater to an audience. Stravinsky's complaint was about injecting non-musical aspects into the music itself.

D: No. While paragraph 4 mentions Stravinsky's involvement in disputes about choreography and instrumentation, it doesn't suggest that he believed choreography had been given too much importance.

4. **D** This is an Inference question.

A: No. Paragraph 4 suggests that his desire to create and present music and his interest in choreography and set design went hand-in-hand.

B: No. While paragraph 2 does suggest that all artists are dependent on others in realizing their vision and managing their career, this doesn't necessarily apply to artistic independence involved in making or creating the music itself.

C: No. Paragraph 2 suggests that Stravinsky believed that interpersonal politics were necessary to some aspects of the process of creation (such as career management), rather than an impediment to it.

D: Yes. Stravinsky expresses a strong attachment to making music in particular ways, untainted by extramusical intentions, and it's hinted in paragraph 5 that he would be unlikely to change his compositions. However, the discussion in paragraph 4 indicates that Stravinsky had learned to compromise artistically and to be open to differing artistic visions.

5. **A** This is an Inference question.

A: Yes. This choice is supported by paragraph 4, where the author describes how Stravinsky benefited from the new experience of collaboration, and yet found himself "engaged in strenuous disputes."

B: No. "Reluctance" contradicts paragraph 4, which suggests that Stravinsky eagerly took on this new opportunity to collaborate, and "destructive" is too extreme to be supported by the author's mention of "strenuous disputes."

C: No. "Onerous" is unsupported; we have no evidence that Stravinsky found these disputes to be burdensome. Furthermore, "ultimately destructive" is too extreme.

D: No. This choice is half-right/half-wrong. "Fruitful" or productive is supported, but the process was not always "harmonious," as indicated in the matter of "strenuous disputes" mentioned in paragraph 4.

6. **D** This is a Retrieval question.

A: No. This choice reflects some points made by the author in paragraphs 2 and 4, but we don't know that Stravinsky shared in this belief. The author states in paragraph 2 that Stravinsky's experience "reveals the extent to which an artist must work with the field that regulates his chosen domain," but not that Stravinsky himself expressed this idea. Note that in paragraph 2, the author states that Stravinsky's life "unintentionally" illustrates the importance of collaboration.

B: No. This choice contradicts Stravinsky's statements in paragraph 5, where he talks about the importance of constraints and obstacles.

C: No. The passage states that he eventually believed in "suppressing whatever revolutionary impulses may have existed in his own person" (paragraph 5).

D: Yes. This is explained in Stravinsky's quote in paragraph 5.

7. **C** This is a New Information question.

A: No. This choice may be tempting, but it takes words out of context from the passage. The author indicates in paragraph 2 that the artist must manage his or her career, but also suggests that this usually requires interaction with, and help from, other people.

B: No. This choice may also be somewhat tempting, but the study would be relevant to evaluating collaboration in the business of the artist's career, including presentation of artistic work to the public, rather than in the essence or fundamental character of the artistic vision itself.

C: Yes. The author's argument in paragraph 2 is that an artist needs to be involved with the business of his or her own career, whether personally or through agents, so a study that indicates that a business manager increases artistic productivity would support the author's argument.

D: No. A study about the effects of business management would not be directly relevant to issues of theatrical production.

Individual Passage Log

Passage # _____   **Time spent on both passages** _____

Q#	Q type	Attractors	What did you do wrong?

Revised Strategy _____

Passage # _____

Q#	Q type	Attractors	What did you do wrong?

Revised Strategy _____

Chapter 8
Refining Your Skills

GOALS

1) To continue the self-evaluation process
2) To further refine your skills
3) To prepare mentally for test day

8.1 CONTINUING THE SELF-EVALUATION PROCESS

At this point in your preparation, you have acquired a variety of tools with which to attack the passages and the CARS section as a whole. Over the remaining time leading up to MCAT day, take the opportunity to further refine those skills, taking your own individual strengths and weaknesses into account. If you don't have a clear list of those strengths and weaknesses (and if you have not been consistently filling out the Individual Passage Logs and Test Assessment Logs), *now* is the time to generate it.

It is still not too late to recognize and correct some of the persistent mistakes you may be making. There is no point in doing passage after passage if you spend little or no time evaluating your performance on those passages. You should spend at least as much time evaluating your performance as you do on doing the passage itself. If not, each passage you do reinforces rather than corrects bad habits and blind spots you may still have.

Consider some of the following things:

- Are you still trying to finish (or almost finish) the entire section and yet are missing a large number of the questions you complete? If so, think about how much time you're spending getting questions wrong. Instead, try two test sections guessing on at least one additional passage, giving yourself more time to carefully consider the questions. See how slowing down affects your overall percentage of correct answers.
- Are you defining the Main Point of each paragraph and articulating the Bottom Line of the passage before addressing the questions? This is one of your most powerful tools. Use it!
- Are you consistently going back to the passage and answering the questions in your own words before evaluating the answer choices?
- Are you actively using POE? Are you approaching the answers skeptically, looking out for traps?

8.2 REFINING YOUR SKILLS

Below are a series of exercises, focusing on the passage, the questions, and the answer choices. They will help you continue to improve your performance in each of those areas, especially on the harder passages.

EXERCISE 1: IDENTIFYING THE AUTHOR'S TONE

Below are four short passages. Read and highlight each as you would work a real MCAT CARS passage, paying close attention to tracking the author's attitude. After working each passage, answer the question or questions regarding the author's tone or attitude. Once you have completed all four, read through the explanations that follow.

1. Formalism, an approach to literary criticism, arose in the early twentieth century. The basic tenet of formalist criticism is that meaning arises from the text itself, and that the intentions of the author are essentially irrelevant. Thus, according to formalism, the appropriate approach to understanding a text relies on close reading of the structure of the work on all levels from sentence structure and grammar to the construction of the work as a whole. Formalism views a text as existing independent from the author; thus, not only the author's intent but also the cultural context within which the work was created (and possible cultural influences on the author) can be largely ignored. The only historical context that may legitimately be seen as potentially relevant is that of previous literary forms to which the given text may be seen as related. In reaction to the strict limits of formalism an alternative approach, reader-response theory, arose in the 1970s. Reader-response theory broadened the possibilities of gaining meaning from a text by examining the various ways in which different readers may interpret a given work. Reader-response theory overcame the limitations inherent in formalism by including within its purview a variety of factors that may in fact provide important insights into the meaning of a work of art. Formalists ineffectually attempted to defend the assumptions at the core of their own school of thought by claiming that while different readers may arrive at different interpretations, those interpretations are irrelevant to gaining a true understanding of the meaning of the text itself, and therefore that reader-response theory belongs in the realm of psychology, not literary criticism.

Question: What is the author's attitude toward formalism? _____

_____

2. Many people see the Denishawn dance company as the founder of modern dance in America. The Denishawn School of Dancing and Related Arts, founded in 1915, based its technique on classical ballet, but included as well influences from other cultures, in particular, India, Spain, Cambodia, and the Middle East. Ruth St. Denis and Ted Shawn, the founders of the company, also incorporated free movement into their teaching and performance; this represented a significant break from classical ballet performance and pedagogy. However others, while recognizing the ground-breaking nature of Denishawn's work, claim that one of Denishawn's students, Martha Graham, is more legitimately seen as the true founder of American modern dance. They claim that she, unlike Denishawn, truly broke with classical ballet by creating an entirely new set of movements that replaced, rather than modified, the traditional choreographical elements on which classical ballet is based.

Question: What is the author's attitude toward who deserves to be called the founder of modern dance?

_____

_____

3. Ethical practice must be fundamentally based on, and judged by, universal duties that apply in all situations. Regardless of the consequences, an action is ethical only if it conforms to these absolute duties. Consider a hypothetical case: you are the driver of a trolley car. As you are driving the car down a hill, the brakes fail and the car cannot be stopped. Ahead, standing on the track, is a group of people who will be hit and killed if you do nothing. However, you can divert the car onto a different track; standing on this track is a single person who will be killed if she is hit by the trolley. There are no other options: you must either do nothing and several people will die, or take action and a single person will be killed. One form of ethical thought, deontological ethics, holds that you have an absolute obligation to take no actions that would result in harming another human being. Therefore, you should do nothing, as taking action would result in the death of a person as a direct result of that action. Another form of ethics, utilitarianism, holds that the ethical decision is the one that results in the least amount of harm. By this way of thought, you should divert the car onto the other track, even though you will be deciding to take an action that directly results in the death of a person, as this action would save the lives of more people.

Question: Based on the passage, what would the author say the driver of the trolley should do? _____

_____

4. The role and power of the president within a political system has been analyzed in various ways. One view, propagated in particular by the political scientist James Barber, focuses on the personality of the president. Barber created a four-part typology of presidential personalities: active-positive, passive-positive, active-negative, and passive-negative. According to Barber, the biography of a president, including his or her childhood, plays a crucial role in determining presidential personality, and any analysis of the nature of a presidency (and of the office itself) must include a consideration of early influences, including family and upbringing. However, in recent decades, Barber's useful analysis has been unfairly discounted in academic fields, and Neustadt's theory based on "the power to persuade" has taken hold. Neustadt provides additional insight by arguing that the power of a president arises in part from his or her domestic and international reputation. Those who take an overly rigid interpretation of Neustadt's argument ignore the influence of formative experiences, and look only at a president's achievements and failures while in office when analyzing the nature of the office of the president as well as the efficacy of individual holders of the office.

Question: What is the author's opinion regarding Barber? _____

_____

Question: What is the author's opinion regarding Neustadt? _____

_____

Explanations for Exercise 1: Identifying the Author's Tone

1) **What is the author's attitude toward formalism?**

Negative

The author states that reader-response theory "broadened the possibilities of gaining meaning from a text" and "overcame the limitations inherent in formalism." The author also states that formalists "ineffectually" attempted to defend their assumptions.

2) **What is the author's attitude toward who deserves to be called the founder of modern dance?**

Neutral

The author discusses the debate without taking sides. Note that while the author does state Denishawn's work "represented a significant break from classical ballet performance and pedagogy," the passage does not indicate that this qualifies Denishawn as the true founder of modern dance. Nor does the author suggest that retaining aspects of classical ballet disqualifies Denishawn as the founder of modern dance, or that creating "entirely new set of movements that replaced, rather than modified, the traditional choreographical elements on which classical ballet is based" (as Graham did) is a necessary condition for being considered as such.

3) **Based on the passage, what would the author say the driver of the trolley should do?**

Stay on the track, rather than diverting in order to save more lives.

The author states at the beginning of the passage that "Ethical practice must be fundamentally based on, and judged by, universal duties that apply in all situations. Regardless of the consequences, an action is ethical only if it conforms to these absolute duties." This put the author in the deontological camp as it is described in the passage, which would hold that taking action to divert the trolley onto the other track, even if this would result in fewer deaths, would be unethical. Be careful not to use your own opinion when analyzing a passage. Even if you think that the ethical standard should be based on weighing the consequences against each other, this is not the author's opinion.

4) **What is the author's opinion regarding Barber?**

Positive

The author states that Barber's analysis is "useful" and that it has been "unfairly discounted."

What is the author's opinion regarding Neustadt?

Positive

Note that the author criticizes those that take an "overly rigid interpretation" of Neustadt's argument, not Neustadt himself. The passage states that "Neustadt provides additional insight" to Barber's analysis. Overall, the author indicates that both Barber and Neustadt have made valid contributions (and does not suggest that they are mutually exclusive, even though others might believe this to be the case).

EXERCISE 2: PARAPHRASING THE PASSAGE

Often, the more difficult passages are characterized by complex, abstract wording. To make your way through these passages with a reasonable level of comprehension (that is, enough to articulate the main point of each chunk and of the passage as a whole), you need to put the author's convoluted, obscure wording into your own clear language.

Read each of the paragraphs below, and write down the main point in the space provided. If you have difficulty with a section of a paragraph (or a paragraph as a whole), don't just go back to the beginning and read it again "harder." Often after multiple readings, a paragraph makes less, not more sense. Instead, pay attention to the structure of the sentence or paragraph. Find an "anchor," or one piece that you understand, and use it to make sense of the rest. Break the reading down into pieces, and the whole will begin to make a lot more sense.

Note: Some of these paragraphs represent the difficulty level of language found in Killer passages. Don't panic, and don't give up; just keep your focus and do the best you can. Practicing on the hardest examples will contribute to your performance on any level of passage. These are not meant to be different paragraphs from the same passage, so don't worry about finding a relationship between them. Explanations follow the exercise.

Paragraph 1

Modern medicine has fixed its own date of birth as being in the last years of the eighteenth century. Reflecting on its situation, it identifies the origin of its positivity with a return—over and above all theory—to the modest but effecting level of the perceived. In fact, this supposed empiricism is not based on a rediscovery of the absolute values of the visible, nor on the predetermined rejection of systems and all their chimeras, but on a reorganization of the manifest and secret space that opened up when a millennial gaze passed over men's sufferings. Nonetheless, the rejuvenation of medical perception, the way colors and things came to life under the illuminating gaze of the first clinicians is no mere myth. At the beginning of the nineteenth century, doctors described what for centuries had remained below the threshold of the visible and the expressible, but this did not mean that, after overindulging in speculation, they had begun to perceive once again, or that they listened to reason rather than to imagination; it meant that the relation between the visible and the invisible—which is necessary to all concrete knowledge—changed its structure, revealing through gaze and language what had previously been below and beyond their domain. A new alliance was forged between words and things, enabling one *to see* and *to say*.

8.2

Note: This is a good example of how a passage about a familiar topic (medicine) may in fact be extremely difficult. When taken as a whole, it is almost impossible to understand. Therefore, take it piece by piece. Find a sentence, or a part of a sentence, that you do understand, and use it to make some sense of the parts around it. Don't get stuck on unfamiliar vocabulary. Do you really need to know what a "chimera" or "millennial gaze" is to get the gist of the paragraph? Do, however, pay attention to the series of contrasts provided (indicated by pivotal words and phrases) to get a sense of what the author is describing.

Main Point: _____

_____

Paragraph 2

We have so far discussed the "absent person" in ads. But since this person is always signified by objects (and above all, the product) in the ad, interchangeable with them in that they represent his absence with their presence, it follows that the other side of the exchange, the product, may likewise be absent from the ad, and signified by the people in it. There is a series of lager ads on TV where the lager itself is never there. In one of these ads, two workers in a factory pick up two empty glasses from the conveyer belt and start drinking "lager" from them.… In another ad the two men come into a pub which turns out not to have this particular brand of lager when they order it. So they take two empty mugs and again "drink" the invisible lager. Although the product is actually absent in these cases, it is sufficiently signified in the ad—by the two men—by their attitude towards it, by their taste, and so on. There is also a definite place for it to fill: the surrounding presence of the mugs makes the actual presence of the lager redundant. Thus with absence in an ad, the thing meant to fill the gap is always defined, not by a simple replacement but by what is contingent: it is what surrounds the gap that determines its shape.

Note: Notice how this paragraph is organized. This structure—a claim followed by one or more examples, and then a further conclusion—is a very common one, and you can use it to help you puzzle through difficult sections of a passage. If you have difficulty with the claims, work backwards from the examples. If you have trouble understanding the examples, start with the claim.

Main Point: _____

_____

Paragraph 3

At a certain point in their historical lives, social classes become detached from their traditional parties. In other words, the traditional parties in that particular organizational form, with the particular men who constitute, represent, and lead them, are no longer recognized by their class (or fraction of a class) as its expression. When such crises occur, the immediate situation becomes delicate and dangerous, because the field is open for violent solutions, for the activities of unknown forces, represented by charismatic "men of destiny."

Note: It is always more difficult to wrap your brain around the abstract than the concrete. If the author doesn't give a specific example or illustration, imagine one of your own to help solidify your understanding of the text.

Main Point: _____

_____

Paragraph 4

As a label, "cyberpunk" is perfection. It suggests the apotheosis of postmodernism. On one hand, pure negation: of manner, history, philosophy, politics, body, will affect, anything mediated by cultural memory; on the other, pure attitude: all is power, and "subculture," and the grace of Hip negotiating the splatter of consciousness as it slams against the hard-tech future, the techno-future of artificial impermanence, where all that was once nature is simulated and elaborated by technical means, a future world-construct that is as remote from the "lessons of history" as the present mix-up is from the pitiful science fiction fantasies of the past that had tried to imagine us. The oxymoronic conceit in "cyberpunk" is so slick and global it fuses high and low, the complex and the simple, the governor and the savage, the techno-sublime and rock and roll slime.

Note: Even sentences that seem like just a cascade of words do have a structure. Try breaking up the long sentences in this paragraph into shorter, more manageable ones before trying to synthesize them into the main idea of the passage.

Main Point: _____

_____

Paragraph 5

But physiologists have also begun to see chaos as health. It has long been understood that nonlinearity in feedback processes serves to regulate and control. Simply put, a linear process, given a slight nudge, tends to remain slightly off track. A nonlinear process, given the same nudge, tends to return to its starting point.

Note: Phrases like *simply put, in other words,* or *that is to say* should be music to your ears. These phrases indicate that the author is going to say it again, in different words, in case it wasn't clear the first time. Make sure you notice and take advantage of these "second chances."

Main Point: _____

_____

Paragraph 6

Western academic philosophy may have a hard time agreeing on its own definition, but any definition must be responsible to certain facts about the application of the concept. In the Euro-American tradition nothing can count as philosophy, for example, if it does not discuss problems that have a family resemblance to those problems that have centrally concerned those we call "philosophers." And nothing that does address itself to such problems but does so in a way that bears no family resemblance to traditional philosophical methods ought to count either. And the Wittgensteinian notion of family resemblance, here, is especially appropriate because a tradition, like a family, is something that changes from one generation to the next. Just as there may be no way of seeing me as especially like my remote ancestors, even though there are substantial similarities between the members of succeeding generations, so we are likely to be able to see the continuities between Plato and Frege only if we trace steps in between.

Note: Another important tool at your disposal is the analogy. Where is an analogy used in this paragraph and what is its relationship to the author's main point?

Main Point: _____

_____

Paragraph 7

This is not to disparage the efforts of the experimenters. They are important as catalysts. For the writer is not alone is his or her endeavor, but is, rather, participating in a collaborative enterprise. The Kriges would not impress us so if it were not for the cooperation of the publishing house (which lends the nobility of its name and ensures that the cloth covers of the book are expensively textured and soberly colored), the librarian (who places the book in the anthropology shelves rather than on those reserved for science fiction) and the teacher (who secures it a place on the anthropology-class reading list). Above all, the Kriges rely on readers' skills in filling out and making sense of scientific discourse, a peculiar one in which data are presumed autonomous, interpretations are either confirmed or disconfirmed by facts that are independently specified, and the discovery of orderliness and the production of definitive accounts are normal and expected.

Note: What is it about this author's writing style that can make this paragraph difficult to read quickly? How might you deal with this "listing" tendency? How could you actually use it to your advantage?

Main Point: _____

_____

Paragraph 8

The aestheticians of painting, especially the modern ones, are the great advocates of "significant form," the movement of the line, the relations of color and tone. Of these critics, the most consistent, the clearest (and the most widely accepted), that I know is the late Mr. Bernhard Berenson. Over sixty years ago in his studies of the Italian Renaissance painters he expounded his aesthetics with refreshing clarity. The merely accurate representations of an object, the blind imitation of nature, was not art, not even if that object was what would commonly be agreed upon as beautiful, for example, a beautiful woman. There was another category of painter superior to the first. Such a one would not actually reproduce the object as it was. Being a man of visions and imagination, the object would stimulate in his impulses, thoughts, memories visually creative. These he would fuse into a whole and the result would be not so much the object as the totality of the visual image which the object had invoked in a superior mind. That too, Mr. Berenson excluded from the category of true art (and was by no means isolated in doing so): mere reproductions of objects, whether actually in existence or the product of the sublimest imaginations, was "literature" or "illustration." What then was the truly artistic? The truly artistic was a quality that existed in its own right, irrespective of the object represented.

Note: What is the importance of the sentence, "That too, Mr. Berenson excluded from the category of true art"? Were you a bit surprised, given what had come before? What role does this statement play in defining the author's main point?

Main Point: _____

_____

Explanations for Exercise 2: Paraphrasing the Passage

Notes: Many of these Main Points are wordier than yours may be (and should be). Remember that you are the only one who needs to understand your own annotation, and therefore complete sentences are unnecessary. You might have written down just a few words to represent these main points.

Paragraph 1

Main Point: Modern medicine developed at the end of the eighteenth century, with the merging of the visible and the invisible in physicians' understanding.

Paragraph 2

Main Point: Advertising sometimes uses the strategy of showing the environment in which a product exists, but not the product itself.

Paragraph 3

Main Point: When the representational party of a social class no longer accurately reflects the perceived reality of that class, violent or drastic actions may be taken.

Paragraph 4

Main Point: The word "cyberpunk" encapsulates all of the contradictory elements present in a postmodern world.

Paragraph 5

Main Point: A nonlinear feedback process can be at least as effective as a linear process, because it has the ability to self-correct.

Paragraph 6

Main Point: Western academic philosophy must trace the steps between generations of philosophical thought in order to accurately include the relevant subject matter.

Paragraph 7

Main Point: The full publication process of this textbook is defined by collaboration.

Paragraph 8

Main Point: Aestheticians of painting (such as Bernhard Berenson) do not judge a painting's beauty on the accuracy of its reproduction of reality, but on a higher level of artistry and creativity.

EXERCISE 3: PARAPHRASING THE QUESTIONS

One common characteristic of hard passages is complexly worded and structured questions. As we discussed in Chapter 4, if you don't understand the question itself, you are likely to spend a lot of time on it, only to arrive at an incorrect answer at the end. For each of the questions below, identify the question category (Specific, General, Reasoning, or Application), question type (e.g., Inference, Strengthen, Evaluate, etc.) and then translate the question into your own words, defining what this question is requiring you to do. Explanations follow the exercise.

1. The information in the passage suggests that the author would be most likely to agree with which of the following statements concerning the use of HDRs as an alternative energy in the event of a failure of other, more traditional recovery systems?

Question category: _____

_____

Question type: _____

_____

Translation: _____

_____

2. The reference to labor negotiation as an example of third party intervention is meant to illustrate which of the following theories in the context of the author's discussion of triadic and quadratic models?

Question category: _____

_____

Question type: _____

_____

Translation: _____

_____

3. The author's claim that the behavior of certain unusual stars has helped "account for previously unexplained phenomena" (paragraph 4) would be most justified by an astronomer's ability to measure the luminosity and pulsation of which of the following types of stars?

Question category: _____

_____

Question type: _____

_____

Translation: _____

_____

4. According to the passage, the author considers each of the following good advice to an owner who has arranged for fast-track construction of a building on his land EXCEPT:

Question category: _____

_____

Question type: _____

_____

Translation: _____

_____

5. The author suggests that the most valid criticism of
the enactment of laws governing large corporations
that encourage aspiration that has been raised by the
advocates of non-regulation is which of the following?

Question category: _____

_____

Question type: _____

_____

Translation: _____

_____

6. It has been argued that when "nation" and "state" are not
viewed as unrelated concepts, methodology takes a back
seat to political concerns in nonacademic arenas. This
claim would be LEAST inconsistent with the author's
argument that:

Question category: _____

_____

Question type: _____

_____

Translation: _____

_____

7. Suppose that a veterinarian specializing in the care of large animals were to experience "differential empathy," as that term is used in the passage. This would be most similar to a lawyer who professed that:

Question category: _____

_____

Question type: _____

_____

Translation: _____

_____

8. In addressing the issue of land reform, Stunwitznow predicted that the unearned benefits accrued to landowners from prior, unregulated transactions would not, in a purely laissez-faire system, be taxed at a higher rate than earned benefits from that same classification or type of transaction given a similar absence of pre-existing regulatory jurisdiction or activity. This prediction would most undermine the author's expectation that:

Question category: _____

_____

Question type: _____

_____

Translation: _____

_____

Explanations for Exercise 3: Paraphrasing the Questions

1. Question Category: Specific
    Question Type: Inference
    Translation: What does the author think about the use of HDR as an alternative energy when traditional recovery systems fail?

2. Question Category: Reasoning
    Question Type: Structure
    Translation: Why does the author use the example of labor negotiation in the discussion of triadic and quadratic models?

3. Question Category: Application
    Question Type: Strengthen
    Translation: The luminosity and pulsation of which type of star would best prove the author's argument regarding the behavior of certain unusual stars?

4. Question Category: Specific
    Question Type: Retrieval EXCEPT
    Translation: What WOULDN'T the author recommend to the owner of land where building is being fast-tracked?

5. Question Category: Specific
    Question Type: Inference
    Translation: What is the most valid criticism raised by the advocates of non-regulation regarding these corporations?

6. Question Category: Application
    Question Type: Weaken EXCEPT (which is not exactly the same as Strengthen)
    Translation: When "nation" and "state" are viewed as related concepts, political concerns take precedence over methodology outside of academia—what part of the author's argument is this most consistent with?

7. Question Category: Application
    Question Type: New Information/Analogy
    Translation: How would "differential empathy" apply to a lawyer (like it does to a large-animal vet)?

8. Question Category: Application
    Question Type: New Information/Weaken
    Translation: Stunwitznow's prediction that the taxation of unearned benefits would be the same as that of earned benefits would undermine what expectation held by the author?

EXERCISE 4: PROCESS OF ELIMINATION

Choose a passage from your practice materials. You can use the Individual Passage Drills at the end of the last few chapters in this book or other printed passages. Put a sheet of paper over the passage, so that only the questions and answer choices are visible. Read each question carefully. Based on your knowledge of question types and common Attractors, eliminate the most suspicious choices and choose what you believe to be the most likely credited response.

For example, consider the following question:

1. The primary purpose of the passage is to:

A) urge consumers to demand quicker development of HDR resources for the production of energy.
B) denounce the federal government for its resistance to necessary changes in its long term energy policy.
C) compare and contrast the energy policies of developed and less-developed nations.
D) discuss the advantages and disadvantages of HDRs as an alternative energy source.

MCAT passage authors rarely call on the reader to take action, nor do they commonly denounce or severely criticize anybody. Thus choices A and B are likely to be inconsistent with the author's attitude and purpose. Choice C is more neutral in tone, but is it really possible to undertake such a wide-ranging study in the course of a few paragraphs? This choice is probably too broad. Choice D is more narrow than choice C, but not too narrow to describe a discussion carried out over 60–70 lines. It is also middle-of-the road in tone, as are most MCAT passages. Thus choice D is the most likely choice. (It is, in fact, the credited response.)

Of course you should never answer the questions without reading the passage on the test! However, after completing this exercise for several passages, you'll be surprised how often you do arrive at the credited response. You'll also increase your sensitivity to, and awareness of, the kinds of suspicious wording that often shows up in Attractors.

EXERCISE 5: WRITING YOUR OWN QUESTIONS

Take a passage from your practice materials. Put a piece of paper or a series of Post-It® Notes over the questions and the answer choices, so that only the passage itself is visible. Read the passage, mapping and annotating as usual. Based on what you see in the passage (for example, comparisons and contrasts, use of examples or lists, unexpected changes in direction, the author's tone or attitude, etc.), predict what questions would likely appear attached to this passage, and what kind of trap answers they will employ.

Now, write your own questions and answer choices, based on those predictions. At this point, feel free to go back to the passage and read it more carefully than you normally would the first time through. Imagine that you are an MCAT writer, trying to confuse the test-taker with complex questions or trick the test-taker into choosing Attractor answer choices. Try to write at least one question from each of the most common question types (Retrieval, Inference, Structure, Strengthen, Weaken, New Information, Main Point/Primary Purpose), but come up with as many, from any category of question, as you can. Now lift up the paper or the Post-It® Notes and work through the questions they give you. How accurately did you predict the questions? Did predicting the questions and trap answer choices help you more effectively answer their questions?

A variation on this exercise is to keep the existing questions but write your own sets of answer choices.

If you are studying with other people, exchange questions on the same passage with each other. Use your knowledge of Attractors to write questions that are defensible but difficult. See how often you fall for each other's Attractors.

You will find that by doing this exercise, you deepen your understanding of how this test is written, and that you are more able to predict and eliminate tricky wrong answers.

EXERCISE 6: QUESTION-TYPE-SPECIFIC PASSAGES

In Chapter 4, you completed a set of passages that included only particular question types. Here is another set of question-type-specific passages. As you attack each passage, keep your focus on employing the strategy appropriate for each particular category and type of question. As you review any questions that you missed, look in particular for mistakes caused by not fully understanding the question task and/or failing to employ the appropriate question strategy.

8.2

PASSAGE I: SPECIFIC—RETRIEVAL AND INFERENCE QUESTIONS

It is good anthropology to think of ballet as a form of ethnic dance. Currently, that idea is unacceptable to most Western dance scholars. This lack of agreement shows clearly that something is amiss in the communication of ideas between the scholars of dance and those of anthropology. The faults and errors of anthropologists in their approach to dance are many, but they are largely due to their hesitation to deal with something which seems esoteric and out of their field of competence. By ethnic dance, anthropologists mean to convey the idea that all forms of dance reflect the cultural traditions within which they developed. Dancers and dance scholars use this term, and the related terms *ethnologic*, *primitive*, and *folk dance*, differently and, in fact, in a way which reveals their limited knowledge of non-Western dance forms.

Despite all anthropological evidence to the contrary, however, [most] Western dance scholars set themselves up as authorities on the characteristics of non-Western (that is, non Euro-American) dance. For example, Terry describes the functions of "primitive" dance, and uses Native Americans as his model. While he writes sympathetically about Native Americans, his paternalistic feelings on the one hand, and his sense of ethnocentricity on the other, prompt him to set aside any thought that people with whom he identifies could share contemporarily those same dance characteristics, because he states "the white man's dance heritage, except for the most ancient of days, was wholly different."

Another significant obstacle to the identification of Western dancers with non-Western dance forms is the double myth that the dance grew out of some spontaneous mob action and that once formed, became frozen. Apparently it satisfies our own ethnocentric needs to believe in the uniqueness of our dance forms, and it is much more convenient to believe that so-called "primitive" dances, like Topsy, just "growed," and that "ethnological" dances are part of an unchanging tradition.

Let it be noted, once and for all, that within the various "ethnologic" dance worlds there are also patrons, dancing masters, choreographers, and performers with names woven into a very real historical fabric. The bias which those dancers have toward their own dance and artists is just as strong as ours. The difference is that they usually don't pretend to be scholars of other dance forms, nor even very much interested in them.

I have made listings of the themes and other characteristics of ballet and ballet performances, and these lists show over and over again just how "ethnic" ballet is. Consider, for example, how Western is the tradition of the proscenium stage, the usual three part performance which lasts for about two hours, our use of curtain calls and applause, and our usage of French terminology. Think how our worldview is revealed in the oft recurring themes of unrequited love, sorcery, self-sacrifice through long-suffering, mistaken identity, and misunderstandings which have tragic consequences.

Our aesthetic values are shown in the long line of lifted, extended bodies, in the total revealing of legs, of small heads and tiny feet for women, in slender bodies for both sexes, and in the coveted airy quality which is best shown in the lifts and carryings of the female. To us this is tremendously pleasing aesthetically, but there are societies whose members would be shocked at the public display of the male touching the female's thighs! So distinctive is the "look" of ballet, that it is probably safe to say that ballet dances graphically rendered by silhouettes would never be mistaken for anything else. An interesting proof of this is the ballet *Koshare* which was based on a Hopi Indian story. In silhouettes of even still photos, the dance looked like ballet and not like a Hopi dance.

The question is not whether ballet reflects its own heritage. The question is why we seem to need to believe that ballet has somehow become acultural. Why are we afraid to call it an ethnic form?

Material used in this particular passage has been adapted from the following source:

J. Kealiinohomoku, "An Anthropologist Looks at Ballet as a Form of Ethnic Dance." © 1970, *Impulse* 20: 24–33.

1. According to the passage, which of the following are aspects of the "ethnic" nature of ballet?

    I.   Common motifs that reflect the perspective of Western tradition
    II. Dance growing out of spontaneous group action
    III. The use of a specific language

A) III only
B) I and II only
C) I and III only
D) I, II, and III

2. Which of the following is implied by the author of the passage?

A) Good anthropology generally regards ethnic dance as a form of ballet.
B) Western dance academics are at odds with anthropologists' perceptions of dance.
C) Western dance scholars are not interested in non-Western dance forms.
D) Some indigenous peoples, such as Native Americans, are considered to be "Western" by dance scholars.

3. The author would most likely disagree with Terry regarding whether or not:

A) dance forms, to some extent, reflect cultural values.
B) ballet has features in common with non-Western dance forms.
C) anthropology is a valuable tool in the analysis of culture.
D) the ballet *Koshare* was based on a Hopi story.

4. Each of the following is stated to be found to be aesthetically pleasing in female ballet performers in the Western tradition EXCEPT:

A) a diminutive head.
B) the lifted body.
C) feet curled in at the toe.
D) the extension of the body.

5. The author implies which of the following to be true of the aesthetic aspects of ethnic dance?

A) They are influenced by certain cultural norms and values of the society in which the dance arose.
B) They reflect universal themes of human experience.
C) They portray the ideals that are most important to the culture in which they were generated.
D) Western and non-Western or "ethnic" dance aesthetics are inconsistent with each other, as evidenced by the failure of *Koshare* to accurately represent Hopi dance.

6. According to the passage, the problem in our understanding of "ethnological" dance forms is that this kind of dance is often incorrectly seen as:

A) shifting and growing through time.
B) deviating from an accepted norm.
C) consisting of a three-part performance.
D) unchanging once established.

7. Based on the passage, which of the following would be LEAST likely categorized as a "folk dance" by dance scholars?

A) The Hopi Powamuya or "bean dance," held in villages every February to prepare for the planting of crops
B) The African American cakewalk, created on Southern plantations before emancipation, perhaps as a way of mocking white slave-owners
C) The Maria Clara dance, done in the Philippines to portray flirtation and courtship
D) The Viennese waltz, which originated in 16th century France and was later imported into the United States, and which was at times seen as immoral because of the closeness of the partners

8.2

PASSAGE II: REASONING—STRUCTURE AND EVALUATE QUESTIONS

The notion that memory can be "distorted" assumes that there is a standard by which we can judge or measure what a veridical memory must be. If this is difficult with individual memory, it is even more complex with collective memory, where the past event or experience remembered was truly a different event or experience for its different participants. Moreover, whereas we can accept with little question that biography or the lifetime is the appropriate or "natural" frame for individual memory, there is no such evident frame for cultural memories. Neither national boundaries nor linguistic ones are as self-evidently the right containers for collective memory as the person is for individual memory.

I take the view that, in an important sense, there is no such thing as individual memory, and it is well for me to make this plain at the outset. Memory is social. It is social, first of all, because it is located in institutions rather than in individual human minds in the form of rules, laws, standardized procedures, and records, a whole set of cultural practices through which people recognize a debt to the past (including the notion of "debt" itself) or through which they express moral continuity with the past (tradition, identity, career, curriculum). These cultural forms store and transmit information that individuals make use of without themselves "memorizing" it. The individual's capacity to make use of the past piggybacks on the social and cultural practices of memory. I can move over great distances at a speed of 600 miles per hour without knowing the first thing about what keeps an airplane aloft. I benefit from a cultural storehouse of knowledge, very little of which I am obliged to have in my own head. Cultural memory, available for the use of an individual, is distributed across social institutions and cultural artifacts.

As soon as you recognize how collective memory, and even individual memory, is inextricable from social and historical processes, the notion of "distortion" becomes problematic. As the British historian Peter Burke writes, "Remembering the past and writing about it no longer seem the innocent activities they were once taken to be. Neither memories nor histories seem objective any longer. In both cases, this selection, interpretation and distortion is socially conditioned. It is not the work of individuals alone." Distortion is inevitable. Memory is distortion since memory is invariably and inevitably selective. A way of seeing is a way of not seeing, a way of remembering is a way of forgetting, too. If memory were only a kind of registration, a "true" memory might be possible. But memory is a process of encoding information, storing information, and strategically retrieving information, and there are social, psychological, and historical influences at each point.

Contest, conflict, controversy—these are the hallmark of studies of collective memory, rather than the concept of distortion. Discovering the attitudes and interests of the present becomes of much greater concern than the legitimate claims of the past upon them. Still, a focus on distortion makes sense in studies of collective or cultural memory. Even the most ardently relativist scholars among us shiver with revulsion at certain versions of the past that cry out "distortion." The most famous example is the flourishing fringe group of Holocaust revisionists who deny that there was ever a plan to exterminate the Jews or that such a plan was ever set in place. The question of what content of the past is not or cannot or should not be subject to latter-day reinterpretation haunts the papers at a 1990 conference at U.C.L.A. on "Nazism and the 'Final Solution': Probing the Limits of Representation" (Friedlander, 1992). The fascination with conflicting versions of the past and the excitement over legitimately revisionist interpretations of once settled and consensual accounts come precisely from the fact that even trained historians (or perhaps especially trained historians) retain strong beliefs in a veritable past. If interpretation were free-floating, entirely manipulable to serve present interests, altogether unanchored by a bedrock body of unshakable evidence, controversies over the past would ultimately be uninteresting. But in fact they are interesting. They are compelling. And they are gripping because people trust that a past we can to some extent know and can to some extent come to agreement about really happened.

Material used in this particular passage has been adapted from the following source:

M. Schudson, *"Dynamics in Distortion of Collective Memory,"* in *Memory Distortion: How Minds, Brains, and Societies Reconstruct the Past.* © 1995 by Harvard University Press.

1. The author provides the example of our capacity to fly in an airplane in order to:

A) indicate that some facts are not open to dispute.
B) illustrate the nature of collective memory.
C) provide a case in which individual memory exists independently of social memory.
D) demonstrate how social memory is more complex than individual memory.

2. Which of the following items of information from the passage provides the best support for the author's argument that there is such a thing as a provable historical fact?

A) It is unclear what the "natural" frame for collective memory might be.
B) A fringe group exists of people who deny that the Holocaust occurred.
C) Memory is inherently selective and therefore distorted.
D) We find controversies regarding past events to be fascinating and compelling.

3. Why does the author cite the historian Peter Burke?

A) In order to support the claim that the concept of distortion is less useful than many claim it to be
B) In order to support the contention that there is no such thing as a "true fact"
C) In order to support the claim that memory is not an entirely factual representation of reality
D) In order to support the contention that institutions encapsulate social memories and make them available to individuals

4. How well supported is the author's claim that, in a sense, individual memory is non-existent?

A) Weakly: the claim is contradicted later in the passage by the author's discussion of how individuals use collective memory
B) Weakly: the claim is simply asserted with no evidence or support
C) Strongly: the author explains with the use of an example how individual memory is shaped by social forces and institutions
D) Strongly: the author directly supports the claim through discussion of revisionist views of the Holocaust

5. Which of the following assertions made by the author is LEAST well supported?

A) The appropriate frame for individual memory is biography or lifetime.
B) Memory is inherently selective.
C) It makes sense to study distortion when considering cultural memory.
D) Our capacity to make use of the past relies on social forms of memory.

6. The author states in the last paragraph that "people trust that a past we can to some extent know and to some extent come to an agreement about really happened," while also stating in the second paragraph that "in an important sense, there is no such thing as individual memory." These two claims are:

A) consistent with each other, because they refer to different aspects of memory.
B) consistent with each other, because the claim regarding the possibility of agreeing on the past provides evidence for the claim regarding individual memory.
C) in contradiction, because it is difficult to justify the notion that historical controversies are gripping if individual memory is absent.
D) in contradiction, because the claim regarding the non-existence of individual memory is logically inconsistent with claim that we can come to agreement about historical memory.

PASSAGE III: APPLICATION—STRENGTHEN AND WEAKEN QUESTIONS

Nobody ever discovered ugliness through photographs. But many, through photographs, have discovered beauty. Except for those situations in which the camera is used to document, or to mark social rites, what moves people to take photographs is finding something beautiful. Nobody exclaims, "Isn't that ugly! I must take a photograph of it." Even if someone did say that, all it would mean is: "I find that ugly thing beautiful."

It is common for those who have glimpsed something beautiful to express regret at not having been able to photograph it. So successful has been the camera's role in beautifying the world that photographs, rather than the world, have become the standard of the beautiful. We learn to see ourselves photographically: to regard oneself as attractive is, precisely, to judge that one would look good in a photograph. Photographs create the beautiful and—over generations of picture-taking—use it up. Certain glories of nature, for example, have been all but abandoned to the indefatigable attentions of amateur camera buffs.

Many people are anxious when they're about to be photographed: not because they fear, as primitives do, being violated but because they fear the camera's disapproval. People want the idealized image: a photograph of themselves looking their best. They feel rebuked when the camera doesn't return an image of themselves as more attractive than they really are. That photographs are often praised for their candor, their honesty, indicates that most photographs, of course, are not candid. A decade after Fox Talbot's negative-positive process had begun replacing the daguerreotype (the first practical photographic process) in the mid-1840s, a German photographer invented the first technique for retouching the negative. The news that the camera could lie made getting photographed much more popular.

The consequences of lying have to be more central for photography than they ever can be for painting, because the flat, usually rectangular images which are photographs make a claim to be true that paintings can never make. A fake painting (one whose attribution is false) falsifies the history of art. A fake photograph (one which has been retouched or tampered with, or whose caption is false) falsifies reality. The history of photography could be recapitulated as the struggle between two different imperatives: beautification, which comes from the fine arts, and truth-telling, which is measured not only by a notion of value-free truth, a legacy of the sciences, but by a moralized ideal of truth-telling, adapted from nineteenth-century literary models and from the (then) new profession of independent journalism….

Freed from the necessity of having to make narrow choices (as painters did) about what images were worth contemplating, because of the rapidity with which cameras recorded anything, photographers made seeing into a new kind of project: as if seeing itself, pursued with sufficient avidity and single-mindedness, could indeed reconcile the claims of truth and the need to find the world beautiful. Once an object of wonder because of its capacity to render reality faithfully as well as despised at first for its base accuracy, the camera has ended by effecting a tremendous promotion of the value of appearances. Instead of just recording reality, photographs have become the norm for the way things appear to us, thereby changing the very idea of reality, and of realism.

The photographer was thought to be an acute but non-interfering observer—a scribe, not a poet. But as people quickly discovered that nobody takes the same picture of the same thing, the supposition that cameras furnish an impersonal, objective image yielded to the fact that photographs are evidence not only of what's there but of what an individual sees, not just a record but an evaluation of the world.

Material used in this particular passage has been adapted from the following source:

S. Sontag, *"The Heroism of Vision," On Photography.* © 1977 by Susan Sontag. Reprinted by permission of Farrar, Straus, and Giroux, LLC, and of The Wylie Agency (UK) Limited.

1. Each of the following would strengthen the author's claim that photography has been successful in beautifying the world EXCEPT:

A) It is quite common for celebrities to have themselves photographed in new clothes before wearing them to important events to ensure that the clothes will look good for the public.
B) Bowing to pressure from parents, many high end private schools now allow families to submit their own professionally produced and retouched yearbook photos as an alternative to having a picture taken at school.
C) A current fad among wealthy home owners is to have a photograph of one's home actually framed on the wall inside the house, making sure that visitors can see the house's features at their best.
D) Because of the extreme realism and the striking uses of light possible in contemporary photography, more and more art museums are devoting sections of their collections to well-known photographers.

2. Which of the following most strengthens the author's suggestion that beauty can be exhausted through overuse?

A) Although in the 1940s Ansel Adams' photographs of the Grand Canyon and of Yosemite Park captured the imagination of the art world, they now, except for their historical value, seem more appropriate to calendars than to museum walls.

B) The huge number of visitors visiting the Sistine Chapel and taking flash photographs has caused certain portions of the glorious paintings to lose their brilliancy and fade, leading officials increasingly to curb the privileges of tourists to take any pictures at all.

C) Despite the fact that almost everyone has seen multiple photographs of Michelangelo's David, seeing the enormous statue in person still generally provokes a powerful sense of awe and wonder.

D) The average career for top models has become shorter and shorter in duration, so that many models now receive top billing for only a single season before magazines and sponsors begin looking for a newer face.

3. The author's explanation of the anxiety many feel around being photographed would be most undermined by which of the following hypothetical examples?

A) After having his privacy repeatedly violated by the paparazzi, a well-known actor becomes extremely anxious and defensive about divulging details of his personal life, and hires guards to travel with him when he goes out in public.

B) A teenage boy measures his popularity, and in essence his worth as a human being, by how many photographs of him get posted online by his friends and acquaintances.

C) A new application for camera phones that automatically removes facial blemishes has the effect of decreasing the value generally placed on photos, as the application provides clear evidence that the accuracy of a photograph cannot be trusted.

D) Confined to a hospital bed, an elderly woman becomes upset when her visiting grandchildren try to take pictures of her, insisting that she doesn't want to be seen looking sick.

4. Which of the following contrasts, if valid, would most weaken the author's claim that there is a significant difference between painting and photography?

A) Unlike a painting, in which the author may portray the subject with total freedom, a photograph is highly limited by the reality of the subject matter.

B) The speed with which one can take a photograph is so much greater than the speed with which one can paint that, viewed from the perspective of the artist, the two practices have essentially nothing in common.

C) To fake a painting is less morally relevant than to fake a photograph, because a counterfeit painting, although a crime against the artist, does not ultimately undermine our collective trust in the accounts we receive of real-world events.

D) Unlike photography, which seeks to achieve both beauty and truth, the only fundamental goal of painting is to portray beauty.

5. Which of the following hypothetical reviews of a photography exhibition would most contribute to the claim that this exhibition has succeeded in the photographic project described in paragraph 5?

A) It is the shadows, the dark spaces in these images, that truly allow the creative imagination of the observer to bring an individual and higher truth, the essence of art.

B) The particular achievement of these photographs is in allowing the eye truly to enjoy the deception brought about through shifts in perspective and clever illusion.

C) The rhythm visible in this succession of images imparts to the viewer a sense of motion much richer than that possible through mere verbal description.

D) In bringing out the subtle hues of moving water, these photographs train our eyes to see water differently, as more varied and more valued than we previously knew.

6. Which of the following statements, if justified, would most undermine a claim that the typical photographer is more "scribe" than "poet" as those terms are used in the passage?

A) Just as different authors describe the same scene in different ways, so different photographers will take pictures of the same scene from different angles.

B) Individual photographer's particular techniques and choices often function as a kind of signature, making his or her photographs instantly recognizable regardless of the subject of the photograph.

C) Tourists at a famous site will frequently observe one another, as each attempts to choose what to photograph based on what, according to his peers, seems the most important or the most beautiful.

D) It is only the rare artist who brings to the practice of photography the vision and skill necessary to reveal in his photographs any meaningful aesthetic decisions or distinctive qualities.

PASSAGE IV:
APPLICATION—NEW INFORMATION AND ANALOGY QUESTIONS

"One Journalism" defines good journalism as the kind of journalism produced at the top of corporate pyramids—the networks and the major national and regional newspapers. This means that journalists address the particular problems and needs of a community in an artificial journalistic context, created and driven from other places. But people practice democratic government in specific locations, in the municipalities and states where they seek to answer the question, "What shall we do?" through deliberation. That process requires shared information and some common values—above all the value of democratic deliberation is the best way to express and experience public life, and that all citizens have a personal responsibility to take part in that process.

The reflexive, value-neutral techniques of One Journalism do not promote democratic deliberation. Rather, their skewed definitions of sources and issues systematically exclude people from democratic deliberation and generate much irrelevant information that does not advance that essential deliberation. One Journalism determines, for instance, that we define "balance" as "both sides" when in fact most issues have multiple sides. It insures the high value we put on conflict as the ultimate illuminator of political discussion. It makes it inevitable that the world we present one day seems disconnected from the world we present the next day. Meanwhile, the culture of detachment denies any journalistic concern or responsibility for what happens, if anything. When citizens see reflected in newspapers and broadcasts a politics of polar extremes that excludes them, when the machinations of experts and absolutists seem beyond their reach, they withdraw into private concerns. They abandon public life. This is a direct threat to journalism, for if people are not involved in public life, they have no need for journalists.

Journalism's authority—its right to be attended to—is disappearing in a cloud of cynicism and loss of credibility brought on by the routine and detached way we go about business. But public journalism offers a solution to this problem. At its core, public journalism suggests a close examination of the alleged overriding value of detachment and seeks to develop more useful journalistic reflexes. Its objective is to find ways for journalism to serve a purpose beyond—but not in place of—telling the news: the purpose of reinvigorating public life by re-engaging people in it. This requires both a change in the perspective of journalists and a change in what they do. It means learning to report and write about public life beyond traditional politics; to write about political issues in ways that reflect the true array of choices; to report the very important news of civic life—including civic successes—that

now occurs outside our pinched definition of news. This can only be done if journalists think of the people by their efforts not as an audience to be entertained or as spectators at an event, but as citizens capable of action.

This response to the decline in public life and journalism conflicts sharply with One Journalism's guiding axiom of detachment. A key tenet of public journalism is that the "line" of detachment defined by One Journalism is a false construct. Traditional journalists speak of "crossing the line" as if three questionable things were true: that a single line defines all possible points of moral, ethical and professional concerns; that every journalist understands precisely where that line lies; and that anything on one side of the line is "good journalism" and everything on the other side is something else.

Think of the line not as a boundary, but as a continuum that runs between two points. One point defines total detachment or non-involvement in what we cover. The other defines total involvement. Journalists exploring public journalism accept the construct of a continuum and seek to operate somewhere beyond total involvement. Precisely where their activity falls is determined by their consciences, their judgment and the needs of their communities. Public journalism is the antithesis of One Journalism.

Public journalism is openly based on broad values as: This should be a better place to live, and people should determine what that means by taking responsibility for what goes on around them. Public life, according to the values of public journalism, requires shared information and shared deliberation; people participate in answering democracy's fundamental question of "What shall we do?" Public journalism opens the possibility that journalists can serve their communities in truly useful ways that go beyond telling the news. It also offers us a chance to regain our lost credibility.

**Material used in this particular passage has been adapted from the
following source:**
D. Merritt, *"Public Journalism—Defining a Democratic Art," Media Studies Journal: Media and Democracy.* ©1995.

1. Suppose that a political analyst wrote the following: "Framing political issues as a conflict between mutually exclusive extremes is the most useful narrative device for engaging the interest of the citizenry in public policy." What would most likely be the passage author's reaction to such a statement?

A) Opposition, because the author believes that a focus on conflict dissuades people from taking an interest in politics

B) Opposition, because the author believes that a focus on conflict undermines the value-neutral stance necessary for good journalism

C) Support, because the author believes that a healthy discussion regarding different policy options is necessary for true democratic deliberation to occur

D) Support, because the author believes that the survival of journalism requires re-engaging the public by presenting the news in an entertaining fashion

2. Suppose that several national surveys showed that the proliferation of different points of view on political issues offered by the spread of blogs and other forms of social media confuses and discourages the public by making politics seem overly complicated. Which of the following claims made in the passage would be most undermined by this information?

A) "One Journalism" defines a balanced story as one that presents two different sides of the issue.

B) Democratic deliberation requires shared information and shared values.

C) The reinvigoration of public life requires that citizens be presented with a true array of options rather than with a dichotomous choice.

D) A culture of journalistic detachment denies that news reporters bear any responsibility for events.

3. Research has shown that under repressive political regimes in which the public has little role in policymaking, people tend to disregard journalistic reports, assuming that news reporters will only present events from a single officially sanctioned point of view. This favors the author's thesis in the passage by suggesting that:

A) the "culture of detachment" fostered by One Journalism discourages engagement in public life.

B) lack of widespread engagement in public life endangers the vitality and relevance of journalism.

C) reporting on positive political outcomes is one way of reengaging people in public life.

D) "good reporting" is defined in part by the motives of the journalist and the relevance of the information to the needs of the community.

4. Which of the following pairs would be most analogous, respectively, to the role of citizens in One Journalism on one hand, and in public journalism on the other?

A) People attending a movie vs. people attending a play

B) People doing their own research into investment opportunities vs. people unquestioningly taking the advice of a financial advisor

C) People investing their own money vs. people investing other people's money

D) People viewing works hanging in a museum vs. audience members going on stage and playing roles within a performance art event

5. Which of the following would be LEAST logically similar to the author's discussion of the correct way to distinguish good from bad journalism?

A) Judging the culpability of a criminal defendant through taking into account her motives, whether or not her actions were reasonable in the situation, and the amount of harm her actions caused to others

B) Judging the artistic merit of a poem by defining whether or not it conforms to clearly defined compositional rules

C) Judging the policies carried out by a mayor by considering the intended and actual effects of the policy on the city

D) Judging the moral character of a historical figure by taking into account the reasonableness of his or her actions within the cultural context in which he or she lived as well as the personal motivations behind his or her actions

6. Which of the following hypothetical examples most closely illustrates the perspective embodied and encouraged by public journalism, as it is described in the passage?

A) A documentary examining the traditional values of detachment and neutrality in the news, detailing how local news stations are trying to change this traditional approach to reporting

B) A magazine article about small town life, written by a national news reporter in New York City

C) An expose on the subversive involvement of corporations in democratic political systems

D) A local newspaper article about a successful community service initiative that cleaned up a polluted town lake

8.2

SOLUTIONS TO PASSAGE I: SPECIFIC— RETRIEVAL AND INFERENCE QUESTIONS

1. **C**   This is a Retrieval/Roman Numeral question.

    I.   **True. Different characteristics of ballet and evidence that ballet is ethnic are discussed in the fifth and sixth paragraphs and different examples are provided. The author mentions "oft recurring themes" such as one-sided love, suffering, and tragedy as examples of things that reveal the Western worldview.**

    II. False. Start with this numeral, as it appears in exactly two answer choices. The idea of dance growing out of spontaneous group action is discussed in the fourth paragraph in the context of myths regarding so-called "primitive" dance, not as part of the discussion of ethnic characteristics of ballet. Hence, it does not answer the question. Strike through this numeral and eliminate any answers that contain it: choices B and D.

    III. **True. The usage of French terminology is specifically referenced as a tradition found in Western ballet (paragraph 5).**

2. **B**   This is an Inference question.

    A: No. This answer is a reversal of passage information and takes the words out of their original context. The passage says that "good anthropology…[thinks] of ballet as a form of ethnic dance" (paragraph 1), meaning that ballet is a specific type of ethnic dance. This does not allow the reverse to be inferred: we don't know that ethnic dance is a specific form of ballet. For Inference questions, be careful to not just match up words from the passage, but instead to look at the meaning as well.

    B: **Yes. The first paragraph references the view anthropology has of ballet as dance, and that dance scholars in the West view this as "unacceptable." In addition, the passage states that there is a "lack of agreement" that shows "something is amiss" between these two groups.**

    C: No. The author indicates that Western dance scholars ARE interested in non-Western dance forms. For example, the author states at the beginning of paragraph 2 that "Western dance scholars set themselves up as authorities on the characteristics of non-Western dance." The problem, according to the passage, is that they misunderstand and misrepresent non-Western dance.

    D: No. The author indicates the opposite to be true. The passage suggests in paragraph 2 that the dance scholar Terry sees Native Americans as performing "non-Western dance."

3. **B**   This is an Inference question.

    A: No. The author of the passage would agree with this statement (paragraph 6) and there is no evidence that Terry would disagree. Terry may or may not belief that ballet reflects any cultural values, but he may agree that some "ethnic" dances do. Therefore, we do not have enough evidence that they would disagree on this point.

    B: **Yes. According to the author, Terry views things from an ethnocentric perspective and "set[s] aside any thought that people with whom he identifies could share contemporarily those same dance characteristics" (paragraph 2). Later, in the third paragraph, the author mentions "double myth[s]" that prevent Western dancers being associated with non-Western dance forms. This suggests that the author believes it possible that ethnic dances (which the author believes includes ballet) can have things in common with other dances including non-Western dances, whereas Terry views Western and non-Western dances as completely different.**

C: No. Although Terry sets himself up as an expert on non-Western dance in opposition to anthropological evidence on the topic, this does not mean that Terry would think that anthropology has no value in studying different cultures.

D: No. The author states that the *Koshare* was indeed based on a Hopi narrative in the second-last paragraph. However, there is no indication in the passage that Terry might disagree with this specific fact.

4. **C** This is a Retrieval/EXCEPT question.

A: No. The sixth paragraph discusses the aesthetically pleasing aspects of the ballet. Small heads are mentioned as an example.

B: No. The author twice explicitly references the lifted body in the sixth paragraph as something pleasing.

C: **Yes. Though feet are mentioned as aesthetically pleasing, it's only in reference to their size ("tiny feet for women"), not the shape of the foot. If anything, the passage suggests the elongated form is more pleasing, not a form that curls inward.**

D: No. The author refers to the long line of the extended body in the sixth paragraph.

5. **A** This is an Inference question.

A: **Yes. The author argues for example that the "lifts and carryings of the female" to us are aesthetically pleasing, but that there are societies whose members would be shocked at the public display of the male touching the female's thighs" (paragraph 6). This indicates that the values of a society can affect what is considered aesthetically pleasing in that society.**

B: No. The author suggests the opposite, that at least some dances reflect the values of particular societies, not values shared by all peoples. For example, ballet, rather than being "acultural" (paragraph 7), reflects the values of "our" society but not all others. The author writes: "Our aesthetic values are shown in the long line of lifted, extended bodies, in the total revealing of legs, of small heads and tiny feet for women, in slender bodies for both sexes, and in the coveted airy quality which is best shown in the lifts and carryings of the female. To us this is tremendously pleasing aesthetically, but there are societies whose members would be shocked at the public display of the male touching the female's thighs" (paragraph 6).

C: No. This choice is too extreme. While the author would say that dance does reflect certain cultural values, the passage does not go so far as to indicate those values are the *most important* values in that culture.

D: No. While the author might say that some Western and some non-Western societies have different values and different "ethnic" dances, the author does not suggest that they are always mutually exclusive. The point made in the discussion of *Koshare* is not that Hopi society was incapable of expressing itself through ballet, but rather that *Koshare* as presented was aesthetically "Western" rather than incorporating true Hopi dance forms.

6. **D**   This is a Retrieval question.

    A: No. The author indicates the opposite to be true; that is, this is a correct view, not a misconception (paragraphs 3 and 4).

    B: No. This is out of scope. The passage does not provide any discussion of moving away from an accepted norm. Deviation would also suggest change, which is the opposite of what the author describes as the myth of ethnological dance.

    C: No. Three parts of a dance are referenced in the sixth paragraph, where the author discusses common Western dance traditions, but not the incorrect assumptions related to ethnological dance.

    D: **Yes. In the fourth paragraph, the author discusses the double myth that pertains to so-called primitive dance and ethnological dance. The author says this myth is that "once formed, [it] became frozen" and that ethnological dances are "part of an unchanging tradition." It's implied that this is incorrect, since it's referred to as a myth that we tell ourselves to fulfill our ethnocentric view of how unique the dance is.**

7. **D**   This is an Inference question.

    Note: In paragraph 1 the author indicates that dance scholars use the terms "ethnic," "ethnologic," "primitive," and "folk dance" more or less interchangeably. In paragraph 2 the author indicates that "non-Western" is equivalent to "non Euro-American" dance. In that same paragraph, the author also indicates that Terry (presented by the author as representative of the views of dance scholars) draws a clear line between "ethnic" and "white-man's" dance. Therefore, the right answer will be the form of dance that as described in the answer choice is least "ethnic" (as that term is used by dance scholars like Terry) and the most "Euro-American."

    A: No. Although a Hopi dance, the *Koshare*, inspired a ballet, the answer choice describes this dance as performed by the Hopi themselves. Therefore, a dance scholar WOULD consider this to be a folk dance.

    B: No. There is no European aspect or influence described here. Also, the dance scholar Terry distinguishes between the dance heritage of the "white man" and that of ethnic dances. Therefore, a dance scholar likely WOULD call this a folk dance.

    C: No. There is nothing "Euro-American" about the Maria Clara, as described in the answer choice. Therefore, a dance scholar likely WOULD call this a folk dance.

    D: **Yes. This dance as described had a European origin and was then brought to the United States. That is, it is a "Euro-American" dance form. There is also nothing in the answer choice that excludes the waltz from the "white-man's dance heritage." Therefore, a dance scholar would most likely NOT call the waltz a folk dance.**

SOLUTIONS TO PASSAGE II:
REASONING—STRUCTURE AND EVALUATE QUESTIONS

1. **B** This is a Structure question

   A: No. This is the right answer to the wrong question. While the author does indicate at the end of the passage that there are historical facts that can in fact be proven, this is not the author's point in this part of the passage. This choice is also attractive based on outside knowledge. It is indisputable that flight in airplanes is possible (and the author would agree that this is true), but again, showing this is not the author's purpose. Rather, the author uses the possibility of flight to illustrate the nature of social memory. When answering Structure questions, make sure to choose an answer that accurately represents not only the passage content, but also the author's purpose in the relevant part of the passage.

   B: **Yes. The author argues in the beginning of the passage that "in an important sense, there is no such thing as individual memory" and that "Memory is social." The author then goes on to describe how forms of collective memory make information useful without individuals themselves having to "memorize" it; the example of air flight illustrates how we can travel in a plane without actually knowing how or why flight is possible. Be careful not to impose your own definitions on terms used by the author; you might not think of a flight as a form of memory, but the author describes it as such.**

   C: No. This choice contradicts the passage. The author states in paragraph 2 that "in an important sense, there is no such thing as individual memory." The rest of the paragraph, including the example of air travel, is intended to illustrate the social, not individual, nature of memory.

   D: No. As with choice A, this is the right answer to the wrong question. In paragraph 1 the author argues that finding a standard by which to judge the truth of a memory is especially complex when dealing with collective memory. Aside from the fact that it is judging the truthfulness of a social memory, not social memory itself, that is "even more complex," in paragraph 2 the author moves on to a different issue: the social nature of all memory. This is the point being illustrated by the example cited in the question.

2. **D** This is a Structure question

   Note: In this form of a Structure question, all the answer choices will generally be paraphrases of statements actually made in the passage (if the statement is not even supported by the passage, the choice is wrong for that reason). The correct answer will be the statement that is offered as direct evidence for the claim cited in the question stem.

   A: No. The author states this in paragraph 1 in support of the claim that judging the truth of a collective memory is even more complicated than judging the truth of an individual memory. This is a different issue than the argument cited in the question stem.

   B: No. This choice is attractive, as the existence of Holocaust deniers is part of the author's argument in the relevant part of the passage (paragraph 4). However, it is not the existence of Holocaust deniers that supports the author's claim about provable facts, but rather the fact that we find such controversies to be fascinating. If Holocaust deniers existed and no one really cared, there would be no support for the author's claim about a provable past.

   C: No. The claim you need to find support for is that there is such a thing as a knowable past exists. The statement in this answer choice is about the other side of the coin; that is, how coming to agreement is challenging because of the inherently distorted nature of memory.

   D: **Yes. In the last paragraph the author gives the example of those who deny the Holocaust, and states that we are fascinated by "conflicting versions of the past." Then, at the end of the passage, the author argues that if there was no such thing as a "veritable" or provable fact, "controversies over the past would be ultimately uninteresting." But, such controversies are interesting to us; therefore, there must be some aspects of the past that are in fact provable.**

3. **C** This is a Structure question

A: No. This choice contradicts the passage. Make sure to take the author's statement that "the notion of 'distortion' becomes problematic" (paragraph 3) in context. When you continue to read paragraphs 3 and 4, you see that the author is not denying that distortion is an important concept. Rather, the author is arguing that distortion is unavoidable, and so presents a problem that should be addressed. For example, directly after the quote from Burke the author states: "Distortion is inevitable. Memory is distortion since memory is invariable and inevitably selective."

B: No. Facts are different from memory, according to the passage. The author indicates at the end of the passage that there are true facts; the author cites Burke in paragraph 3 in order to make the argument that memory inherently distorts factual reality.

C: **Yes. First, note the wording used by the author to introduce the quote; when the author says "As the British historian Peter Burke writes," the word "as" indicates that the author agrees with Burke. According to Burke, and as therefore also according to the author, "Neither memories nor histories seem objective any longer." The author goes on to make the point even more strongly directly after the quote: "Distortion is inevitable. Memory is distortion since memory is invariably and inherently selective."**

D: No. This is the right answer to the wrong question. While this statement is supported by the second paragraph (where the author discusses the institutional nature of social memory), it is not the claim being supported by the quote from Burke (which is about the inaccuracy of memory). To the extent that the two claims are related, their relationship is reversed; it is in part the social (including institutional) nature of memory that distorts it (given that memory "is inextricable from social and historical processes (paragraph 3)), rather than the distortion of memory that makes it institutional.

4. **C** This is an Evaluate question

A: No. The author's discussion of how individuals use collective memory (paragraph 2) supports rather than undermines the claim. When answering an Evaluate question, make sure that the answer choice correctly describes the logic and direction of the author's argument.

B: No. The author provides extensive explanation for the claim in the second paragraph, including the use of an example (air travel). Make sure to read above and below the relevant passage reference, and take into account how other parts of the paragraph and passage as a whole relate to the cited claim.

C: **Yes. The second paragraph provides a detailed discussion of why the author believes that individual memory is always essentially shaped by institutions and social practices.**

D: No. While the claim is strongly supported, the purpose of the Holocaust example is not to support the claim about individual vs. social memory, but rather to bolster the case for taking the concept of distortion of memory seriously. When answering an Evaluate question, make sure that all parts of the answer choice are consistent with the content and logical structure of the passage.

5. **A** This is an Evaluate question

A: **Yes. The author states this in the first paragraph, but never supports or explains it; the passage immediately moves on to discuss the greater complexity of collective memory.**

B: No. The author goes on to explain that "memory is a process of encoding information, storing information, and strategically retrieving information, and there are social, psychological, and historical influences on this process."

C: No. The much of the last paragraph, including the example of revisionist versions of history and our interest in them, supports this claim.

D: No. The example of how we can fly in a plane without understanding how a plane actually works directly supports this claim.

6. **A**   This is an Evaluate question

A: **Yes. When the author argues in the second paragraph that individual memory does not exist, he means that all memory is essentially shaped by social forces and institutions, not that individuals literally have no memory or knowledge of the past. The author's point in the last paragraph is that historical facts do exist, and it seems that there must be some way within our collective memory of coming to an "agreement about what really happened."**

B: No. The answer choice reverses the relationship between the two statements in the passage. The author's claim that individual memory does not exist is based on the argument that all memory is collective or social. This supports the claim (rather than being supported by) at the end of the passage that there appears to be some way of coming to agreement about history based on our collective memory. When answering any Reasoning question, make sure that the answer you choose accurately represents the logical relationship between the relevant points in the passage.

C: No. There is no inconsistency between the two claims. The author argues in the second paragraph that all memory, including so-called individual memory, is shaped by social forces. In the last paragraph, the author claims that because historical controversies are gripping, we must believe that there is a knowable past within our social memory. In sum, the "absence" (that is, the social nature) of individual memory is part of, not inconsistent with, the author's argument in the last paragraph.

D: No. This choice has the same problem as choice C. If individual memory is non-existent because all memory is essentially social or collective, and if it is within or through our social memory that we can come to some agreement about the past, the two claims cited in the question stem are consistent, not in contradiction, with each other.

SOLUTIONS TO PASSAGE III:
APPLICATION—STRENGTHEN AND WEAKEN QUESTIONS

1. **D**   This is a Strengthen question in the EXCEPT/LEAST/NOT format

Note: The incorrect answers to this question type and format will Strengthen the relevant part of the passage. The correct answer will weaken it, or have no impact on it, or strengthen it less than the other three choices.

A: No. The author explains the claim that photography beautifies the world by asserting that photography determines for us what qualifies as beauty and that we measure beauty according to our ability to see it in photographs. Photographing clothes to determine whether they are sufficiently attractive would strengthen this claim.

B: No. The author explains the claim that photography beautifies the world by asserting that photography determines for us what qualifies as beauty and that we measure beauty according to our ability to see it in photographs. Increasing significance being attributed to attractive yearbook photos would strengthen this claim.

C: No. The author explains the claim that photography beautifies the world by asserting that photography determines for us what qualifies as beauty and that we measure beauty according to our ability to see it in photographs. The idea that seeing a photograph of the house (in addition to the actual house) will impress visitors would certainly strengthen this claim.

D: **Yes. The author explains the claim that photography beautifies the world by asserting that photography determines for us what qualifies as beauty and that we measure beauty according to our ability to see it in photographs. Although the photographs in museums may be beautiful, there is no indication here that they are altering the way anyone perceives reality. So this answer choice does not strengthen the claim.**

8.2

2. **A**   This is a Strengthen question.
    A: **Yes. The idea that beauty can be exhausted through overuse suggests that after seeing too many photographic representations of something, one's capacity to find it beautiful will fade. The example of these Grand Canyon photos shows that images once seen as fresh and beautiful have, after years of public attention, come to seem more mundane and amateurish. This does strengthen the claim.**
    B: No. The idea that beauty can be exhausted through overuse suggests that after seeing too many photographic representations of something, one's capacity to find it beautiful will fade. The fading described in the Sistine Chapel example is a physical change, not a change in perception, through the influence of light rather than of over-exposure.
    C: No. This choice is the opposite. The idea that beauty can be exhausted through overuse suggests that after seeing too many photographic representations of something, one's capacity to find it beautiful will fade. The David example would weaken the claim, suggesting that in this case much exposure has not caused the experience of beauty to fade.
    D: No. The idea that beauty can be exhausted through overuse suggests that after seeing too many photographic representations of something, one's capacity to find it beautiful will fade. The passage describes this process as one that happens over generations, not over a single season. The magazine example suggests a pursuit of novelty but not necessarily the idea that familiar models are not regarded as beautiful.

3. **C**   This is a Weaken question.
    A: No. The author attributes contemporary anxiety towards being photographed to a fear of looking bad in the picture (the camera's disapproval). It is loss of privacy, not a fear of looking unattractive that troubles this actor.
    B: No. The author attributes contemporary anxiety towards being photographed to a fear of looking bad in the picture (the camera's disapproval). The boy in this example is concerned with the frequency of pictures, not with their quality or his appearance.
    C: **Yes. The author attributes contemporary anxiety towards being photographed to a fear of looking bad in the picture (the camera's disapproval). This application might, accordingly, be expected to reduce anxiety. However the answer choice says that it causes dissatisfaction, weakening the claim that people want photographs to look better than reality.**
    D: No. The author attributes contemporary anxiety towards being photographed to a fear of looking bad in the picture (the camera's disapproval). This grandmother fears having a poor appearance in a picture, so this answer choice strengthens rather than weakens the claim.

4. **A**   This is a Weaken question.
    A: **Yes. In paragraph 4 (and first sentence of paragraph 5) the author contrasts photography with painting, claiming that for the former "lying" is more important because reality itself is at stake. This answer choice contradicts the passage and weakens that claim in suggesting that photography cannot deceive as readily as can painting.**
    B: No. This choice is consistent with the author's argument. The author describes quicker speed of photography in paragraph 5, and suggests that this represents an important difference between photography and painting.
    C: No. This choice strengthens rather than weakens the author's argument. In paragraph 4 (and first sentence of 5) the author contrasts photography with painting, claiming that for the former "lying" is more important because reality itself is at stake. This answer choice strengthens the claim that photography and painting are different by emphasizing that the distinction the author describes, between reality and the history of art, is indeed a real and an important one.

D: No. This choice is not inconsistent with the passage. The author herself argues that photography is concerned with both truth and beauty (paragraph 4). While the author does not discuss painting's concerns, the claim in this choice that painting is only concerned with truth supports a contrast between painting and photography.

5. **D** This is a Strengthen question.
A: No. The project, as described in the passage, is to reconcile the claims of truth and beauty with the effect of changing how we actually view reality. Truth, as portrayed in this context, refers to the accurate portrayal of reality. There is nothing in this answer choice to suggest that the photographs are accurate; rather, they are obscure. There is also nothing to suggest that the photograph affects our view of reality.
B: No. The project, as described in the passage, is to reconcile the claims of truth and beauty. Focused on deception, the photographs in this answer choice do not appear to value truth, nor do they affect our view of reality.
C: No. The project, as described in the passage, is to reconcile the claims of truth and beauty. The contrast between image and word in this answer choice perhaps hints at the scribe vs. poet contrast in the passage, but there is nothing in this answer choice that directly relates to truth or beauty.
D: **Yes. The project, as described in the passage, is to reconcile the claims of truth and beauty. According to the author, this entails "changing the very idea of reality, and of realism." The description in this choice suggests that the photographs capture "true" (unaltered) images of water but impart to it a new beauty, and by so doing change our vision of the real nature of water.**

6. **B** This is a Weaken question.
Note: The author herself rejects this claim in the last paragraph. She writes: "The photographer was thought [emphasis added] to be an acute, but non-interfering observer—a scribe, not a poet. But as people quickly discovered that nobody takes the same picture of the same thing, the supposition that cameras furnish an impersonal, objective image yielded to the fact that photographs are evidence not only of what's there but of what an individual sees, not just a record but an evaluation of the world."

The correct answer will be consistent with the view we have come to have of photography by indicating that the photographer is not necessarily just a scribe, but can also be a poet.

A: No. This choice, while tempting, doesn't go far enough to weaken the claim. The fact that different photographers choose different angles does not by itself indicate that they are not just recording reality.
B: **Yes. The scribe, as described in the passage, is a non-interfering observer and recorder of "what's there," whereas the poet brings artistry and self-expression. The fact that many photographers have a distinctive style that separates them from all others indicates that these photographers are not simply recording, but are interpreting or evaluating, reality.**
C: No. The scribe, as described in the passage, is a non-interfering observer, whereas the poet brings artistry and self-expression. This answer choice suggests that amateur photographers make their choices based on other people rather than on an artistic vision. This choice provides no reason to believe that photographers go beyond recording "what's there."
D: No. The scribe, as described in the passage, is a non-interfering observer, whereas the poet expresses a personal and subjective view of the world. The statement in this answer choice suggests that most photographers do not express a unique aesthetic vision, which is consistent with the view that the typical photographer is a mere scribe.

SOLUTIONS TO PASSAGE IV:
APPLICATION—NEW INFORMATION AND ANALOGY QUESTIONS

1. **A**   This is a New Information question

    A: **Yes. The author argues in paragraph 2 that placing a high value on conflict disengages the public from journalism and from public life.**

    B. No. This choice is half-right but half-wrong. While the author would oppose the political analyst's claim—the author argues in paragraph 2 against focusing on conflict— the author also opposes the idea that journalism should take a value-neutral stance (paragraph 2).

    C: No. This choice is half-right but half-wrong. On one hand, the author would most likely agree that healthy discussion is necessary for democratic deliberation in the service of answering the question "What shall we do?" (paragraphs 1 and 6). On the other hand, however, the author believes that a focus on conflict between polar extremes dissuades people from taking part in that discussion (paragraph 2).

    D: No. Both parts of this answer choice are wrong. The author would oppose the statement; the passage argues that conflict, and framing issues in terms of opposing extremes, discourages people from paying attention to public concerns (paragraph 2). Furthermore, the author argues at the end of paragraph 3 that people can be reengaged in public life only if "journalists think of people by their efforts not as an audience to be entertained or as spectators at an event, but as citizens capable of action."

2. **C**   This is a New Information/Weaken question

    A: No. The effect of social media (which would not, by the author's description in the passage, qualify as part of "One Journalism") has no relevance to this part of the author's definition of One Journalism.

    B: No. The new information in the question stem is relevant to whether or not public journalism would encourage public engagement in democratic deliberation, not to the necessary conditions for the deliberation itself.

    C: **Yes. The author claims in the passage that the limited range of information and points of view offered through One Journalism discourages engagement in public life (paragraph 2), and that presenting "the true array of choices" would reengage the public (paragraph 3). If credible evidence exists that the public is confused and discouraged by the presentation of multiple options and ideas, it would undermine this part of the author's argument in the passage.**

    D: No. The new information in the question stem is not directly relevant to the author's argument about responsibility. It is possible for both claims to be true; that is, that public journalism confuses people, and One Journalism denies journalistic responsibility.

3. **B**   This is a New Information/Strengthen question

    A: No. The author describes the "culture of detachment" as the supposed value-neutral and "balanced" nature of One Journalism (paragraph 2). However, the reporting described in the question stem is anything other than value-neutral. Rather, it presents only one value or point of view (that of the political regime). Therefore, the new information and the passage information are describing two significantly different factors that would discourage public interest in journalism.

B: Yes. The author argues in paragraph 2 that when citizens feel excluded from the life reported in the news, they "withdraw into private concerns" and that this is a "direct threat to journalism." The new information in the question stem describes a different cause of exclusion from public life, but that exclusion has the same result—people see journalism as irrelevant. Therefore, the new information would strengthen the causal connection drawn by the author between engagement in public life and the perceived relevance of journalism.

C: No. The new information in the question stem describes a form of "positive" reporting that discourages, not encourages, engagement in public life. Furthermore, the successes discussed by the author are "civic successes" that occur "outside our pinched definition of the news" (paragraph 3); that is, the successes brought about by active citizens (not a by repressive regime).

D: No. While the journalism described in the question stem might not qualify as good journalism or reporting by the author's standards, it has no impact on the validity of the author's discussion in paragraphs 4 and 5 of how to evaluate what constitutes good reporting.

4. **D** This is an Analogy question

Note: The author indicates that within One Journalism, people play a passive role "as an audience to be entertained or as spectators at an event," whereas public journalism treats the public as "citizens capable of action" (paragraph 3). Therefore, the correct answer will show a contrast between a passive viewer or consumer on one hand, and an active participant on the other. Look out for wrong answers that reverse the relationship ("respectively" in the question stem means in the same order), or that show no contrast between the two sides.

A: No. Both parts of this choice describe a passive audience.

B: No. This choice reverses the relationship; doing one's own research would be more active, while taking advice without question would be more passive.

C: No. In both cases people are actively involved; there is no reason to think that investing someone else's money would entail more active involvement than investing one's own money.

D: Yes. In the first case, people are passively viewing art with no role in actually creating the art. In the second case, the audience members become an active part of the performance.

5. **B** This is an Analogy question in the EXCEPT/LEAST/NOT format

Note: The author discusses distinguishing good from bad journalism in paragraphs 4 and 5. The author rejects the method used by One Journalism, which is to draw a clear line between good and bad. According to One Journalism, if you cross that clearly defined line, you are creating bad journalism, and if not, you are writing good journalism. The author argues that instead we should judge journalists in terms of where their work lies along a spectrum, taking into account a variety of factors such as "their consciences, their judgment, and the needs of their communities" (paragraph 5). The correct answer will be most similar to the unitary standard used by One Journalism, or at least significantly different from the author's approach, while the wrong answers will be more similar to the author's proposed method of evaluation.

A: No. This method of judgment takes a variety of factors into account, including the motives or conscience and the judgment of the defendant, and the effect of her actions on others (which would be comparable to considering the needs of the community). Therefore, this case is similar to the standard of judgment proposed by the author.

B: Yes. This method of evaluation assumes that a clear standard (compositional rules) exists, and does not take a variety of factors into account. Therefore, this case out of the four choices is the least similar to the author's proposed method.

C: No. In this case, a variety of factors are taken into account and weighed against each other, including the effect on the community and the mayor's intentions. Unlike in choice B, there is no suggestion of the existence of a single clear standard or line that can be used to evaluate the merit of the mayor's decisions.

D: No. There is no suggestion in this choice of a single line or standard that can be used to judge a person. Instead, a variety of factors are taken into account including how reasonable his or her actions were within a particular historical context, and his or her motivations (which could include judgment and conscience).

6. **D** This is an Analogy question

Note: This is a twist on a standard Analogy question. It has aspects of an Inference question in that the answer choices are all about the same topic as the passage. However, the answer choices also include new information that is or is not logically similar to what is described in the relevant part of the passage.

The author states in the passage that the objective of public journalism is reengage people in public life and to "find ways for journalism to serve a purpose beyond—but not in place of—telling the news." This includes reporting on "the very important news of civic life—including civic successes—that now occurs outside our pinched definition of news" and treating people as "citizens capable of action" (paragraph 3). The correct answer will be the closest among the four choices to this description.

A: No. While this story reports on the actions of journalists trying to change how reporting is done, there is no indication of citizen involvement or civic successes.

B: No. The author states in paragraph 1 that One Journalism addresses "the particular problems and needs of a community in an artificial journalistic context, created and driven from other places." Therefore, while this article is about small town life, the fact that it is written by a national news reporter in New York puts this closer to One Journalism than to public journalism.

C: No. This choice jumbles together a variety of words and concepts from the passage (including corporations and democracy) but does not suggest that the story represents or encourages citizen involvement or civic successes.

D: **Yes. This locally written story depicts a civic success achieved through active involvement of the citizenry. Therefore, of the four choices, it is the most logically similar to the perspective encouraged by public journalism.**

8.3 MANAGING STRESS:
PREPARING FOR THE DAY OF THE TEST

There are a variety of things you can do in the time remaining to make the day of the MCAT as comfortable and familiar as possible.

- Make peace with your anxiety. Everyone experiences it, including the highest scorers. Feel free to be nervous on test day and the several days (or weeks) before. Even if you don't sleep well the night before the test, you'll be fine. Nervousness can be a good thing; adrenaline intensifies your ability to concentrate intensely.
- Let go of the need to be perfect. You don't need to complete every question, or get every question that you complete correct, to get a high CARS score.
- This is not the time to quit smoking (do that *after* the MCAT) or give up caffeine, but take care of your health. Keep eating well and exercising up until the test date. And, don't turn to drugs or alcohol for stress management, and definitely don't start experimenting with black-market ADHD drugs! Maintain a habit of 7–8 hours of sleep (per night, not per week).
- Get up roughly at the same time each morning as you will on test day, and go to bed at the same time that you will the night before the test. If you are in the habit of staying up until 2 A.M., but need to go to bed at 10 P.M. in order to get a reasonable amount of sleep the night before the test, you won't be able to magically change your sleeping habits at the last minute. Get into a good sleep schedule at least the week or two before the test, and you will thank yourself on test day!
- Whenever possible, practice CARS at the same time of day as the real test.
- Make a plan for getting to your testing site, and practice it. What time will you get up? What will you eat? What route will you take to the test site? Make sure that you plan to leave in plenty of time to get there a little early. Travel to the site at the same time as you will on the day of the test to see how long it takes you.
- Visualize success. Elite athletes, before each competition, visualize themselves going through each step of a successful performance. This both calms their nerves and focuses them on the task at hand. Remember a time in which you worked through a passage or set of passages with good results, and mentally run through the steps you took. Recall the sense of control and confidence you have when you stay calm and focused, use the techniques you've learned, and take charge of the material. If you begin to feel stress or anxiety, close your eyes and remember that feeling.

Chapter 8 Summary

- Continue to evaluate your performance and diagnose reasons for mistakes. Focus on correcting bad habits, rather than on doing as many practice passages as possible.

- Continue to hone your skills in the three basic areas: working the passage, translating the questions, and POE.

- Monitor your stress level and find ways to relax. Don't wait to feel overwhelmed; build "vacations" into your weekly study schedule.

CHAPTER 8 PRACTICE PASSAGES

Individual Passage Drills

You may wish to use these passages for Exercises 3 and 4 from this chapter. If not, do them back-to-back, timed, at the pace you have determined works best for you (for most people, this will be approximately 10–11 minutes per passage).

Once you have completed the passages and checked your answers, fill out the Individual Passage Logs. Focus in particular on identifying continuing patterns in the mistakes you are making, as well as identifying times when you successfully implemented appropriate strategies.

CHAPTER 8 PRACTICE PASSAGE 1

We all start out as animists, as toddlers vaguely uncertain about whether our beloved doll or pull-toy puppy might be a living being. When I was a child, my favorite cartoons were those that played in to that confusion, films in which toasters or teapots or slippers sprouted legs and faces and revealed their true natures as menacing agents of mayhem and chaos.

In time, we learn to distinguish the creature from the object, and, later, consumer society conditions us to detach ourselves from our stuff so effectively that we can dedicate ourselves to the perpetual quest for nicer stuff and embrace the necessity of regularly exchanging older models for newer ones. But some vestige of the child remains, evidenced by the tenacious hold material things have over us, as objects of desire and, more mysteriously, as personal mementos and totems—as clues to our secret selves and as signposts along the circuitous route that has taken us from the past into the present. Objects survive because we need them, or because we are convinced that we need them. The unreconstructed animist will see a Darwinian triumph in the rapidity with which a crumpled boarding pass evolves into an all-important and indispensable detail in the narrative of some meaningful chapter in our lives.

One such chapter is the subject of *Important Artifacts and Personal Property from the Collection of Lenore Doolan and Harold Morris, Including Books, Street Fashion, and Jewelry*. A series of captioned photographs, Leanne Shapton's ingenious book does a deadpan imitation of the auction catalogues that often accompany the sale of an estate or private collection, catalogues that constitute a peculiar genre in themselves. Typically, the detritus of dead movie stars and the obsessions of rich eccentrics crowd the pages of these paperbound volumes designed to persuade potential bidders that the auction is a purely professional, emotionally neutral transaction, and not, as one might suspect, a thinly disguised *memento mori*, an indication that something has ended—a life, someone's fiscal solvency, or, in the best case, an acquisitive passion.

Shapton presents and describes the artifacts that once belonged to a couple, now broken up. Someone (one or both of the lovers) is jettisoning everything (or almost everything; some lots have been removed from the sale, for unspecified reasons) that the pair possessed or acquired over a relationship that lasted four years, more or less. There are cake stands, blankets, sports equipment, snapshots, T-shirts, clippings, hand-lettered menus from celebratory dinners for two, unopened bottles of wine — and many of these humble items will turn out to signal a plot turn in the history of a romance.

A slightly charred backgammon set, a souvenir of a summer the lovers spend in the country, precedes a handwritten message from Hal: "I want this to work, but there are sides to you I just can't handle sometimes. Chucking the backgammon board into the fire was the last straw." The phone number of a couples' therapist appears on the back of a business card, and we realize that the crisis has escalated when we see a photo of Morris's white-noise machine, which appears to be smashed by a hammer.

Just as the concept of *Important Artifacts* is amusing in itself, so is its central conceit: Although the bidding estimates assigned to the lots fall well within the range that a provident auction house might term "sensibly" or "reasonably" priced, the fact is that a large percentage of what is being auctioned off is basically crap that no sensible person would want, not even for free. The seriousness beneath the joke is that these scraps of paper, used clothes, and borderline garbage were formerly objects of incalculable worth; indeed, they once meant everything to this fictional couple.

Reading the final pages of *Important Artifacts*, I found myself reflecting that the cartoonists whose work I so loved as a child might have been right about the potentially subversive or maniacal ways that objects would behave, if only they could. It may not be true that the furious teapot is plotting to grab a soup spoon and chase us around the house, but it seems inarguable that the deceptively innocent tea cozy could say far more than we would ever want strangers—or anyone, really—to know about who we are, what we did, what was done to us, and how we felt when it happened.

Material used in this particular passage has been adapted from the following source:

F. Prose, *"Love for Sale: Appraising the Relics of a Relationship," Harper's Magazine,* © 2009, Francine Prose.

1. All of the following items are listed in the passage as relics of Doolan and Morris's relationship EXCEPT:

A) a white-noise machine.
B) bottles of wine.
C) a crumpled boarding pass.
D) T-shirts.

2. The author's attitude toward Shapton's book is:

A) predominantly critical but balanced.
B) effusive with praise and superficial.
C) approving and contemplative.
D) disparaging and plaintive.

3. Which of the following statements best summarizes the author's central purpose?

A) To express her appreciation of *Important Artifacts* and to explain how it gave her an elevated awareness of the meaning of objects
B) To praise Shapton's defense of animism inherent in the pages of *Important Artifacts*
C) To laugh at the irony that the objects that once meant so much to Doolan and Morris as a couple become, after their breakup, objects of little to no worth
D) To heighten the reader's awareness of everyday objects and those objects' potential to speak for us and tell stories of the events of our lives

4. Why does the author present the example of the backgammon set in paragraph 5?

A) To provide proof of Lenore Doolan's bad temper as the reason for the decline of the couple's relationship
B) As a piece of evidence for her claim that objects photographed for the book signal plot turns in the couple's relationship
C) To support her point that worthless objects acquire sentimental value when people are in relationships and are therefore invaluable
D) To suggest that objects only acquire meaning after they are altered in some form

5. The author most likely believes that:

A) her toaster is plotting grand schemes to reveal her darkest secrets.
B) it was not right of Shapton to expose a couple's private life the way she does in her book.
C) Doolan and Morris' relationship was doomed to failure.
D) we turn certain objects into significant and necessary documents of memorable parts of our lives.

6. According to the author, auction catalogues are generally designed to create what sort of impression for potential bidders?

A) A belief that the lives of movie stars and rich eccentrics are more fascinating than our own
B) An acknowledgment that something has ended—a life, someone's fiscal solvency, or an acquisitive passion
C) A wistful imagining of the stories and secrets those objects can potentially reveal
D) An appearance of impartiality and professionalism

CHAPTER 8 PRACTICE PASSAGE 2

One difficulty in following Adam Smith's account of self-interest is that he had discussed the matter thoroughly in the *Theory of Moral Sentiments*, and he assumed that the reader of the *Wealth of Nations* would not think that he, Smith, considered self-interest the only or even the main motive, or virtue, of humanity. His teacher, Hutchenson, indeed, had taught that the only virtue was benevolence; but Smith, while agreeing that this was the major virtue and the one which aimed "at the greatest possible good," felt strongly that the system of benevolent ethics was too simple and left no room for the "inferior virtues." Therefore he devoted himself to a more naturalistic theory of morals, in which man's nature was accepted as it was.

In the *Wealth of Nations*, Smith combined the two doctrines: God's providential benevolence and man's earthly self-interest. The result is his famous "invisible hand" theory in which the individual, intending only his own gain, is led "to promote an end which was no part of his intention," the well-being of society. The view that personal self-interest is the best regulator of public affairs had been put forward before: it is expressed in Bernard de Mandeville's, *Private Vices, Public Benefits*. When Smith wrote, this view was already familiar to eighteenth-century thinkers. What Smith did was to give it a reasoned economic exposition which made it acceptable and, so to speak, respectable. From then on, the inevitable benefits of self-interest become a doctrine to which rising manufacturers and owners of newly enclosed land constantly appealed. However, he was constantly inveighing against the farmers, the workers, the manufacturers, and the banks, complaining that they did not understand their own particular interests. He chided the mercantilists that their very cupidity, by imposing a heavy duty on certain goods, called into being a smuggling of the goods which ruined their business. Country gentlemen were told that in their demand for a bounty on corn "they did not act with that complete comprehension of their own interest" which should have directed their efforts.

Smith's method was to form out of experience an abstract principle, to state this as a general rule and to give evidence and examples to support it. Thus, he and his science of economics could show "how" and "in what manner." In order to discover such a science of economics, however, Smith had to posit a faith in the orderly structure of nature, underlying appearances and accessible to man's reason. This, in our judgment, is what Smith really meant by the "invisible hand"; that, so to speak, an "order of nature" or a "structure of things" existed which permitted self-interest, if enlightened, to work for mankind's good.

Man's task, therefore, was to understand the nature or structure of things and to adjust himself harmoniously to the necessary results of this structure. On one level, this might mean the acceptance of a "natural" price of things (reached when the supply, whether of goods or of labor, exactly equaled the demand). On another level, Smith applied his faith in a structure of things when he said: "A nation of hunters can never be formidable to the civilized nations in their neighbourhood. A nation of shepherds may." This is true, he thought, because the nature of hunting is such that large numbers cannot indulge in it; the game would be exterminated. On the other hand, shepherds can grow in number as their flocks grow: and can carry war into the hearts of civilized nations because they carry with them their food supply.

What effect did Smith's work actually have? First, it gave the rising manufacturers and merchants a rationale for their desire to change existing government policy. (Existing policy, as we have pointed out, favored the older trades, methods, and classes against the new "Lunar Society" type of individual and enterprise.) Thus, for example, it helped Pitt to pass a free-trade agreement, the Eden Treaty of 1786 with France, through Parliament.

The second effect of Smith's work was in the shaping of thought. His influence in introducing historical method into political economy was far-reaching. He made the foundation of all subsequent economics the notion that wealth was created by labor. But, more than any of these things, he introduced science into the study of economics. Although he talked much about the "invisible hand" and the "natural course of things," Smith really freed man from the tyranny of chance by forming for him the analytical tools with which he might learn to control his economic activities.

Material used in this particular passage has been adapted from the following source:

J. Bronowski and B. Mazlish, *The Western Intellectual Tradition*. ©1960 by HarperCollins Publishers.

1. The authors state that Smith draws which of the following relationships between nature and economics?

A) Humans are selfish and always take as much from the marketplace as they can.
B) Humans are inherently communal beings and share all their resources.
C) Humans fundamentally act in their own interest.
D) Humans are generous and act in defense of others.

2. Which of the following statements, if true, would most *undermine* the authors' characterization of Smith?

A) Smith extrapolated his theories from real-life observations.
B) Smith's work was wholly theoretical.
C) Smith based part of his work on an older idea.
D) Smith's theory influenced the work of later economists.

3. Which of the following items of information from the passage most supports the authors' claim that Smith believed that the economy can be not only studied but influenced by human actions?

A) Smith felt that the system of benevolent ethics was too simple and left no room for the "inferior virtues."
B) Smith combined two doctrines to create his "invisible hand" theory.
C) Smith introduced a historical method into the study of economy.
D) Smith criticized businessmen who did not act in their own best interest.

4. According to the information provided, the attitude of the authors toward Smith's theories can best be described as:

A) exuberant support.
B) informed approval.
C) qualified praise.
D) inexplicable disappointment.

5. A reasonable supposition from passage information about Smith and de Mandeville is that they agreed that:

A) individual motivation can provide a benefit to society.
B) benevolence is the only virtue.
C) a naturalist theory of morals would prove the most accurate.
D) economics is a science.

6. The term "invisible hand" in Smith's economic theory is most defined by the principle that:

A) there is a "natural" price of things.
B) individual action can influence society.
C) economics can be quantified through analytical tools.
D) manufacturers can change existing government policy.

7. According to the authors, Smith's most important contribution to economics was:

A) identifying benevolence as man's only virtue.
B) identifying the role of nature in economics.
C) identifying self-interest as the best regulator of public affairs.
D) identifying a method by which to analyze economic activity.

SOLUTIONS TO CHAPTER 8 PRACTICE PASSAGE 1

1. **C** This is a Retrieval question.
    A: No. This item is mentioned in paragraph 5.
    B: No. This item is mentioned in paragraph 4.
    C: **Yes. While a crumpled boarding pass is mentioned in paragraph 2, this is a hypothetical example and not tied explicitly to the relationship.**
    D: No. This item is mentioned in paragraph 4.

2. **C** This is a Tone/Attitude question.
    A: No. Nowhere in the passage does the author say anything critical about the book.
    B: No. While the author praises Shapton's book at a few points in the course of the passage, "effusive with praise" is too extreme. Also, the opening and closing ruminations on the relationship of objects to people's lives mean the author is not superficial in her treatment of the subject matter.
    C: **Yes. This comes closest to capturing the author's tone. She calls the book "ingenious" in paragraph 3, and in paragraph 6, she calls the book's concept and central concept "amusing." The author clearly enjoys the book and has given its ideas some thought (which supports "contemplative") as evidenced by the first and last paragraphs.**
    D: No. This is overly negative. The author never criticizes or disparages the book. Also, there is no mournfulness about, or lamenting of, anything regarding the book, which invalidates "plaintive."

3. **A** This is a Main Idea/Primary Purpose question.
    A: **Yes. While the author does not mention Shapton's book immediately, her early discussion about objects leads into a discussion and appreciation of *Important Artifacts*; the last paragraph shows the author's elevated understanding of the meaning of objects after reading the book.**
    B: No. While the author mentions animism in paragraph 1, she does not indicate that Shapton's book explicitly deals with this concept.
    C: No. This choice puts too negative a spin on the author's tone. While the author is interested in the difference between the dollar value and the emotional investment in objects (paragraph 6), she is not discussing these things to laugh at Doolan and Morris or their possessions.
    D: No. While this answer contains correct information, it makes no reference to Shapton's book, which is central to the author's understanding and explanation of the relationship between people and objects.

4. **B** This is a Structure question.
    A: No. The author is not interested in analyzing the reasons for the decline of the relationship; she is only interested in how the objects that belonged to the couple tell the story of their romance. Also, the word "proof" is too strong.
    B: **Yes. At the end of paragraph 4, the author suggests that objects signal plot turns in the couple's relationship. The backgammon example immediately following is illustrative, along with Hal's note, of this point, since it is evidence of a negative turn for the couple. This is furthered by the author's assertion in paragraph 5 that the smashed white-noise machine helps us "realize the crisis has escalated."**
    C: No. This is a point made in paragraph 6 where the author discusses the central conceit of the book. The example of the backgammon set is given to support a different idea in paragraph 5: the connection between changes in the couple's relationship and these objects.
    D: No. The author does not suggest that things must be altered in order to acquire significance.

5. **D** This is an Inference question.

    A: No. This takes the reference in paragraph 1 out of context. While the author mentions cartoons she watched as a child in which objects would sprout limbs and move, and in the final paragraph she suggests that a tea cozy may have a lot to say about one's personal life, she would not go so far as to believe her toaster capable of plotting schemes. Note in the final paragraph she says "if only they could," referring to the fact that objects are unable to enact or consider plots on their own.

    B: No. The author makes no negative judgment about Shapton; besides, the author mentions that the couple is fictional (paragraph 6), so real lives are not actually being exposed.

    C: No. The author does not weigh in on whether the relationship had chances of survival or not; she is merely interested in how the objects from that relationship tell its story.

    D: Yes. See the final sentences of paragraph 2. This answer fits well with the author's assertion that objects become "all-important and indispensable" details in the narratives of chapters of our lives.

6. **D** This is a Retrieval question.

    A: No. There is nothing in the passage that contrasts the lives of famous people with those of regular people in terms of fascination.

    B: No. This choice directly contradicts the passage. In paragraph 3, the author states that the catalogues are not designed to give "an indication that something has ended."

    C: No. See paragraph 3. While the author herself expresses this attitude, she does not suggest that the catalogues do so.

    D: Yes. In paragraph 3 the author says, "Typically, the detritus of dead movie stars and the obsessions of rich eccentrics crowd the pages of these paperbound volumes designed to persuade potential bidders that the auction is a purely professional, emotionally neutral transaction."

SOLUTIONS TO CHAPTER 8 PRACTICE PASSAGE 2

1. **C** This is a Retrieval question.

    A: No. This overstates Smith's contention that self-interest is the primary motivation of humans. While one might call acting in one's self interest "selfish," the authors do not indicate that self-interest always involves taking as much as one can. For example, in the second half of paragraph 2 the authors suggest that self-interest is more complex.

    B: No. Although the passage mentions benevolence (paragraph 1) and Smith's acceptance of it as "the major virtue," this answer choice misrepresents how Smith saw human nature as fundamentally self-interested (paragraphs 1 and 2).

    C: Yes. The authors most directly discuss the relationship between nature and economics in paragraph 3: "In order to discover such a science of economics, however, Smith had to posit a faith in the orderly structure of nature...This...is what Smith really meant by 'the invisible hand'; that...an 'order of nature' or a 'structure of things' existed which permitted self-interest, if enlightened, to work for mankind's good." Also, in paragraph 1 and the beginning of paragraph 2 the authors discuss how Smith believed that humans are motivated by their own self-interest, which grows out of man's very nature.

    D: No. Despite the mention of benevolence in paragraph 1, the passage does not indicate that humans are fundamentally generous, nor that they act in defense of others as a general rule.

2. **B**   This is a Weaken question.

  A: No. The authors characterize Smith as forming an abstract principle out of real-life experience (paragraph 3.) Therefore, this choice is consistent, not inconsistent, with the passage.

  B: Yes. The authors stress the real-life evidence formulating Smith's theories, and the real-life impact they had (see paragraph 2 for examples). Therefore this statement, if true, would undermine the authors' characterization of Smith.

  C: No. Smith did base his work in part on the work of Hutchenson and de Mandeville (see paragraphs 1 and 2). This choice is consistent with the passage.

  D: No. The authors state that Smith's work laid the foundation of all subsequent economic studies (see paragraph 6). This choice is consistent with the passage.

3. **D**   This is a Structure question.

  Note: This question asks you to decide which of the four statements cited in the choices is most directly used within the passage as support for the authors' claim that Smith believed the economy can be influenced.

  A: No. This statement represents the inspiration for Smith's theory, but does not demonstrate that Smith feels that the economy can be influenced.

  B: No. The fact that the "invisible hand" theory combines two different elements (the doctrines of "God's providential benevolence and man's earthly self-interest" (paragraph 2) does not show that Smith feels that the economy can be influenced. These are two separate issues in the passage.

  C: No. This answer speaks to how the economy is now studied (paragraph 6), but has no direct relevance to whether or not the economy can actually be influenced.

  D: Yes. The fact that Smith actively tried to get farmers, workers, and manufacturers to act in their own best interest (and not just their perception of it) clearly indicates that by changing their behavior, he feels that he can change the marketplace (see paragraph 2). Therefore, out of the four choices (all of which are from the passage), this information most acts to give support for the claim cited in the question stem.

4. **B**   This is a Tone/Attitude question.

  A: No. This answer is too extreme. The authors do give Smith's work credit, but in a balanced manner.

  B: Yes. The authors provide concrete reasons for their support of Smith's work.

  C: No. There is no qualification of, or stepping back from, the praise that the authors have for Smith's work.

  D: No. The passage is complimentary towards Smith and gives no indication of disappointment.

5. **A**   This is an Inference question.

  A: Yes. As we can see in paragraph 2, they both believe that "personal self-interest is the best regulator of public affairs."

  B: No. This is Hutchenson's idea, not de Mandeville's. Also, we know from paragraph 1 that Smith does not agree with this idea, because his work is based on a modification of it.

  C: No. We are not told how de Mandeville (mentioned only in paragraph 2) would feel about such a statement.

  D: No. According to the passage, it was Smith who "introduced science into the study of economics" (paragraph 6); we have no way of knowing whether de Mandeville would agree or not.

6. **B**   This is an Inference question.

A: No. While Smith does believe in the possibility of a "natural" price of things (see paragraph 4), this is not the primary principle underlying his "invisible hand" theory. The idea of the "natural" price level creates a backdrop within which Smith's "invisible hand" (human self-interest) may act.

B: Yes. Smith believes that people acting in self-interest will have an inadvertent effect on the "well-being of society" (see paragraph 2). This is at the heart of Smith's theory of the "invisible hand."

C: No. Although Smith did introduce analytical tools to the study of economics (paragraph 6), the idea of quantification is not presented as an underlying principle of the "invisible hand" theory.

D: No. While paragraph 5 explains that Smith's theory provides manufacturers a rationale for desiring change in government policy, the authors do not present this very specific possibility as an underlying principle (nor do we know that the manufacturers were successful).

7. **D**   This is a Retrieval question.

A: No. This was Hutchenson, not Smith (see paragraph 1).

B: No. Smith used the term "nature" but the passage does not suggest that he was the first to connect human nature (or the nature of things in general) to economics, or that this was the most important aspect of Smith's work.

C: No. This was an aspect of his contribution, but the author specifically describes the "science" that Smith provides as his most important contribution to the study of economics (paragraph 6).

D: Yes. The authors stress that his lasting and most important contribution was introducing a scientific methodology to economics (paragraph 6).

Individual Passage Log

Total time spent _____

Passage # _____

Q#	Q type	Attractors	What did you do wrong?

Revised Strategy _____

Passage # _____

Q#	Q type	Attractors	What did you do wrong?

Revised Strategy _____

Chapter 9
Final Preparation

GOAL

•   To stay relaxed and focused

9.1   MENTAL PREPARATION

Yes, the MCAT is very important to your future. Medical schools put a lot of emphasis on the MCAT score and therefore you're likely to feel a great deal of pressure and anxiety about the test. We know this. You know this.

More importantly, however, the AAMC knows this. In fact, they are counting on it to "standardize" you. They want you to become nervous about finishing, to wonder how well you are doing compared to the person next to you, and to start watching the clock, rushing, and re-thinking your strategy.

However, having completed your entire CARS preparation with us, you will be much better prepared for the test than most of your peers. Nobody else will have had a more rigorous experience. You've learned about how the test is put together, you've practiced the types of reading strategies needed for the exam, you've evaluated your strengths and weaknesses, and you have un-learned the habits the AAMC is counting on to standardize you. In other words, you are as well-prepared as humanly possible to beat the odds and to score well on the MCAT.

Take time to prepare mentally also. Visualize yourself calm and confident on the day of the exam. See yourself alert and rested. Imagine beginning the test with confidence because you have seen and practiced on dozens of tests just like it.

Your main job in the last week before the exam is to keep yourself relaxed and focused. Don't burn yourself out at the end. Taper off the hours you spend per day on homework as you approach the test day. Continue to practice your stress reduction techniques. Make time for some enjoyable activities.

Here are some suggestions for the day before—and of—the MCAT.

•   Do not study the day before the test. Try to do some light exercise (don't overdo it), eat well, watch a funny movie, and get to bed at your regular set time.
•   Don't rush. Make sure that you set your alarm—or better still, alarms!—to ensure that you have time to eat a good breakfast, take a shower, and do what you need to do before you leave the house. Most importantly, NO CRAMMING! Aside from doing a quick warm-up (see below), don't open your MCAT books on the day of the test, and don't bring any books or notes with you to the test center.
•   Warm up before the test. Get your mind working in the right direction before you leave home. That could mean just reading through some MCAT-like material, or doing a passage or two (best to redo passages you have already done) untimed. You are not trying to learn anything new; you just want to get your mind into "MCAT mode."

- Use music to set a good tone. Have a playlist selected ahead of time. As you get ready to leave the house, or as you make your way to the testing center, use music to either calm down or rev up.
- While waiting to be seated, if other test-takers are gathered together talking frantically about their fears or, on the other hand, about their superior preparation, step away. Don't let anyone make you nervous or negatively influence your calm, confident state of mind.
- Once the test begins, follow the strategy that you have outlined for yourself. Work calmly and methodically. Do not re-think your strategy or your career choice at this point! If you feel that the test is very hard and that you do not have enough time to finish it, then you are doing it correctly—this is not a reason to panic.
- During the test, take the breaks you are given. You have a long testing day ahead of you. If you power through the first couple of sections without taking advantage of your rest periods, you will burn out at some point. Use the breaks to eat and hydrate, but also to clear your mind, refresh your eyes, and shift gears for the next section.
- Put things into perspective—do not overestimate the importance of the results of this particular test. It is not the only thing in your admissions packet. Yes, the test is a big deal, but schools look at a large array of things when evaluating candidates.
- Plan to reward yourself after the test. Make plans with friends or family to do something that you like to do. You deserve a reward!

CHAPTER 9 PRACTICE PASSAGES

Individual Passage Drill

On the following pages are two final individual passages. Do them timed, but with an intense focus on maximizing both your accuracy and your efficiency. After completing the passages and checking your answers, fill out the Individual Passage Logs.

Identify continuing patterns in the mistakes you are making, as well as identifying times when you successfully implemented appropriate strategies.

CHAPTER 9 PRACTICE PASSAGE 1

Basketball, a game of constant movement and a thousand actions, is a difficult game to remember; Leonard Koppett makes this and other excellent points in *All About Basketball*. Football is a series of set plays, as clear in our minds as moves in chess; and the high drama of a baseball game is often distilled in a single pitch, catch, throw, or hit. We remember baseball and football actions as though the players were etched upon our minds like figures on a distant green. In basketball, by contrast, we remember movement, style, flair, but only occasionally a single play. Perhaps we recall the seventh game of the Lakers-Knicks playoff on May 8, 1970, after the Lakers had pounded the Knicks in the sixth game. Willis Reed was injured and out, it seemed, for the season; and we may remember Reed walking stiffly to the floor for that final game just minutes before warm-ups were concluded; remember the sustained ovation; remember his stiff jumps as he put the first two shots of the game through and then had to leave the game in pain; remember that the Knicks, lifted high by his courage, went on to win game seven, bringing to New York basketball a new perspective. But it is hardly ever, even here, individual plays one remembers. A basketball game plays past like a river, like a song.

In basketball as in no other sport, Koppett also notes, the referee is part of the drama. Decisions of the scorer and the timer are critical and affect the outcomes of countless games every year. But the referee is an agent, an actor; he affects the changing tissue of the drama every instant. He cannot call every infraction, but he must control the game. He needs to gain the players' and the crowds' attention, respect, and emotional cohesion. Thus, referees like Pat Kennedy, Sid Borgia, and Mendy Rudolph in the NBA became better known than many of the players. Each blew the whistle in a range of different tones and styles; each had a repertoire of operatic gestures; each had an energy and physical exuberance that added to the total drama. All won respect for coolness under withering emotion.

Basketball players are visible in every action, Koppett notes, and easily singled out by the spectators as football players are not. They handle the ball scores of times and are physically involved in every moment of offense and defense, as baseball players are not. They are subject to many more flukes than baseball or football players, for they pass and run at high speed constantly, forcing dozens of errors, breaks, and opportunities. "Don't shoot!" the coach screams in despair, his voice trailing off to "Nice shot" as he sits down.

Teams move in patterns, in rhythms, at high velocity; one must watch the game abstractly, not focusing on any single individual alone, but upon, as it were, the blurred and intricate designs woven by the paths through which all five together

cast a spell upon an opposition. The eye watches five men at once, delighting in their unity, groaning at their lapses of concentration. Yet basketball moves so rapidly and so depends on the versatility of each individual in escaping from the defense intended to contain him that the game cannot be choreographed in advance. Twelve men are constantly in movement (counting two referees), the rebounds of the ball are unpredictable, the occasions for passing or dribbling or shooting must be decided instantaneously; basketball players must be improvisers. They have a score, a melody; each team has its own appropriate tempo, a style of game best suited to its talents; but within and around that general score, each individual is free to elaborate as the spirit moves him. Basketball is jazz: improvisatory, free, individualistic, corporate, sweaty, fast, exulting, screeching, torrid, explosive, exquisitely designed for letting first the trumpet, then the sax, then the drummer, then the trombonist soar away in virtuosic excellence.

The point to stress is the mythic line of basketball: a game of fake and feint and false intention; a game of run, run, run; a game of feet, of swift decision, instantaneous reversal, catlike "moves", cool accuracy, spring and jump. The pace is hot. The rhythm of the game beats with the seconds: a three-second rule, a ten-second rule, a rule to shoot in twenty-four seconds. Only when the ball goes out of bounds, or a point is scored, or a foul is called does the clock stop; the play flows on. Teams do not move by timeless innings as in baseball, nor by set, formal, single plays as in football. Even when a play is called or a pattern is established, the game flows on until a whistle blows, moving relentlessly as lungs heavy and legs weary. It is like jazz.

Material used in this particular passage has been adapted from the following source:

M. Novak, *The Joy of Sports.* © 1955 by Madison Books, Incorporated.

1. We can justifiably infer from this passage that the appearance of Willis Reed at the seventh game of the Lakers-Knicks playoff in 1970:

A) brought New Yorkers a new perspective on the significance of physical injury.
B) played some part in the Knicks' victory.
C) was at the insistence of his coach.
D) was necessary to the Knick's victory.

2. As it is used in the context of the passage, word "operatic" in paragraph 2 most nearly means:

A) classical.
B) musical.
C) comedic.
D) histrionic.

3. Which of the following would most *undermine* Koppett's position on the difference between basketball and other sports like football and baseball?

A) Days after a basketball game, commentators cite a memorable play made in the third quarter.
B) After a football game, commentators cite a memorable play made in the last few moments of the game.
C) Following a basketball game, commentators discuss the contrasting playing styles of team members.
D) After a basketball game, commentators discuss a particular team member's strengths and weaknesses.

4. The author most likely compares basketball to jazz primarily in order to:

A) claim that because of the fast-paced and unpredictable nature of the sport, basketball players are among the most skilled athletes.
B) suggest that, like jazz, basketball allows for flexibility and individual excellence within a set format.
C) assert that basketball is a newer and more dynamic sport than football or baseball.
D) indicate that basketball requires athletes to be fast.

5. The primary purpose of the passage is most nearly:

A) to describe the unique characteristics and challenges of the sport of basketball.
B) to defend the ideas offered in Leonard Koppett's *All About Basketball* against his critics.
C) to compare and contrast basketball players and musicians.
D) to describe the crucial role of the referee in a basketball game.

6. The role of the individual athlete during a basketball game as described by the author is most analogous to:

A) the role of the solo instrumentalist in an orchestra.
B) the role of the director of a film.
C) the role of a member of a selective think-tank in a brainstorming session.
D) the role of an average student in a class.

7. The author describes the reaction of the coach in paragraph 3 in order to do all of the following EXCEPT:

A) provide an illustration of the various emotions that can be inspired by the game.
B) contrast the limited role of the coach with the central role of the referee.
C) indicate a limitation on the role of the coach during the game.
D) communicate the unpredictable nature of the game.

CHAPTER 9 PRACTICE PASSAGE 2

It is not easy to define Benjamin Franklin's religious and moral beliefs; yet it is important to do so, because they are representative of a large body of men of his time, whose worldly success certainly derived from their beliefs. D. H. Lawrence, who was angered by all success, treats Franklin as a hypocrite who found the rules which lead to success and turned them into a religion. This analysis is certainly false, but even if it were true, it would not take us far enough. For it would not tell us what made Franklin respected by men as different as his American friends, his English enemies, and his French admirers. There was something in Franklin's beliefs which had a symbolic quality for them all.

The charge that Franklin was a hypocrite can be presented simply. He advocated many virtues at a time when he undoubtedly lapsed into some vices. He began his marriage in 1730 by bringing an illegitimate son into the house. Indeed, he may never have been very vigorous in resisting the temptations of the flesh. These lapses from the conventions of family life would not have outraged D. H. Lawrence if they had not been coupled with a certain priggishness in many of the household maxims which Franklin popularized. In 1732, Franklin began publishing *Poor Richard's Almanac*, which was by far the most successful work that he wrote, and in some ways the most influential. Like other almanacs, this is stuffed with those plums of wisdom which most people like to taste and few to digest—"hunger never saw bad bread," and "well done is better than well said." It is these crystallized plums, so eminently homely and homemade, which have made Franklin's beliefs seem commonplace.

But this criticism confuses the manner in which Franklin expressed himself—and expressed himself at all times—with the content of his thought. Franklin had a special gift for putting a thought into a simple and earthy sentence. This is a gift of expression: a rare gift, but Franklin had it to perfection. The gift has a drawback, however. In this form, Franklin's isolated thoughts do indeed wear a simple and sometimes a commonplace air. But it is a crude error to suppose therefore that the totality of Franklin's thoughts, the system into which the isolated thoughts lock and combine, is commonplace. In this respect, the simplicity of Franklin's sentences is as deceptive as the simplicity of Bertrand Russell's, and the outlook which they make up all together is equally complex.

The informality with which Franklin wrote and spoke is, however, just to his thought in one respect: he was opposed to formality and rigidity of belief. It is not merely that he did not care for the fine points of dogma; he thought it wrong in principle to wish to formulate religion in fine points. He did

not acknowledge any sectarian monopoly of truth. For example, when, at the age of 83, he stated his belief in God, he coupled it with another belief, "that the most acceptable service we render Him is doing good to His other children."

At bottom, it is this tolerance in Franklin's make-up which we must understand. He was tolerant of others because he recognized in them the same humanity that he knew in himself. He never hid his motives from himself, but neither did he belittle the motives of others. We should recognize him as honest because he judges others exactly as he judges himself, with a realistic and generous sense of what can be expected of human beings. Sustained by humanity, he could gain the respect of those as religiously diverse as the anticlerical Tom Paine and the evangelist George Whitefield.

Material used in this particular passage has been adapted from the following source:
J. Bronowski and Bruce Mazlish, *The Western Intellectual Tradition*. ©1960 by HarperCollins Publishers.

1. Which of the following statements best expresses the main point of the passage?

    A) Benjamin Franklin's writings were distinctive in his day for arguing against religious dogma and in favor of tolerance, thereby attracting much criticism from other authors.
    B) The simplicity of Benjamin Franklin's writing, although somewhat at odds with the sophistication of his thought, was connected to the broad-mindedness that gained him the respect of many of his contemporaries.
    C) Despite being accused of hypocrisy, Benjamin Franklin became successful because of his gift for simple speech and to his impressive tolerance.
    D) Benjamin Franklin's deep insights into moral and religious questions, although gaining him the respect of many, contrasted sharply with the simplicity of his writing style.

2. It is reasonable to infer from the passage that D. H. Lawrence:

    A) was more critical of Franklin's writings than of his behavior.
    B) upheld in his own household and writings the accepted conventions of family life.
    C) was envious of Benjamin Franklin's wealth and popularity.
    D) believed that successful religions are usually hypocritical.

3. In the context of the passage, the word "vigorous" most nearly signifies:

    A) healthy.
    B) vociferous.
    C) diligent.
    D) tolerant.

4. According the passage, the relationship of Franklin's writing style to his ideas is most analogous to which of the following?

    A) A symphony which alternates between fast and slow sections.
    B) An intricate painting composed entirely of basic geometric shapes.
    C) A novel advocating virtues that the author does not uphold in his own personal life.
    D) A movie showing the same events from different perspectives, each of which is equally valid.

5. The authors probably quote Franklin in paragraph 2 in order to:

    A) illustrate his simple and unpretentious style.
    B) contrast Franklin's and Lawrence's moral outlook.
    C) deride the trite expressions common to his more popular writings.
    D) emphasize his preference for action over speech.

6. Which of the following statements, if true, would most call into question the authors' characterization of Benjamin Franklin's attitude towards religion?

    A) Although Franklin often attended religious services, he did not claim formal membership in any religious institution.
    B) Like D. H. Lawrence, Franklin was greatly intrigued by Eastern religions, helping to bring Buddhist and Hindu lecturers to Boston and Philadelphia.
    C) Franklin was influential in removing "sacred and undeniable" from Thomas Jefferson's first draft of the Declaration of Independence and in replacing these words with "self-evident."
    D) Active with the Freemasons, Franklin published pamphlets denouncing the beliefs of the Catholic Church.

7. It may be inferred from the passage that each of the following describes Benjamin Franklin's writings EXCEPT:

    A) they attracted some readership outside the United States.
    B) they at times addressed controversial religious topics.
    C) they were notable for their somewhat commonplace style.
    D) their style reflected in a certain fashion Franklin's attitude towards religion.

SOLUTIONS TO CHAPTER 9 PRACTICE PASSAGE 1

1. **B** This is an Inference question.
   A: No. While the author does ask us to "remember that the Knicks, lifted high by his courage, went on to win game seven, bringing to New York basketball a new perspective," choice A goes too far by appending the idea of "physical injury" to that new perspective.
   B: Yes. The author says in paragraph 1 that "the Knicks, lifted high by his courage, went on to win game seven."
   C: No. This choice goes too far, since we do not know from the passage what Reed's motive was, or whether or not the coach was involved in his decision to play.
   D: No. The word "necessary" makes this choice too strong. Remember that when dealing with inferences, it is best to stick with answers that do not stray too far from the passage. It is impossible to say with certainty that the Knicks would have lost had it not been for Reed's appearance. This makes B a better supported answer than choice D.

2. **D** This is a an Inference question.
   A: No. While "classical" as in classical music or as in traditional or elegant (which are other possible interpretations of the word "classical") may come to your mind when you think of opera, there is nothing in the passage to support this interpretation of the word.
   B: No. As in choice A, this may fit your own interpretation of "operatic," but there isn't anything in this part of the passage to suggest a connection or relationship to music.
   C: No. "Comedic" does not fit the author's description of the referees as respected, cool under pressure, and dramatic. It also doesn't fit the author's relatively serious tone in this passage.
   D: Yes. Be careful not to eliminate a word just because you don't know what it means. "Histrionic" is a synonym for "dramatic" and thus best fits the author's context.

3. **A** This is a Weaken question.
   A: Yes. Koppett posits in paragraph 1 that "basketball, a game of constant movement and a thousand actions, is a difficult game to remember" and that "it is hardly ever...individual plays that one remembers." Because it is fast-paced and relies on action from multiple players, the author of the passage points out, fewer single plays stick out in our minds. In order to weaken Koppett's position, our credited response should describe a memorable singular moment. Choice A does this. While this choice doesn't destroy Koppett's argument, it is the only one of the four answers that is at all inconsistent with it.
   B: No. Choice B describes a memorable moment in a football game, in a way that is consistent with Koppett's claim about the difference between basketball and football.
   C: No. This answer actually strengthens Koppett's position, since the passage points out that we remember the "movement, style, [and] flair" of basketball players (paragraph 1).
   D: No. As in choice C, this answer is consistent, not inconsistent. According to paragraph 4, "the versatility of each individual" is crucial, and "each individual is free to elaborate as the spirit moves him." Therefore, a discussion of an individual's strengths and weaknesses would fit with Koppett's position.

4. **B** This is a Structure question.
   A: No. This choice goes too far, since the author never tells us baseball and football are not challenging in their own way.
   B: Yes. The author tells us that "basketball players must be improvisers. They have a score, a melody; each team has its own appropriate tempo, a style of game best suited to its talents; but within and around that general score, each individual is free to elaborate as the spirit moves him" (paragraph 4). This answer choice is the best paraphrase of this idea.

C: No. This option takes the metaphor too literally and is too judgmental in tone towards football and baseball. Furthermore, nothing in the passage suggests that basketball is a newer sport.

D: No. While the author does mention speed in paragraph 4, this is not the primary purpose of the metaphor, but only one of many aspects within it. The main theme of the comparison is how basketball, like jazz, relies on individual action and creativity within the context of a group or team endeavor.

5.   **A**   This is a Main Idea/Primary Purpose question.

A: **Yes. This choice can include all of the author's major points, without going beyond the scope of the passage.**

B: No. This option is too narrow; also, the author never makes mention of any critics of Koppett's ideas.

C: No. This answer might be tempting, since so much of the passage is devoted to comparing basketball and jazz. But since the answer frames it in terms of "comparing and contrasting basketball players and musicians," it misrepresents the focus of the passage, which is on the sport of basketball itself not just the players.

D: No. This choice is too narrow. Referees are discussed only in paragraphs 2 and 4, and the rest of the passage isn't written in support of the author's claims about referees in those paragraphs.

6.   **C**   This is an Analogy question.

A: No. The soloist may be virtuosic, but not an equal member of a team. This choice also fails to capture the theme of constant interaction in the passage.

B: No. The director of a film is in charge of the other "players" rather than being on equal footing with the rest of the team.

C: **Yes. Novak describes basketball players as all being virtuosic in their own way, but working together, all players being equally necessary to success. A member of a think tank involved in a brainstorming session would play a similar role, including the constant interaction and responsiveness to new scenarios that is described in the passage.**

D: No. We don't have any indication in this choice that an average student would be virtuosic in his or her own way, and yet in constant interaction with the rest of the class, improvising as the class progressed in unpredictable ways.

7.   **B**   This is a Structure/EXCEPT question.

A: No. This choice is supported by the passage. The coach's reaction demonstrates varied emotions in response to the unexpected twists and turns of the game.

B: **Yes. This choice is not supported by the passage, and so is the correct answer to an EXCEPT question. This answer is too extreme; we don't know from the passage that the coach's role overall is limited, just that at times the coach's instructions are invalidated by rapid changes in the game as it plays out. Also, the there is no suggestion in the passage that the purpose of the reference is to contrast the role of the coach with that of the referee in terms of their relative importance.**

C: No. This statement is supported by the passage. While we don't know that the coach plays a limited role overall, his or her role during the game is constrained, such that the command "Don't shoot" is invalidated by the rapidly changing nature of play on the court.

D: No. This statement is supported by the passage. The coach's scream of "Don't shoot" is contradicted by an unpredictable shift in the game which leads to a successful shot.

SOLUTIONS TO CHAPTER 9 PRACTICE PASSAGE 2

1. **B** This is a Main Idea/Primary Purpose question.

   A: No. This choice may be eliminated because, although Franklin and Lawrence are contrasted, the passage makes no general claim that Franklin's writings were distinctive or much criticized. In fact, paragraph 1 suggests that his beliefs were shared by a wide range of other people.

   B: Yes. Both paragraphs 1 and 5 address the respect with which Franklin was viewed. Franklin's simple writing style also relates to the tolerance (paragraph 4) which the authors describe as central to his character.

   C: No. The only reference to Franklin's success is in paragraph 1, which suggests that his worldly success derived from his beliefs. While tolerance may have been one of these beliefs, the passage as a whole is not about the reasons for his success in life, but about the beliefs themselves, and how they related to his style of writing.

   D: No. This choice is attractive in appearing to draw on many components of the passage. However, the authors do not claim that Franklin had deep insights into religious and moral questions. Complexity of thought (paragraph 3) is not necessarily the same as deep insight. Furthermore, this answer choice says nothing about Franklin's tolerance, which is a major theme in the passage. Finally, it was this complexity, not the deepness of his insight, which contrasted with Franklin's simple writing style.

2. **A** This is an Inference question.

   A: Yes. Paragraph 2 emphasizes that D. H. Lawrence was not outraged by Franklin's behavior but by the apparent hypocrisy of his publications, which the authors describe as described as "priggish" and "commonplace" in paragraph 2.

   B: No. We know nothing of Lawrence's own family life.

   C: No. Like choice B, this reaches beyond the available information since, although Lawrence was angered by success, there is nothing in the passage to indicate envy.

   D: No. This answer may be attractive because it draws on language in paragraph 1. However, Lawrence believed Franklin was hypocritical in his success; we don't know how Lawrence felt about "successful religions" in general.

3. **C** This is an Inference question.

   A: No. "Healthy" may be one literal definition of "vigorous," but it doesn't fit in the context of the passage, which is about Franklin's lack of will rather than his health.

   B: No. "Vociferous" means outspoken. The issue in the passage is about Franklin's behavior, not his expressed opinions (which were at odds with his behavior).

   C: Yes. The authors suggest that Franklin's lapses were somewhat common and that Franklin did not make any great effort to uphold family norms.

   D: No. Tolerance is not discussed until paragraph 5, and it is not directly relevant to this discussion of Franklin's failures to live up to his own standards of virtue in his private life.

4. **B** This is an Analogy question.

   A: No. There is no alternation or back and forth (that is, first one, then the other, then back again to the first) between Franklin's style and ideas.

   B: Yes. The principle relationship (paragraph 3) is that Franklin's simple words, taken singly, may deceptively mask the complexity of his overall thought.

C: No. This choice is attractive because it points to the charge of hypocrisy brought against him in paragraph 2. However, the question asks about the relationship between Franklin's style and his beliefs, not about a relationship between his beliefs and his private life.

D: No. While this choice may reflect Franklin's tolerance towards other beliefs (paragraphs 4 and 5), it doesn't match the relationship between his writing style and his beliefs.

5. **A** This is a Structure question.

A: Yes. These words make Franklin's beliefs seem commonplace or simple.

B: No. There is no reference to different moral positions in this paragraph.

C: No. While the authors do say that Franklin's maxims show a certain "priggishness" and commonplace nature, the passage goes on in paragraph 3 to show that the simple and commonplace nature of Franklin's individual statements hides to some extent the true complexity of his thought. Therefore, the authors are not deriding or mocking his expressions, or calling them "trite" or trivial.

D: No. Although this is a paraphrase of the second maxim, it does not relate to the authors' purpose in including the quotation, which is to illustrate the simplicity of Franklin's sayings.

6. **D** This is a Weaken question.

A: No. The authors make no claim concerning Franklin's formal affiliation. The passage's characterization of Franklin's attitude toward religion, or of his self-professed "belief in God," doesn't rest on an assumption that Franklin was affiliated with a particular church.

B: No. This choice would strengthen, not weaken, the authors' claim that Franklin was tolerant towards other religious beliefs.

C: No. This answer is consistent with the authors' claim that Franklin denied any "sectarian monopoly of truth" and that he resisted dogma (paragraph 4).

D: Yes. The authors characterize Franklin's attitude as tolerant of other beliefs. As part of this argument, the authors state that Franklin, because of his tolerance, was respected by other diverse religious figures (paragraph 5). If Franklin denounced the beliefs of the Catholic Church, this would significantly undermine the authors' characterization. Notice the difference between choice C and choice D. Choice C involves resistance to incorporating language that suggests religious dogma into the Declaration, but does not involve criticizing any particular beliefs themselves.

7. **B** This is an Inference/EXCEPT question.

A: No. Paragraph 1 demonstrates that Franklin's work was known internationally.

B: Yes. Although Franklin spoke of God (paragraph 4), there is no evidence that his writings addressed religious topics, especially controversial religious topics. Also, the fact that D.H. Lawrence claimed that Franklin "found the rules which lead to success and turned them into a religion" (paragraph 1) can't be interpreted to mean that Franklin literally wrote about religion itself. Because you cannot infer this answer to be true based on the passage, it is the correct answer to an EXCEPT question.

C: No. Their commonplace style is discussed in paragraphs 2 and 3. Note the more moderate wording of this choice as compared to choice B.

D: No. This is a paraphrase of the first sentence of paragraph 4. Note the difference between choice B and choice D. Choice D says that the style of Franklin's writings reflected religious attitudes, but choice B states that his writings directly addressed religious topics.

Individual Passage Log

Passage # _____   Time spent on passage _____

Q#	Q type	Attractors	What did you do wrong?

Revised Strategy _____

Passage # _____   Time spent on passage _____

Q#	Q type	Attractors	What did you do wrong?

Revised Strategy _____

CARS Appendix

A.1 APPLYING CARS TECHNIQUES TO THE SCIENCE PASSAGES

The challenges posed by the science sections of the MCAT differ in a number of important ways from those posed by the CARS section. Indeed, the differences must seem all too obvious. Most striking is the amount of information you need to bring with you to the test; even the brightest and most alert reader would be lost in Physics or Biology without an understanding of the basic scientific principles and a good grasp of the fundamental definitions and nomenclature. It's also the case that you must engage in a lot more problem-solving for the sciences than you do for CARS, where your primary task is to *find* answers rather than to calculate them. CARS passages tell you almost everything you need to know, while the science passages require you to know much more before you read them.

Nevertheless, there's a great deal of overlap in the skills required to do well on these apparently dissimilar sections. *You will not score very high in the sciences if you merely try to plug numbers into formulas or to spit back information that you've stuffed into your memory; you also need to be able to draw inferences from the passages, to extrapolate answers from the information provided to you.* You need to work quickly, wasting no time on calculating answers that can be taken directly from the text—or, conversely, on searching a passage for information that isn't there. Most important, you need to mobilize your scientific "common sense," your intuitive understanding of what is and isn't likely to be true for any described scenario involving the physical world. You also need to apply that common sense to the answer choices, eliminating those that are not likely ever to be true. For all of these tasks—looking for specific information, drawing inferences, evaluating the plausibility of answer choices—your CARS skills will be invaluable.

In short, to do well on the MCAT, you need to think both scientifically *and* strategically. Many people feel that they *must* work out the answer to every last question. There is something very noble in this endeavor, but it is not smart test-taking. Remember: you don't get extra points for the tougher questions. Use your knowledge of the test to help you find the correct answers.

For one thing, you should know when the passage information can help you and when it cannot. There are, broadly speaking, three types of MCAT science questions.

1) **Memory ("Pure Science") Questions**
   These are based entirely on information that you bring with you to the test; there is nothing in the passage that will help you solve them, or, there is no passage attached to the questions.
2) **Explicit ("Retrieval") Questions**
   Less common than the other two question types, these require only that you *find* an answer in the passage.
3) **Implicit ("Application") Questions**
   The most common question type, these require you to apply your scientific knowledge to the information in the passage.

Recognizing the question types will affect your solution strategy. You should answer all Explicit/Retrieval questions. Their answers are right in the passage; just use the same techniques you would for CARS Retrieval questions, checking your final answer choice to make sure that it matches the information in the passage.

Implicit/Application questions will vary in difficulty, depending on the amount and type of outside information involved. Some will require that you apply a quite basic principle; for example, that gases expand as they warm. Others call for more precise knowledge of, say, the function of a particular endocrine gland. Most questions will be Implicit or a hybrid of Implicit and Explicit (even Explicit/Retrieval questions require some knowledge to recognize the answer). Your strategy here is to determine how much help the passage will give you, and to pass quickly over those questions for which you lack sufficient outside knowledge.

Finally, Memory/"Pure Science" questions are freestanding, or they deal with the passage *topic* but refer only nominally to the passage itself. You can skip a pure science question if you cannot work out the answer, coming back to it at the end of the section if you have time. Such a strategy doesn't work for CARS, because the questions are so closely based on the passages, and because once you've left a passage, you will most likely forget most of it. Pure Science questions, however, don't rely on context and can be solved at any point.

Solutions to Some Sample Passages

The following pages contain four passages from General Chemistry, Physics, Biology, and Psychology/Sociology and outline the ways in which you can use CARS strategies to tackles these types of passages. Note that these techniques are less useful for Organic Chemistry passages, which tend to have much less text, often consisting of little more than a few chemical equations. Solutions to all four passages can be found at the end of this Appendix.

MCAT G-Chem Drill: Solubility

Oxygen is transported from the lungs to the capillaries where it is released into the tissues. The oxygen in the circulatory system of mammals is bound to hemoglobin, a protein found in red blood cells.

Hemoglobin has a complex quaternary structure since it is composed of four separate polypeptide chains. Each polypeptide serves as a giant ligand for the single iron(II)-heme unit, the location of oxygen fixation. The oxygen-binding strength of the heme unit and transport efficiency are directly related to blood pH level.

Unlike oxygen, the carbon dioxide which is released into the capillaries by the surrounding tissue is transported by two different mechanisms. Foremost, carbon dioxide is rather soluble in water due to the following equilibria:

$$(1) \quad CO_2 + H_2O \rightleftharpoons H_2CO_3$$

$$(2) \quad H_2CO_3 \rightleftharpoons H^+ + HCO_3^-$$

Therefore, some carbon dioxide immediately dissolves into the blood plasma and is transported to the lungs as bicarbonate ion. Most mammals have an enzyme, carbonic anhydrase, to catalyze Reaction (1), because under normal conditions, CO_2 and carbonic acid cannot reach equilibrium fast enough for efficient transport.

In the second mechanism, CO_2 may react with the N-terminus of the protein chains of hemoglobin, forming a carbamate functional group:

$$(3) \; Hb\text{—}NH_2 = CO_2 \rightleftharpoons Hb\text{—}NHCOO^- + H^+$$

Once in the lungs, the Hb-carbamate decomposes to release CO_2, and Hb NH_2 is restored.

1. Carbon dioxide is much more soluble in water than is oxygen. Why?

A) Oxygen has a greater dipole moment.
B) Carbon dioxide has a greater dipole moment than oxygen.
C) Carbon dioxide is a polar molecule.
D) Carbon dioxide is reactive to nucleophilic attack.

2. The expiration of CO_2 from the bloodstream in the lungs:

A) increases blood pH.
B) decreases blood pH.
C) decreases the oxygen content of the blood.
D) None of the above

3. Acidosis—a condition characterized by a decrease in blood pH—rapidly develops after cardiac arrest because tissues continue to load the capillary plasma with more and more CO_2. If the blood pH is not buffered (reset to normal), the patient may die, even after cardiac revival. Why?

A) Too much CO_2 can cause a cell's lipid bilayer to decompose.
B) High concentrations of bicarbonate can cause insoluble salts to precipitate out of the plasma.
C) The nervous system can no longer function properly.
D) Hemoglobin cannot effectively transport O_2.

4. If the enzyme carbonic anhydrase were added to a glass of soda pop which had been allowed to reach equilibrium with the atmosphere, it would:

A) produce a large number of carbon dioxide bubbles.
B) produce a large amount of oxygen.
C) form more carbonic acid.
D) have no effect on the equilibrium.

5. Which one of the following will decrease the solubility of CO_2 in water?

A) Increasing the external pressure of CO_2
B) Increasing the temperature of the water
C) Increasing the pH of the water
D) None of the above

6. What is the electron configuration of the iron(II) ion?

A) [Ar] $3d^6$
B) [Ar] $4s^2\, 3d^4$
C) [Ar] $4s^2\, 3d^6$
D) [Ar] $4s^2\, 3p^{10}$

CARS Strategies for MCAT G-Chem Drill: Solubility

This passage deals with aspects of oxygen transport in the blood. It consists of four paragraphs, two of which include chemical reactions. Although it begins by referring to hemoglobin (paragraphs 1 and 2), the bulk of the questions have to do with plasma CO_2.

1) Oxygen/hemoglobin introduction
2) Structure and functionality of hemoglobin
3) Chemical reactions re: CO_2 solubility (especially re: carbonic acid)
4) CO_2/hemoglobin reaction

1. Nominally, a **Memory** question—but you can make a good guess by treating this as a Retrieval question. See 3: "Foremost, carbon dioxide is rather soluble in water *because of* the following equilibrium reactions…" [emphasis added]. Since the passage states that the solubility of carbon dioxide is due to a chemical reaction, look for an answer choice that refers to a chemical reaction. This leads you to the correct answer, which is D.

2. An unusual example of an **Explicit** question: the answer is really in the next question! You are asked what happens to the blood when CO_2 is expired by the lungs. Question 3 tells you that when plasma CO_2 goes up, blood pH goes down. Hence, when CO_2 goes down (via the lungs), blood pH must go up. This gives you A, the correct answer.

3. See paragraph 2: O_2 binding and transport is proportional to blood pH. Thus low pH = low oxygen transport = a dead person (answer choice D, in other words). This is mostly an **Explicit** question.

4. See paragraph 3: **Apply** your knowledge of what "equilibrium" means to the information that carbonic anhydrase speeds up the reaction—until it reaches equilibrium.

5. **Memory:** The answer comes only from your own outside knowledge, not from passage information.

6. **Memory:** The answer comes only from your own outside knowledge, not from passage information.

MCAT Physics Drill: Force

Near the surface of the earth, the density of air is approximately 1.2 kg/m³. A hot-air balloon with total mass M (including passengers) and volume V will float motionless if there is no wind and the buoyant force (magnitude F_B) due to the air is equal to the weight of the balloon and passengers: $F_B = Mg$, where g is the magnitude of the acceleration due to gravity near the surface of the Earth.

The strength of the buoyant force may be altered by heating the air inside the balloon, thereby changing its volume. The total weight of the balloon may be decreased by equipping the balloon with sandbags that can be dropped to the ground.

Many hot-air balloons are equipped with propellers that drive air backward and allow the balloon to travel horizontally. All balloons have a maximum achievable volume which depends on the extent to which the air inside can be heated as well as on the elastic limits of the material used to construct the balloon.

1. A balloon, moving upward and eastward, casts a shadow that moves along the ground at a speed of 10 m/s. What is the balloon's total speed if its velocity vector makes an angle of 60° with the horizontal?

    A)   5 m/s
    B)   17 m/s
    C)   20 m/s
    D)   34 m/s

2. A balloon of total mass M sits motionless 40 m above the ground. A sandbag of mass m is dropped out of the balloon. What is then the net force on the balloon?

    A) Mg
    B) $(M - m)g$
    C) mg
    D) $(M + m)g$

3. Two unladen hot-air balloons are weighed and measured. Their masses and volumes are as follows:

    Balloon I: Mass = 1200 kg; Volume = 1600 m³

    Balloon II: Mass = 1100 kg; Volume = 1200 m³

    Which of these balloons could be used to carry four people whose average mass is 100 kg each?

    A)   I only
    B)   II only
    C)   I and II
    D)   Neither balloon could carry such a load.

4. Which of the following best illustrates the flow of air inside a closed-top balloon as the air is heated by a flame directly beneath the opening at the base of the balloon?

    A)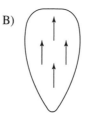

    B)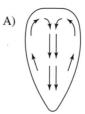

    C)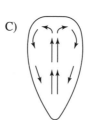

    D)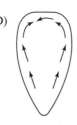

5. A balloon is moving upward at constant velocity. Which one of the following equations involved the magnitudes of the gravitational force, F_G, the drag forces due to air resistance, F_D, and the buoyant force of the air, F_B, is correct?

A) $F_D + F_B > F_G$
B) $F_D + F_B = F_G$
C) $F_D + F_G < F_B$
D) $F_D + F_G = F_B$

6. A balloon for a county fair is designed to carry four 100-kg passengers when it is expanded to its maximum volume. The designers assumed the balloon would operate in ordinary spring temperatures. If, on the day of the fair, the temperature reaches a record-breaking maximum:

A) the balloon will not be able to achieve its maximum volume.
B) more sandbags will be needed for proper operation of the balloon.
C) the total weight the balloon is able to carry will be reduced.
D) once in flight, the balloon cannot be lowered until the ambient temperature drops.

7. A balloon has a mass of 1500 kg with no passengers. A typical passenger weighs 100 kg. A balloon with 5 passengers is floating motionless high above the ground when a 2 kg pelican lands on the balloon. Making which of the following adjustments would allow the balloon to remain floating motionless?

A) Increase the volume of the balloon by 0.1%
B) Slightly cool the air in the balloon
C) Drop a 4-kg sandbag from the balloon
D) None of the above

8. Four 100-kg people are holding a 1200-kg inflated balloon by means of four ropes. Three people let go and the balloon accelerates upward at 2 m/s². What is the tension in the rope that the last person is holding?

A) 200 N
B) 400 N
C) 800 N
D) 1200 N

MCAT CRITICAL ANALYSIS AND
REASONING SKILLS REVIEW

CARS Strategies for MCAT Physics Drill: Force

Three short paragraphs about hot-air balloons. Notice that almost all of the useful information is contained in paragraph 1.

1) Useful stuff: density of air, forces acting on the balloon, etc.
2) How to make a balloon go up (gee, Toto…)
3) Balloon propellers, elasticity

1. **Memory.** It doesn't matter if it's a balloon, a pelican, or the space shuttle that's moving upward and eastward; just mobilize your math here.

2. **Implicit.** Use your understanding of "net force" and apply it to paragraph 1. If it's motionless, there's no net force. If you dump a sandbag of mass m, what has changed?

3. **Implicit/Explicit.** Be canny about this one. You're given the density of air. You aren't given any other information (e.g., the mass of air *inside* the balloon, the temperature of the air inside or outside of the balloon, etc.). Don't panic, thinking this is one of those questions where you need to remember some complicated physics formula or something. With what you've been given, you must be able to answer this one by calculating the mass of air displaced by the balloon, and then seeing if it's more or less than the combined mass of the balloon and the passengers.

4. **Memory.** Or pure common sense: where is the hot air going to go? And what is it going to do when it gets there? As for A, what would make the stream of hot air split into two? As for D, why would the air circulate counterclockwise as opposed to clockwise?

5. **Implicit.** See paragraph 1 and note that answer choices A and B can't be right because F_G and F_D have to go on the same side of the equation.

6. **Implicit.** Use your knowledge of what happens to air when it gets hot (it expands and its density decreases) to answer this one.

7. **Implicit**—but a little common sense would help, too. B makes no sense; you know what happens to balloons as they cool and shrink. C makes no sense because the pelican only weighs 2 kg. As often happens, you're left with two plausible answer choices—and, in a time crunch, you might want to abandon the calculations and figure that there *is* a way to adjust to one crummy bird landing on the balloon, so answer choice D is rather unlikely.

8. **Memory.** The answer cannot be found in the passage.

MCAT Biology Drill: Embryology

The events that contribute to successful fertilization have been intensively studied in the soil nematode *Caenorhabditis elegans*. This organism has several advantages for developmental biology. First, at 1 mm in length, it is small enough to easily culture, and yet the embryos are large enough to see under a compound microscope. Second, its three-day life cycle makes it ideal for genetic studies. Third, *C. elegans* is a self-fertilizing hermaphroditic species—its two sexes are 1) male and 2) self-replicating hermaphrodite. Heterozygous mutations can easily be made homozygous by allowing the hermaphrodites to self-fertilize. Finally the males are missing an X chromosome, and can thus be crossed to normal XX hermaphrodites, facilitating genetic studies.

The entire developmental process from fertilization to adulthood can be observed under the compound microscope. Fertilization takes place in the hermaphrodites as the oocyte passes through the spermatheca, which is where the sperm are stored. If the embryos are collected at this point, the following events can be observed in the light microscope: After the entry of the sperm into the posterior end of the egg, the oocyte nucleus, having been suspended in diakinesis of meiotic prophase I, now completes the meiotic divisions. The excess genetic material is extruded as polar bodies, and the eggshell is secreted, forming an impermeable barrier that protects the developing embryo. The cytoplasmic rearrangements that follow begin with the female pronucleus migrating toward the male pronucleus. A pseudocleavage is observed, where a cleavage furrow appears but disappears without cell division. The pronuclei fuse in the posterior end of the cell, rotate, then move toward the center. At this point, the nucleus of the embryo is formed. Finally, the first division occurs, producing a smaller posterior (P) cell and a larger anterior cell (AB).

Another event that can be observed is the migration of granules from the cytoplasm of the fertilized embryo into the P cell — hence their name, P-granules. As the zygote develops by mitosis into a full organism, the P-granules become sequestered by the cells destined to become the germ line. The function of the P-granules is not known. Exposing the developing embryos to microtubule inhibitors (such as colcemid) blocks the migration of the pronuclei, but does not affect P-granule movement. The inhibitor of actin polymerization, cytochalasin B, has the opposite effect, preventing P-granule segregation, but allowing pronuclei to migrate. The entire process of fertilization, from entry of the sperm to the first cell division, takes about 35 minutes.

Material used in this particular passage has been adapted from the following source:

W.B. Wood, *The Nematode, Caenorhabditis elegans,* (Cold Spring Harbor Monograph Series 17), © 1988 by Cold Spring Harbor Laboratory Press.

1. Which of the following would be the least appropriate organism for studying developmental processes such as fertilization and the ensuing cell divisions?

A) The bacterium, *Escherichia coli*
B) The fruit fly, *Drosophila melanogaster*
C) The African clawed toad, *Xenopus laevis*
D) The human being, *Homo sapiens*

2. Since male nematodes arise as a result of nondisjunction in the XX hermaphrodite, what is their genotype?

A) XY
B) XXX
C) XO
D) XYY

3. What is the ploidy of the fertilized egg?

A) n
B) $2n$
C) $3n$
D) $4n$

4. The spermatheca is where:

A) the progenitor cells of the sperm enter meiosis.
B) sperm are stored in the hermaphrodite.
C) sperm received their protein coat.
D) sperm are stored in the males.

5. Which one of the following accurately describes pseudocleavage?

A) The embryo divides into two cells, which then fuse.
B) A cleavage furrow forms then disappears.
C) A cell membrane begins to form then disappears.
D) Polar bodies are formed.

6. When the pronuclei fuse, which of the following event(s) must occur for cell division to proceed?

    I.   Homologous chromosomes pair
    II. Recombination events occur
    III. Nuclear membranes are reorganized

A) I only
B) I and II only
C) III only
D) I, II, and III

7. The effects of colcemid and cytochalasin B on the embryo suggest that:

    I.   Microfilaments are involved in P-granule migration.
    II. Microfilaments are involved in pronuclear migrations.
    III. Microtubules are involved in pronuclear migrations.
    IV. Microtubules are involved in P-granules migration.

A) I and III only
B) I and IV only
C) II and III only
D) II and IV only

CARS Strategies for MCAT Biology Drill: Embryology

This passage is long and dense; let's map it. There are only three paragraphs here, but each is long and filled with detail. Annotate this passage so that you can find where important categories of information begin and end.

1) Nematode sex
   Research advantages:
   - size
   - 3-day life cycle
   - self-fertilizing hermaphrodite
   - males missing X chromosome
2) Development from fertilization to adulthood
   Map separate events after *oocyte* passes through *spermatheca*
3) Migration of P-granules
   (Note: "P cell" is defined at the end of paragraph 2)

1. **Memory.** Don't sweat this one: how much fertilizing do bacteria do?

2. **Explicit.** See paragraph 1: the hermaphrodite is XX, and the male is missing an X chromosome; $2 - 1 = ?$

3. **Implicit.** Apply your knowledge of the meaning of "ploidy" and "diakinesis of meiotic prophase I" to the information in paragraph 2.

4. **Explicit.** You can read the definition of "spermatheca" exactly from paragraph 2.

5. **Explicit.** "pseudocleavage" is defined in paragraph 2.

6. **Implicit.**

7. **Implicit/Explicit.** See paragraph 3: everything is spelled out for you except the role of microfilaments in pronuclear migration.

MCAT Psychology/Sociology Drill: Global Health Trends

Across the globe, income and health outcomes are positively correlated. As gross domestic product (GDP) increases, so do certain standard measures of a population's health (such as longevity), while others (such as infant mortality) decrease. Taking multiple standard measures into account, each country is assigned an overall health score, meant to use aggregate health data to reflect the population's general health (or, as a predictor of any given individual's health). The wealthiest countries consistently receive the highest overall health scores, while the poorest countries consistently receive the lowest. This can also be seen at the individual level; as a general rule, the lower a person or family's income, the more likely they are to develop certain health problems and the less likely they are to have access to care for these problems.

Obesity is one of the few measures that defies this global health trend. In recent years, obesity rates have been skyrocketing in the countries with the highest GDPs. The most extreme example of this is the United States, which has an obesity rate that far exceeds every other country (Figure 1). Many experts predict that by the year 2020, obesity (and obesity-related health problems) will trump cancer and heart disease as the number one risk factor for premature death in the U.S. And in almost all cases, obesity is completely preventable.

Country	GDP per capita in thousands (converted to U.S. dollars)	% population with BMI > 30 in 2012
United States	55.6	31.5
Canada	46.0	19.4
Sweden	40.4	12.3
Belgium	38.3	15.8
South Africa	10.1	20.6
China	6.5	10.3
India	1.5	9.3

Figure 1 Prosperity (measured by Gross Domestic Product or GDP in U.S. dollars) and obesity (measured by percent of the population exceeding a BMI of 30) in selected countries in 2012

Body Mass Index (BMI) is used as a rough, non-invasive way to assess body fat. BMI is calculated using weight and height, and is a fairly reliable indicator of body fat for most people. For U.S. adults, a BMI of less than 18.5 corresponds to "underweight status;" between 18.5 and 24.9 corresponds

to "normal weight status;" between 25.0 and 29.9 corresponds to "overweight status;" and a BMI over 30 is considered obese. The U.S. National Health Statistics Center conducted a 30-year longitudinal study of BMI rates for adults and children per state based on a representative sample of the total population for each state. These data were also used to calculate national averages. The state with the highest rate of adult and childhood obesity is Mississippi, and the state with the lowest rate of adult and childhood obesity is Colorado (Figure 2).

Percentage of population with BMI >30 from 1980 to 2010

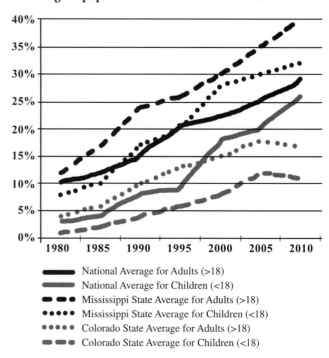

Figure 2 Percentage of the population with a BMI over 30 for the state with the highest rates of obesity (Mississippi), lowest rates of obesity (Colorado), and the national averages, from 1980 to 2010.

Based on this study, the Mississippi Department of Health implemented mandatory health screenings for third graders and eighth graders in 2011. Preliminary data suggest that third graders are more than twice as likely to be diagnosed with type-II diabetes, and about three times as likely to be diagnosed with other hormonal imbalances, when compared to national health statistics for children the same age. Eighth graders are almost four times as likely to be diagnosed with type-II diabetes and over five times as likely to be diagnosed with other hormonal imbalances compared to national health statistics for children the same age. Based on these preliminary results, the state of Mississippi is considering implementing new laws concerning school-based activity minimums and school lunch calorie maximums.

1. Catecholamine derivatives that act as agonists for a specific neuronal receptor have been shown to help prevent obesity in many severely overweight patients. These derivatives also promote neuroprotection from Parkinson's disease. What is a possible mechanism of action for this process?

A) For people suffering from a food addiction, eating excessive high fat food triggers the dopamine reward system in the brain (similar to a drug addict). The catecholamine derivative acts as an agonist for dopamine, thus stimulating the dopamine reward center without the presence of food, and leading to a decrease in overeating.

B) Catecholamine derivatives stimulate the parasympathetic nervous system, thus increasing the activity of the gut. Therefore, despite consuming a highly caloric diet, food is processed more quickly, leading to weight loss.

C) Acetylcholine is responsible for muscular contractions. Since catecholamine derivatives are the precursors to acetylcholine, the presence of these derivatives in the body stimulates the musculoskeletal system, thus burning additional calories and leading to weight loss.

D) Catecholamine derivatives block the release of cortisol, a known contributor to stress-related over eating and weight gain.

2. Obesity is considered a marker of poor health. According to Figure 1, which country most aligns with the general global health trend described in the first paragraph concerning the relationship between GDP and population health?

A) Canada
B) South Africa
C) China
D) India

3. Which of the following is NOT a known environmental risk factor for developing obesity in individuals below the poverty line in the U.S.?

A) Limited access to health care
B) Presence of "food deserts" (areas where healthy food is hard to find)
C) Genetic predisposition
D) Lack of green space for exercise or other physical activity

4. Which of the following weight-loss strategies would a neobehaviorist most endorse?

A) A combination of group therapy and prescription medication to help people lose as much weight as possible in a short time frame.
B) For every five pounds a person loses, they are given a non-food reward such as money or praise/attention from others.
C) Whenever a person gains weight they are publicly criticized by others.
D) A group exercise class where the exercises become increasingly more difficult over time.

5. Which of the following does NOT demonstrate how social networks can influence weight?

A) Research shows that joining an online weight-loss community is successful at helping people lose weight.
B) Kids who participate in group sports are less likely to be obese than those who prefer solitary activities, such as reading or playing video games.
C) Teenage girls who report having at least one friend with an eating disorder are more than twice as likely to also experiment with disordered eating behaviors such as binging and purging or extreme calorie restriction.
D) Multiple studies have shown that people eat roughly the same amount when they are dining out as they do when dining alone at home.

CARS Strategies for MCAT Psychology/Sociology Drill: Global Health Trends

The passage includes four paragraphs and two figures relating to the relationship between GDP and health and to national and state trends in obesity. Here is the map of the passage.

1) Positive correlation between health and wealth of nation—also individual level
2) Obesity is exception—opposite relationship
3) BMI: categories and study results
4) Mississippi: children's poor health, state response

And here are the questions.

1. **Memory.** For this question, you really do have to know something about catecholamine neurotransmitters, the parasympathetic nervous system, and Parkinson's disease.

2. **Explicit.** Once you define what the question is asking for—high GDP + low obesity/better health or vice versa—all you need to do is use the data in Figure 1. Make sure to read the question carefully; you are not looking for the relationship discussed in paragraph 2, which tells you that high GDP is correlated with high levels of obesity.

3. **Implicit.** While the question appears to require you to use your knowledge of specific environmental risk factors to eliminate choices B and D, and to use either your own knowledge or information from paragraph 1 to eliminate choice A, all you really need to do is read the question stem carefully. Once you see that it is asking which is NOT a known environmental risk factor, look for a non-environmental factor in the answer choices.

4. **Memory.** For this question, you do need to know the basics of neobehaviorism.

5. **Memory.** Even if you don't know much about social networks, this question is doable if you just read the question stem carefully. It asks which answer does NOT demonstrate how social networks influence weight. Look for any choice that either does not discuss social/group influence on behavior, or that suggests that social factors do not play a causal role.

Final Notes

In general, using CARS techniques on the science passages will increase your speed and accuracy, and help you to make the most of your scientific knowledge. The MCAT does not demand an exhaustive understanding of biology, chemistry, and physics; rather, it requires you to have a sound basic knowledge of chemical and physical principles, and of the ways in which organisms function. Combine your scientific common sense with your critical reading skills to raise your science scores.

Use your understanding of the three types of science questions (Memory, Implicit, and Explicit) to shape your solution strategies; make the information in the passages work for you. Don't waste your time working out a solution that the passage spells out for you; conversely, don't bother to search a passage for information that your map indicates isn't there.

Solutions to MCAT G-Chem Drill: Solubility

1. **D** The first three choices are false. O_2 and CO_2 are nonpolar (i.e., have no dipole). As a consequence of the electronegativity of the oxygen atoms, the carbon in carbon dioxide has a slight positive charge and is therefore attracted to any atom with a negative charge. Organic chemists use the term electrophile for an atom or molecule which has some positive charge and nucleophile for an atom or molecule with a negative charge. The oxygen in water is a mild nucleophile.

2. **A** Based upon the first two equilibrium reactions in the passage, if the concentration of CO_2 were decreased, the first equilibrium would shift to the left. The subsequent reduction in the concentration of H_2CO_3 would cause the second equilibrium to also shift to the left, hence the concentration of H^+ would decrease and blood pH would increase.

3. **D** The last sentence of paragraph 2 indicates that the transport efficiency of O_2 is directly related to the blood pH. Therefore, as blood pH decreases, so too does the ability of hemoglobin to transport oxygen. Choice A is incorrect because lipid bilayers are only unstable under extreme conditions. If this statement were true, drinking a glass of soda would be a painful experience. Bicarbonate is one of the most soluble anions, so choice B is not plausible. The passage does not provide any insight as to how the nervous system (choice C) would be impacted by acidosis.

4. **D** A catalyst increases the rate at which a reaction reaches equilibrium. The addition of a catalyst to a system that is already at equilibrium, like this one, will have no effect.

5. **B** The solubility of a gas in a liquid decreases with increasing temperature (as illustrated by the fact that CO_2 readily erupts from a bottle of warm soda). Choices A and C will increase the solubility of CO_2 gas in water.

6. **A** Whenever dealing with electron configuration questions, first eliminate any choices that have the wrong number of electrons. A neutral Fe atom has twenty-six electrons, so Fe^{2+} must have twenty-four electrons. Choices C and D are eliminated because they account for twenty-six and thirty electrons, respectively. Choice A is the correct answer because transition metal elements always lose their valence s electrons (here the $4s$ electrons) before losing any d electrons (choice B is eliminated).

Solutions to MCAT Physics Drill: Force

1. **C** The question says that the horizontal component of velocity, $v_x = v \cos \theta$, is 10 m/s. Since $\cos 60° = 1/2$, the total velocity v must be 20 m/s.

2. **C** As explained in the passage, dropping a sandbag does not change the buoyant force, but it does change the gravitational force. When the sandbag is dropped the gravitational force drops by mg while the buoyant force stays the same. Since the two forces originally balanced, the buoyant force is now bigger by mg. Note that the buoyant force is a constant Mg pointing up, while the gravitational force is originally Mg pointing down and then $(Mg - mg)$ pointing down after the sandbag is dropped.

3. **A** For a balloon to float, its density has to be less than that of air. So if the mass in kg divided by the volume in m^3 is less than 1.2 (the density of air), then the balloon floats. If you add the mass of the four people (total = 400 kg) to the mass of the balloon and divide by the volume, you get a value of less than 1.2 for Balloon I only.

4. **C** The upward buoyant force (acting along the central axis of the balloon, directly above the flame) on the warmer, less dense air propels it upward. When it reaches the closed top of the balloon, it will be deflected downward. As the warmed air makes its journey, it cools, returns downward, and the cycle repeats.

5. **D** The buoyant force makes it go up; gravity and the drag force hold it back. The net force is zero since its velocity is constant ($a = 0$), so the upward forces are equal to the downward forces, as stated in choice D.

6. **C** Warmer air is less dense than cooler air. Less dense air will give a smaller buoyant force and the balloon will be able to carry less weight.

7. **A** The pelican is 2 kg added on to 2000 kg for the balloon and passengers. This is a 0.1% increase in mass and therefore a 0.1% increase in gravitational force. Increasing the volume by 0.1% will result in a compensating increase in the buoyant force (which is $\rho g V$, where ρ is the density of the air).

8. **D** The rope is pulling a 100-kg person at an acceleration of 2 m/s², so the tension (the force on the person exerted by the rope) is just $T = m(g + a) = 100(10 + 2) = 1200$ N.

Solutions to MCAT Biology Drill: Embryology

1. **A** Since bacteria are unicellular and reproduce asexually through binary fission, they do not undergo fertilization, and would not be appropriate organisms to study that process. All the other organisms listed reproduce sexually; they can be (and have been!) used for developmental studies (choices B, C, and D can be eliminated).

2. **C** The question states that the males are the result of nondisjunction in the hermaphrodite. Nondisjunction is the failure of the chromosomes to separate properly during cell division. Since the hermaphrodite has two X chromosomes and no Y chromosomes, and the male arises from the hermaphrodite, the males cannot contain Y chromosomes (choices A and D are wrong; do not always assume male organisms have Y chromosomes). Furthermore, the passage states that the males are missing an X chromosome, not that they have gained one (choice B is wrong).

3. **C** The sperm nucleus is $1n$ (choice A is wrong), and because the oocyte has not yet completed meiosis I (it is suspended in prophase I), its nucleus is $2n$ (choice B is wrong). Therefore, the ploidy of the fertilized egg is $3n$ ($1n$ sperm + $2n$ oocyte, choice D is wrong).

4. **B** The passage states that sperm are stored in the spermatheca (choices A and C are wrong) and that this is found in the hermaphrodite (choice D is wrong).

5. **B** The passage describes pseudocleavage as an event where a cleavage furrow appears, then disappears without cell division (choice A is wrong). Formation of a cleavage furrow does not require the formation of a cell membrane (the existing membrane simply pinches inward, choice C is wrong), and polar bodies are formed during the meiotic division of the oocyte following fertilization (choice D is wrong).

6. **C** The cell division that occurs after fusion of the pronuclei is mitosis. Pairing of homologous chromosomes (numeral I) and recombination events (numeral II) occur during meiosis, so these statements are false (choices A, B, and D can be eliminated). Only numeral III is true; nuclear membranes must be reorganized both when the pronuclei fuse and when the (now) embryonic nucleus disintegrates during prophase.

7. **A** The passage states cytochalasin B inhibits actin polymerization (actin filaments are also called microfilaments) and prevents P-granule movement, thus movement of the P-granules must depend on microfilaments; numeral I is true (choices C and D can be eliminated). However, cytochalasin B does not affect migration of the pronuclei, so that process must not depend on microfilaments; numeral II is false. The passage also states that colcemid inhibits microtubules and prevents migration of the pronuclei, thus migration must depend on microtubules; numeral III is true (choice B can be eliminated). However, colcemid does not affect P-granules movement, so that process must not depend on microtubules; numeral IV is false.

Solutions to MCAT Psychology/Sociology Drill: Global Health Trends

1. **A** The catecholamine neurotransmitters are dopamine, norepinephrine, and epinephrine. Therefore, a catecholamine derivative that acts as an agonist would somehow act on a pathway involving one of these three neurotransmitters (choices C and D are wrong). The primary neurotransmitter of the parasympathetic nervous system is acetylcholine, so choice B is also wrong. In Parkinson's disease, neurons in the brain that make dopamine and control muscle movement begin to die. Therefore, even without necessarily knowing which of the catecholamine neurotransmitters is involved in obesity, the most reasonably correct answer is choice A.

2. **B** The first paragraph describes a relationship where high GDP correlates to better public health and low GDP correlates to worse public health. The only country in Figure 1 that roughly reflects this relationship and that also appears in the answer choices is South Africa; with the second highest percentage of the population with a BMI above 30 (reflecting worse public health) and a relatively low GDP, this is the only country where a low GDP corresponds to worse health (choice B is correct). Canada has a high GDP and a moderately high percentage of the population with a BMI above 30 (indicating poor health, choice A is wrong), and China and India both have low GDPs and low percentages of the population with a BMI above 30 (indicating better health, choices C and D are wrong).

3. **C** Genetic predisposition to obesity is not an environmental risk factor for developing obesity, it's a biological risk factor (choice C is the correct answer choice); for those living below the poverty line in the U.S., limited access to health care (choice A), limited access to healthy food (choice B), and a lack of green space to exercise (choice D) are all environmental risk factors contributing to the development of obesity. Therefore, choices A, B, and D can all be eliminated.

4. **B**   Neobehaviorists believe that behavior can be modified by rewards or punishments. There- fore, if someone exhibits a desired behavior, providing a reward after that behavior will encourage the behavior to happen again (positive reinforcement). When a person exhibits an undesirable behavior, the application of a punishment will discourage that behavior from happening again (positive punishment). Choice A is wrong because it does not describe any type of reward or punishment. Choice B describes positive reinforcement, and choice C describes positive punishment; neobehaviorists believe that the most effective way to modify behavior is with positive reinforcement. Therefore, choice B is right and choice C is wrong. Choice D seems to be describing the implementation of a punishment (exercises getting harder) in response to a desired behavior (exercise). This would be the opposite of a strategy that a neobehaviorist would endorse, and choice D is incorrect.

5. **D**   Social networks involve an individual and any of the various other individuals, groups, or organizations that an individual might interact with; by definition, social networks will influence the behavior of the individual in some way. Since the question asks which choice does NOT demonstrate the influence of social networks on weight, all of the answer choices that demonstrate that an individual is somehow influenced by others should be eliminated (choices A, B, and C indicate that weight is somehow influenced by groups or individuals, and can be eliminated). Choice D, however, indicates that there is no difference between eating around others and eating alone (choice D does not demonstrate how social networks can influence weight and is the correct answer choice).

A.2   INTERVIEW AND PERSONAL STATEMENT PREPARATION QUESTIONS

The following list of questions will help prepare you for your interviews and inspire your personal state- ments. Try to answer a few each week. Answers that are written out will be the most fully formed and the ones you are likely to remember.

1)   Where did you grow up and go to school? What was your town/community like? How did this shape your views?
2)   What was your family life like? What do your parents do?
3)   How is your relationship with your parents and siblings now? How did your family life shape you as a person?
4)   Was one particular person an inspiration to you in your life? Why?
5)   Why did you choose your undergraduate major?
6)   How have you tried to achieve breadth in your undergraduate education?
7)   How has your undergraduate research experience, if any, better prepared you for a medical career?
8)   If you get into medical school, you will be making a huge time commitment. What *won't* you give up in order to be successful in your medical career?
9)   How have the jobs, volunteer opportunities, or extracurricular experiences that you have had made you better prepared for the responsibilities of being a physician?
10) How do you envision using your medical school education?
11) You have stated many humanistic and socially responsible ideals in your essays. What have you done so far to demonstrate those ideals in practice?

12) How would you describe yourself in terms of your greatest strengths and weaknesses?

13) In the broad sense, what travels have you taken, and what exposure to cultures other than your own have you had?

14) Thinking of examples from your recent past, how would you assess your empathy and compassion?

15) What excites you about medicine in general?

16) What do you know about the current trends in our nation's health care system?

17) Tell me what you believe to be the most pressing health issues today. Why?

18) What do you feel are the social responsibilities of a physician?

19) What is the most important social problem facing the United States today, and why?

20) How do you think national health insurance might affect physicians, patients, and society?

21) In what manner and to what degree do you stay in touch with current events?

22) What books, films, or other media come to mind as having been particularly important to your non-science education?

23) What is "success," in your opinion? After practicing medicine for 20 years, what kind of "successes" do you hope to have achieved?

24) What qualities do you look for in a physician? Can you provide an example of a physician who exemplifies these ideals? How does he or she do this?

25) What kind of experiences have you had working with sick people? What have you learned from these experiences?

26) If you could invite four people from the past to dinner, who would they be, and why? What would you talk to them about?

27) Do you have any "blemishes" on your academic record? If so, explain the circumstances.

28) If you are a minority candidate, how do you feel your background uniquely prepares you to be, and will influence you as, a physician?

29) If you are not a minority, how do you feel prepared to meet the diverse needs of a multiethnic, multicultural patient population?

30) To what extent do you feel that you owe a debt to humanity? To what extent do you owe a debt to those less fortunate than you?

31) Who has been influential in your decision to pursue a medical career?

32) What special qualities do you feel you possess that would set you apart from other medical school candidates? What makes you unique or different as a medical school candidate?

33) What sort of expectations will you hold for your classmates?

34) What are the three most important properties you think the ideal medical student should have?

35) What kind of medical schools are you applying to, and why?

36) Pick any specific medical school that you are applying to, and tell the interviewer about it. What goes on there, and what makes it particularly desirable to you?

37) What general and specific skills would you hope an "ideal" medical school experience would give you? How might your ideal school achieve that result?

38) When did you decide to become an MD, and why?

39) Why did you decide to choose medicine and not some other field where you can help others, such as nursing, physical therapy, pharmacology, psychology, education, or social work?

40) How have you tested your motivation to become an MD? Please explain.

41) Where do you see yourself in five years? In ten years?

42) Have you decided what to specialize in? How did you reach this decision?

43) What will you do if you are not accepted to medical school this year? Do you have an alternative career plan?

44) Is there anything else we have not covered that you feel the interviewer should know about you or your interest in becoming a physician?

GOOD LUCK ON THE MCAT AND IN MEDICAL SCHOOL!

Passage Permissions Information

Passage Permissions Information

NOTES

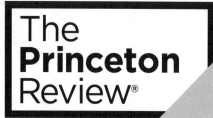
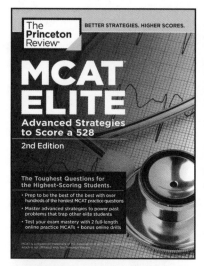
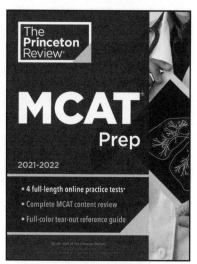
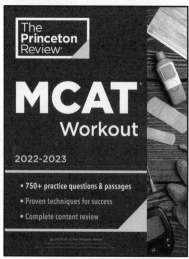
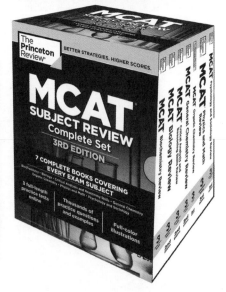